The Art of Computer-Guided Implantology

THE ART OF COMPUTER-GUIDED IMPLANTOLOGY

Edited by

Philippe B. Tardieu, DDS

Adjunct Associate Professor
Division of Reconstructive Comprehensive Care
College of Dentistry
New York University
New York, New York

Private Practice
Dental Implantology and Aesthetic Dentistry
Dubai, United Arab Emirates

Alan L. Rosenfeld, DDS, FACD

Professor
Department of Periodontology
College of Dentistry
University of Illinois
Chicago, Illinois

Private Practice
Periodontics and Dental Implantology
Park Ridge, Illinois

quintessence books

Quintessence Publishing Co, Inc

Chicago, Berlin, Tokyo, London, Paris, Milan, Barcelona,
Istanbul, Moscow, New Delhi, Prague, São Paulo, and Warsaw

Library of Congress Cataloging-in-Publication Data

The art of computer-guided implantology / edited by Philippe B. Tardieu, Alan L. Rosenfeld.
p. ; cm.
Includes bibliographical references and index.
ISBN 978-0-86715-477-1 (hardcover)
1. Dental implants. 2. Computer-assisted surgery. I. Tardieu, Philippe B. II. Rosenfeld, Alan L.
[DNLM: 1. Dental Implantation--methods. 2. Software. 3. Surgery, Computer-Assisted--methods. WU 640 A681 2009]
RK667.I45A78 2009
617.6'9--dc22
2009013578

quintessence books

Quintessence Publishing Co, Inc
4350 Chandler Drive
Hanover Park, IL 60133
www.quintpub.com

Editors: Kathryn Funk and Lisa C. Bywaters
Production: Sue Robinson and Patrick Penney

Printed in China

CONTENTS

Foreword vi
Preface vii
Contributors viii

1 **Introduction** 1

2 **Imaging Techniques and Diagnostics** 5
R. Anthony Reynolds

3 **The Dynamic Nature of SimPlant Software** 21
Alan L. Rosenfeld

4 **Scanning Appliances and Virtual Teeth** 47
Philippe B. Tardieu

5 **Axial Image Conversion and Segmentation** 59
Ellen Dhoore

6 **SurgiGuide Options** 67
George A. Mandelaris and Alan L. Rosenfeld

7 **Computer-Guided Implant Treatment Pathway** 89
Richard Mecall

8 **Clinical Cases** 113
George A. Mandelaris, Alan L. Rosenfeld, and Philippe B. Tardieu

9 **SAFE System and Immediate Smile** 177
Philippe B. Tardieu and Veerle Pattijn

10 **Advanced Case Planning with SimPlant** 193
Scott D. Ganz

11 **Oral-Maxillofacial Surgery Software** 211
Benoît L. Philippe

Index 223

FOREWORD

Innovations in implant dentistry have allowed the profession to progress at a very fast rate. One technique now commonly used for diagnostics in implant therapy is the computed tomography (CT) scan. Although the technology has been available since 1987, the ability to use this radiographic knowledge in a method that integrates the restorative treatment plan with the surgical placement of implants has only recently been standardized to its proper level. Drs Tardieu and Rosenfeld have been true pioneers in the field and have been working for years to improve the use of CT scans for clinical dentistry. I have known them both for over 20 years, and during that time they have been actively involved with this and related technology. It is wonderful to see their collaboration on this fine textbook.

This book is very timely since so many new techniques are now available to the clinician. It is particularly relevant to show how the restorative dentist can now have an important dialogue with the implant surgeon. All too often, the surgeon has paid little attention to the actual desires of the restorative dentist or did not know how to incorporate them into the surgical treatment. Those days should be over, and this book will help the team to better communicate with each other before any surgery is performed. In fact, with the use of surgical guides described in the book, the accuracy of the work performed will now be superior to what is being done today.

The use of guides will greatly benefit the patient as well as the dental team. The work performed should be more accurate with less discomfort than in regular cases. The ability to transfer the desired angle and location of placement of the implants from the working models to the mouth has made this a reality. This textbook allows the reader to proceed step by step in the understanding and implementation of this new and exciting technology. It is no longer only for the most highly trained specialists. Indeed, the clarity of the writing along with the diagrams and case reports in the book will allow all implant teams to improve their ability to design better cases and surgically place implants. This is therefore a timely book with benefits for both restorative and surgical practitioners.

However, the real benefit will be to our patients. The increased precision and speed of treatment, along with reduced discomfort, all add up to a must read for clinicians. I congratulate my two friends on this wonderful work.

Dennis P. Tarnow, DDS
Professor and Chairman
Department of Periodontology and Implant Dentistry
New York University College of Dentistry
New York, New York

PREFACE

This book is the first to introduce a radiographic paradigm shift in implant therapy that provides an accurate method for transferring the patient's prosthetic needs into a resin-based surgical template designed to guide implant placement.

Computed tomography (CT) was introduced to the dental profession in 1987 to facilitate radiographic examination of the jaws and implant treatment planning. It allowed the dental profession for the first time to evaluate anatomic structures and the effects of postextraction resorptive patterns with submillimeter accuracy. Because there was no mechanism for introducing prosthetic information into the CT dataset, however, the value of this technology was limited to diagnostic applications.

In 1999, real-time 2D-3D interactive imaging software was developed, allowing the prosthetic outcome to be transferred to the CT dataset with the use of an appropriate scanning appliance. This technologic breakthrough facilitates a direct link between anatomic interpretation, treatment planning, and precise surgical execution. Through computer-guided implantology, preoperative rather than intraoperative planning drives treatment decisions.

This book has been organized to allow the clinician an opportunity both to survey the field as a broad overview and to implement the critical-thinking skills necessary to navigate the complexities of patient treatment. While the technology in this field will undoubtedly continue to advance, the fundamental principles presented in these 11 chapters will remain the cornerstone of patient care. All of the contributors share a common belief that technology is not a substitute for clinical experience and wise judgment and that the implementation of computer-guided implantology should be predicated on the unique experiences of each clinician and not what is therapeutically fashionable at the moment.

We wish to thank our families for their support and understanding during the extensive period of time we devoted to the completion of this book. We also express our gratitude to the members of our office staff and to dental colleagues who have contributed to the contents of this book through their participation in collaborative patient care. Without their support, this book could not have been written.

CONTRIBUTORS

Ellen Dhoore, MSc
Clinical Research Engineer
Materialise Dental
Leuven, Belgium

Scott D. Ganz, DMD
Assistant Clinical Professor
Department of Prosthodontics
University of Medicine and Dentistry of New Jersey
Newark, New Jersey

Private Practice
Prosthodontics, Maxillofacial Prosthetics, and Implant Dentistry
Fort Lee, New Jersey

George A. Mandelaris, DDS, MS
Private Practice
Periodontics and Dental Implantology
Park Ridge, Illinois

Richard Mecall, DDS, MS
Private Practice
Periodontics and Dental Implantology
Las Vegas, Nevada

Veerle Pattijn, MSc Eng, PhD
Application Engineering Manager
Materialise Dental
Leuven, Belgium

Benoît L. Philippe, MD
Private Practice
Pre-implant Maxillofacial Surgery and Implantology
Paris, France

R. Anthony Reynolds, MSc, PhD
IDT Dental Products
London, England

Alan L. Rosenfeld, DDS, FACD
Professor
Department of Periodontology
College of Dentistry
University of Illinois
Chicago, Illinois

Private Practice
Periodontics and Dental Implantology
Park Ridge, Illinois

Philippe B. Tardieu, DDS
Adjunct Associate Professor
Divison of Reconstructive Comprehensive Care
College of Dentistry
New York University
New York, New York

Private Practice
Dental Implantology and Aesthetic Dentistry
Dubai, United Arab Emirates

1

INTRODUCTION

Philippe B. Tardieu, DDS
Alan L. Rosenfeld, DDS

Background

With the introduction of dental computed tomography (CT) in 1987, the method by which patients were evaluated for the placement of dental implants changed dramatically.[1,2] For the first time, the dental implant surgeon was able to understand regional anatomy and its influence on surgical decision-making preoperatively. This radiographic modality was superior to all other forms of dental radiographs in both accuracy and anatomic insight. However, two significant problems needed to be addressed. First, no prosthetic information was available in the CT study; since early implant placement was surgically driven, there continued to be a lack of prosthetically driven implant diagnostic analysis. Second, there was no means to transfer the prosthetic information and treatment plan directly to the patient at the time of surgery, and this disconnect between diagnostics and treatment prevented broader professional acceptance. Nevertheless, as the demand for more esthetic and life like restorations increased, clinicians worldwide used surgical guides to facilitate more accurate placement of dental implants. And despite a lack of uniformity in the design of the guides and lack of transferability to the patient, from 1987 to 2000, more clinicians used CT scans than ever before.

Meanwhile, the concept of true prosthetically directed surgical guides made little progress. In fact, surgical guides were treated as little more than "wish lists" or documented treatment plans and often were never used at the time of surgery. Despite improvements in evaluating surgical and prosthetic requirements for successful implant treatment, the inability to physically transfer a plan from the CT scan to the patient was a major shortcoming. This shortcoming is the single most significant reason why many clinicians continue to use analogue radiographic modalities instead.

Purpose

This book is designed as a self-instruction guide to diagnosis, treatment planning, and the development of a surgical strategy that allows accurate control of osteotomy and implant placement. With the use of specialized scanning appliances, prosthetically relevant information is transferred to the CT study and becomes the basis by which a prosthetically directed surgical treatment plan, manufactured into a resin-based (plastic) surgical guide, is physically and precisely transferred to the patient. The surgical guide referred to herein is an actual template that is placed in the patient's mouth at the time of implant placement. This template helps direct the precise placement, direction, and depth of the implant(s). The most experienced clinicians from around the world share their knowledge and experiences using computer-guided implant surgery to achieve predictable prosthetic outcomes based on a preoperative treatment plan.

History and Evolution of Computer-Guided Implantology

The authors have been involved with computer technology using the SimPlant software program since 1993. The original software program was developed by Columbia Scientific to help dentists plan surgical implant treatment in 2D reconstructions derived from raw CT data. Compared to classic, noninteractive analogue CT scan films, this format supported interaction through navigation within the bone volume, which allowed the selection of cross-sectional reconstructions that are still used today. By incorporating holes or by removing the lingual or palatal portion, the scanning appliance became the surgical guide, which was then used during implant surgery (albeit as more of a visual rather than a true surgical guide).

To convert a computer plan for use in actual patient treatment required a revolution. The breakthrough that we needed was the result of two major studies. The first was the PHIDIAS Project, which targeted the development of a dedicated system based on laser photopolymerization for the production of medical models. The second was the PISA Project, which validated the transfer of information from the computer to the mouth using surgical guides fabricated from medical-grade resin with the use of stereolithographic modeling. This transfer methodology formed the missing link by allowing a prosthetically directed treatment plan to be developed within the SimPlant software and transferred directly to the patient at the time of surgery. A brief synopsis highlighting the milestones of these projects follows.

Laser Photopolymerization Models Based on Medical Imaging: A Development Improving the Accuracy of Surgery (PHIDIAS) Project and Network (1993–2002)

The research in this project targeted the development of a dedicated system based on laser photopolymerization for the production of medical models. It was carried out in five discrete stages, each targeting a specific goal:

1. Develop a scan mode on existing medical scanners to gather data with the accuracy needed for model production.
2. Develop software that allowed the radiologist to gather data with the accuracy needed for medical models.
3. Develop a material low in toxicity and colorable for the laser photopolymerization process.
4. Adapt the laser photopolymerization equipment for use in the medical field and produce colored and biocompatible models.
5. Perform analysis of clinical trials to validate the results of the study by a task force of surgeons from different specializations.

The outcome of this project proved that it was possible to produce accurate medical models based on medical image data. Selective coloring of medical models has been developed so that relevant information derived from the images can be

Advantages for Patients

The growth of computer-aided implantology has been attributed, in part, to the favorable experiences of surgeons and patients alike. Patient satisfaction relates to shorter and less painful surgical experiences, and an appreciation for state-of-the-art treatment. Following are five ways in which patients benefit by the use of this technology:

1. **Enhanced security for greater planning accuracy and better implant location.** There is no question that guided implant placement is more accurate than manual placement. In 2000, cadaver studies revealed an average deviation of 3.71 mm in manual implant placement. This degree of deviation is sufficient to cause injury to important regional anatomy, such as the inferior alveolar nerve. A computerized approach can considerably enhance the ability to place implants within submillimeter accuracy.[8]
2. **Improved patient comfort.** Knowing the requirements for implant placement prior to surgery allows the clinician to reduce the size of the surgical field. Implant placement through a 4-mm opening without bone exposure reduces the risk of postoperative swelling, pain, infection, and complications.
3. **Improved efficiency in implant planning and simplified treatment.** When specific instruments are used to drill and guide the implants into their precise planned positions, implants can be immediately placed into fresh extraction sites with greater confidence.
4. **Accuracy in the fabrication and delivery of a fixed prosthesis.** "Immediate Smile" is the name of a unique procedure whereby the prosthesis is fabricated based on computer data prior to implant placement, without a traditional impression. The implants and prosthesis are placed during the same appointment without pain and, in many instances, without flap elevation. When the focus is on accuracy, there is no need for expensive and complex components.
5. **Improved esthetics to meet the rising demand by patients.** Accuracy facilitates the development of appropriate prosthetic emergence through the soft tissue. The 10-degree average deviation associated with manual implant placement is reduced to 1 degree with guided implantology.

transferred to the surgeon. Improvements have been made to the images generated with spiral CT, which is the format most suitable for medical model data acquisition. Noise levels and artifacts due to spatial inhomogeneities have been reduced. Image-based segmentation has also been investigated and implemented, resulting in a more user-friendly environment for the medical data processing. Special image techniques to enhance segmentation clarity have been developed. Most important, the quality of the resulting image is improved.

The treatment of medical images can be controlled by the clinician. Medical and technical software have the capability to produce models with selected colored regions. Low-toxicity resin (FDA Class 6–approved) was developed to produce medical models that can be safely used during surgical treatment. This resin can be used on commercially available stereolithographic equipment. Achieving this was essential so that special manufacturing equipment would not be required for medical application.

Validation of the results has been performed at both technical and clinical levels. From a technical point of view, the accuracy of the medical models is limited only by the accuracy of the medical images and scanning equipment. It is possible to overcome the resolution limitation of the scanner with intelligent interpolation approaches. Accuracy up to several tenths of a millimeter can be achieved, allowing medical prostheses to be custom designed on stereolithographic models. From a clinical point of view, the PHIDIAS Network has been the first study to go beyond individual case reports. A validation study was started in 1999, and a total of 253 cases were evaluated.[3–7]

Medical Image–Based Personalized Implants and Surgical Aids (PISA) Project (1997–2001)

As noted above, validation of rapid prototyping and its application in medical treatment was achieved by the PHIDIAS project. The purpose of the PISA project was to create and validate a system that would integrate computer-aided design and medical imaging in order to allow segmentation of data. Several European companies and universities were involved: Ceka (Belgium), DePuy International (UK), Materialise (Belgium), OBL (France), Philips Medical Systems (the Netherlands), Katholieke Universiteit Leuven (Belgium), and the University of Leeds (UK).

A generic system was developed that allowed for the design of custom prostheses and individualized surgical guides. These patient-specific surgical guides fit perfectly on the internal structure of patients and enabled the surgeon to be guided during surgical operations, directing the surgical instrumentation to the exact position based on a preoperative plan. This system also helped resolve the image-to-patient registration inaccuracy, which was a serious limitation in the use of this technology. Another goal of the PISA project was also to produce and convert the prototyping techniques into a reliable, cost-effective, fast, one-of-a-kind production methodology for medical devices.

The applicability and validity of the products developed in the project were investigated in oral, craniofacial, orthopedic, and spinal surgery applications. Experienced surgeons from each of these fields were enlisted to participate. The studies were validated first on cadavers, then on simulators, and finally in limited patient trials.

Within the 4-year study, technical support surgical guide templates were developed for the placement of atlanto-axial screws in cervical vertebrae, pedicle screws in the lumbar vertebrae, glenoid components of the shoulder prostheses, and dental implants. In a clinical validation study, the atlanto-axial drill guides showed submillimeter accuracy while the pedicle screws were placed within a 2-mm range. These studies and the possibility of guided surgery became attractive to oral implantology because they facilitated a fast and secure method for placing dental implants. After 3 years, more than 100 patients were treated in the framework of the PISA project, due in large part to the collaboration between clinicians and educators. To disseminate this revolutionary information, workshops were organized and products were released. This was the true beginning of stereolithographic surgical guides in oral implantology.

6. **Such precision reduces the need for expensive components to correct angulation abnormalities and re-establish good emergence.** Finally, the cost of treatment can be predicted based on a prosthetically directed treatment plan. There is a reduction in laboratory expenses by using SurgiGuides to place implants compared to manual placement.[9] This is an important and valuable benefit.

Advantages for Clinicians

This book covers current developments, accuracy research, surgical applications, surgical devices, and surgical protocols. Our objective is to simplify the use and understanding of the new technology to help surgeons and restorative dentists provide better care to their patients.

Step-by-step procedures assist the reader in a complete understanding of the process, and clinical cases illustrate how to apply the technology. One of the procedures described is the placement of implants, such as trans-sinusal and zygomatic implants, in surgically inaccessible areas without bone exposure.[10] In addition, the delivery of an immediate prosthesis and application of the Immediate Smile technique can facilitate prosthetic treatment opportunities only dreamed about previously. This book also covers procedures and techniques still in research and development, such as assisted virtual implant planning and soft tissue imaging.

The editors have assembled clinicians and educators from around the world who have extensive experience with computer-guided implantology. It is our hope that the reader will gain the knowledge and confidence to embark upon a personal and professional journey into the realm of this new and exciting technology.

References

1. Schwarz MS, Rothman SL, Chafetz N, Rhodes M. Computer tomography. Part II. Preoperative assessment of the maxilla for endosseous implant surgery. Int J Oral Maxillofac Implants 1987;2:143–148.
2. Schwarz MS, Rothman SL, Chafetz N, Rhodes M. Computer tomography. Part I. Preoperative assessment of the mandible for endosseous implant surgery. Int J Oral Maxillofac Implants 1987;2:137–141.
3. Popat AH. Rapid prototyping and medical modeling. Phidas Newsletter 1998;1:10–12.
4. Swaelens B. Drilling templates for dental implantology. Phidas Newsletter 1999;3:10–12.
5. Poukens JM, Haex JK, Verdonck H, Riediger D. Study on the accuracy of stereolithographic surgical guides in dental implantology. Phidas Newsletter 2002;8:8–14.
6. Wouters K. Colour rapid prototyping. An extra dimension for visualizing human anatomy. Phidas Newsletter 2001;6:4–7.
7. Wulf J, Vitt KD, Gehl H-B, Busch LC. Anatomical accuracy in medical 3D modeling. Phidas Newsletter 2001;7:1–2.
8. Sarment D, Sukovic P, Clinthorne N. Accuracy of implant placement with a stereolithographic surgical guide. Int J Oral Maxillofac Implants 2003;18:571–577.
9. Beckers L. Positive effect of SurgiGuides on total cost. Materialise Headlines 2003;1:3.
10. Vrielinck L, Politis C, Schepers S, Pauwels M, Naert I. Image-based planning and clinical validation of zygoma and pterygoid implant placement in patients with severe bone atrophy using customized drill guides. Preliminary results from a prospective follow-up study. Int J Oral Maxillofac Surg 2003;32:7–14.

2

IMAGING TECHNIQUES AND DIAGNOSTICS

R. Anthony Reynolds, MSc, PhD

The primary purpose of imaging before implant placement is to identify bone quantity (width and height), bone quality (cortical plate thickness and trabecular density), and the exact location of anatomic structures to be avoided (inferior alveolar nerve canal, incisive foramen and canal, maxillary sinuses, etc). It is equally important to identify unerupted teeth, submerged roots, sinus disease, and other pathologic conditions.

The ideal imaging technique for planning dental implants should provide (*1*) accurate distance measurements in buccolingual, mesiodistal, and superior-inferior directions; (*2*) a quantitative assessment of bone density; and (*3*) an overview of patient anatomy and pathology using images of diagnostic quality.

There are a number of imaging modalities available (see Table 2-1 for a comparison of their key properties), and each has its place in the implant-planning and placement process. However, only computed tomography can meet all three of the criteria identified above.

Computed Tomography

Computed tomography (CT) provides the most detailed images available. It combines high measurement accuracy (freedom from geometric distortion) with high contrast for visualizing both soft tissue and bony structures.

CT produces cross-sectional images in which the grayscale pixel values are computed directly from a set of raw data collected by the x-ray apparatus. Unlike conventional tomography, the computed pixel values are a direct representation of the x-ray attenuation at each point of the body, and there is no blurring from out-of-focus structures.

To produce a CT image, the x-ray apparatus uses a row of electronic detectors to make a set of x-ray attenuation measurements covering the entire field of view (Fig 2-1). Each detector gives rise to a single attenuation measurement, taken along a line (called a *ray*) traced back to the x-ray source. Because there may be 500 or more detectors, at least 500 attenuation measurements (comprising a *view*) are made for each position of the x-ray source. However, the x-ray tube and detector system rotate rapidly around the patient, so the process is repeated for a large number of angular positions of the tube/detector system. Suppose a set of measurements is taken every half a degree: There will be 360 / 0.5 = 720 views, each resulting in 500 rays. (720 × 500 = 360,000 attenuation measurements per rotation.) It is not hard to see that at least in principle, the computer has sufficient information to calculate the 512 × 512 = 262,144 pixel values making up a typical CT image (called a *slice*).

The earliest CT scanners worked in exactly this way, calculating the pixel values needed to give rise to the measured attenuation data through an iterative process.[1] Contemporary CT scanners use a different mathematical process known as *filtered backprojection* or *convolution and backprojection*, which achieves equivalent results with greater speed and improved image quality.[2]

Table 2-1 Comparison of various dental imaging modalities

	Periapical (Paralleling technique)	Lateral skull (Cephalometric technique)	Dental panoramic tomogram (DPT)	Complex motion tomography	Computed tomography (MSCT)
Distance measurements					
Mesiodistal accuracy	< 1.0 mm	NA	Unreliable	Same as for DPT	< 0.5 mm
Bone height accuracy	< 1.0 mm	Midline only	Unreliable	< 1.0 mm	< 1.0 mm
Bone width accuracy	NA	Midline only	NA	< 1.0 mm	< 0.5 mm
Bone quality assessment					
Cortical plate thickness	NA	NA	NA	< 1.0 mm	< 0.5 mm
Cortical plate density	Qualitative	Unreliable	Unreliable	Qualitative	< 0.5%
Trabecular density	Qualitative	Unreliable	Unreliable	Qualitative	< 0.5%
General overview					
Anatomy and pathology	Local only	Good	Good	Same as for DPT	Very good
Identification of possible implant sites	Local only	Unreliable	Good	Same as for DPT	Very good

CT scanners

There are currently four types of scanners available for dental CT scans.

Single-slice sequential CT

While the patient lies perfectly still on a table, the x-ray tube/detector assembly rotates once around the patient, and an image of a very thin cross-sectional slice (typically 1 mm thick) is acquired. Then the table moves a short distance (typically 1 mm) into the gantry, and another thin cross-sectional slice is taken. In this way the entire volume is imaged one slice at a time.

Because of the need to stop and start the motion between each slice, these scanners are very slow. Each slice can take up to 6 seconds, thus an entire mandible (consisting of 50 slices 1 mm apart) could take up to $6 \times 50 / 60 = 5$ minutes. Given these limitations, single-slice sequential CT scanners should be avoided for dental scans if possible.

Spiral or helical CT

Spiral and *helical* refer to an acquisition mode in which the tube and detector assembly rotates continuously around the patient, and the table moves continuously into the gantry.

Helical acquisition results in much more rapid scanning (a complete mandible might take 50 seconds or less), but the computer algorithms are considerably more complicated. This has a number of unexpected and counterintuitive consequences:

- The interpolated slices can be any desired distance apart. This is advantageous as it leads to improved resolution in the Z (longitudinal) direction.
- Acquisition of a large number of interpolated slices does not result in an increase in radiation exposure.
- The process leads to helical artifacts, which in some cases make the images less clear.
- An "overrun" occurs at the start and end of each acquisition process. Typically, the patient is irradiated for half a rotation of the tube/detector assembly, for which no images are produced. This effect must be taken into account when calculating the radiation dose.

Multislice CT

Multislice CT (MSCT) is also called *multidetector CT* because the detector comprises multiple rows. As the tube/detector assembly and the patient table move continuously in helical mode, multiple sets of measurements are

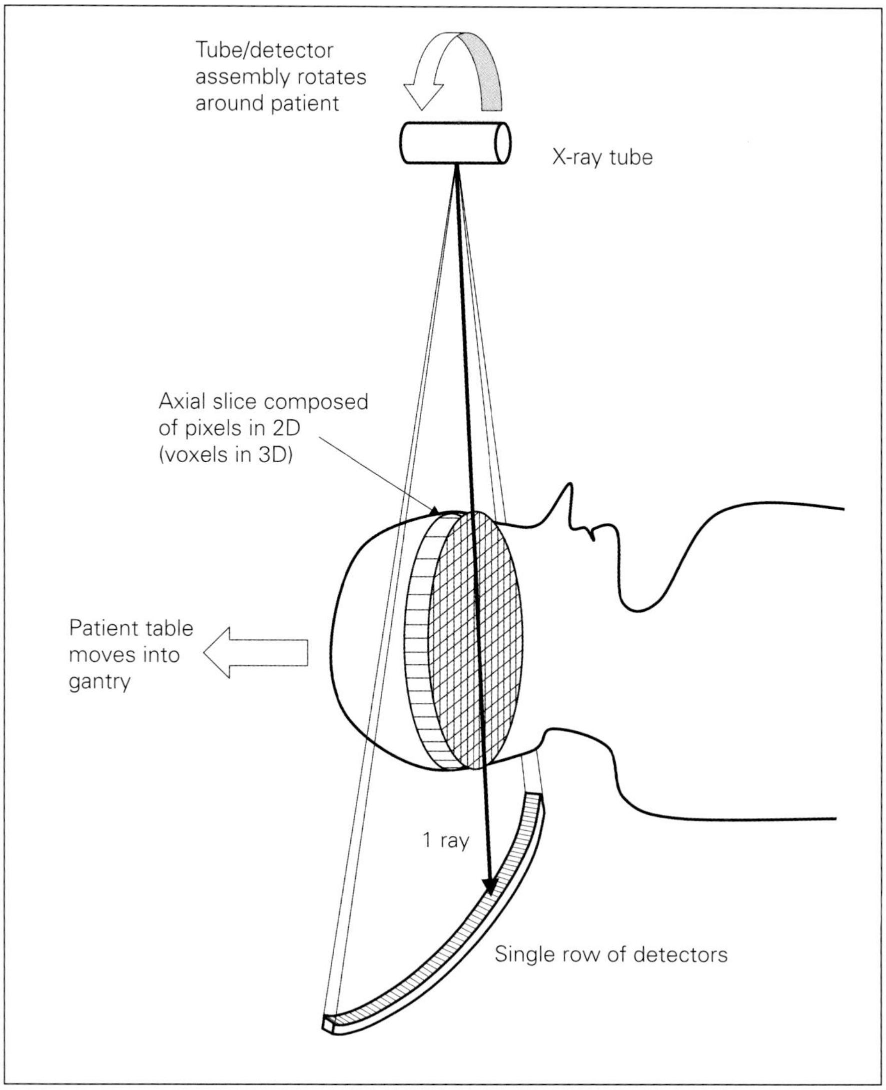

Fig 2-1 Single-slice sequential CT. A set of x-ray attenuation measurements is made, one for each ray (detector position) making up a view. With enough rays and views, it is possible to calculate all of the pixel values making up a slice. When one slice is complete, the patient table (not shown) moves into the gantry (not shown), and another slice is acquired.

acquired simultaneously. Currently, up to 320 sets of data can be acquired at once, resulting in very fast scan times.

Because of the overrun effect, the volume irradiated may be larger than that for which useful images are produced. For a 16-slice scanner, the overrun typically is 2 to 3 mm at each end of a 50-mm mandible or maxilla acquisition, with an increase in radiation of up to 12%, which is borderline acceptable. (Collimation issues must also be taken into account.[3]) The overrun may be considerably higher with scanners that obtain a greater number of slices simultaneously, and therefore great care must be taken when using these scanners.

A 16-slice MSCT scanner can capture an entire mandible or maxilla in 5 to 10 seconds, producing an image quality and radiation dose comparable to that of a single-slice sequential CT scanner. This speed is sufficiently fast for most dental applications, and there is little advantage in acquiring more slices simultaneously with a potentially higher radiation dose.

Cone beam CT

In cone beam CT (CBCT), a two-dimensional (2D) detector is used, permitting an entire volume to be captured in a single rotation. These machines use a beam of x-rays emanating in a cone shape from the x-ray source to capture the teeth and facial bones with a single rotation while the patient assumes a natural sitting position (Fig 2-2). Originally developed for cardiac examinations,[4] CBCT

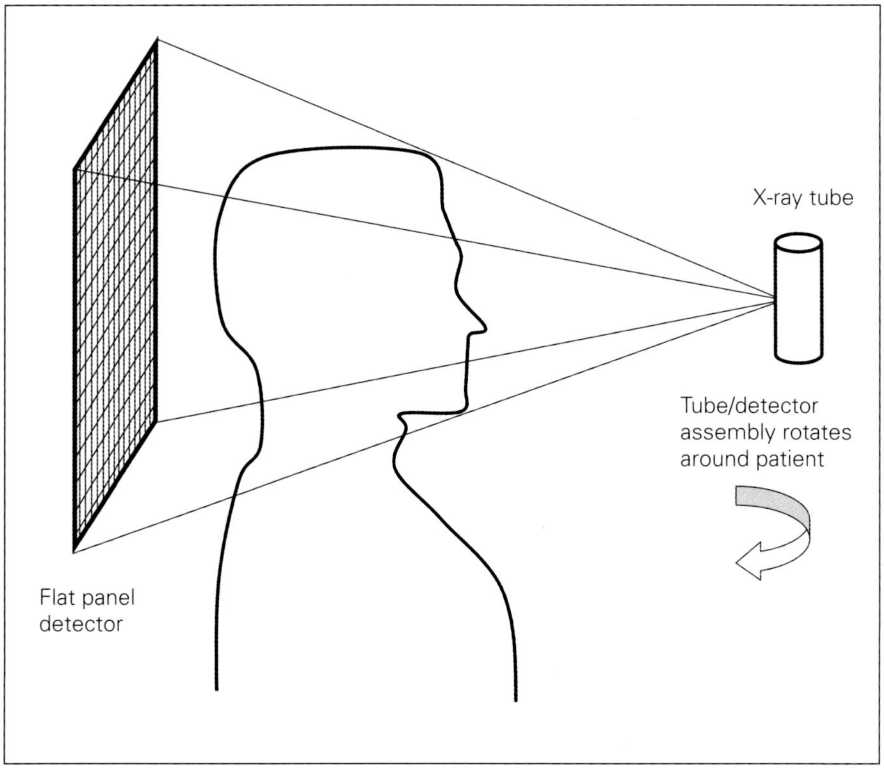

Fig 2-2 Cone beam CT. The patient is usually imaged sitting up. A large area detector captures most or all of the head in a single rotation. Special reconstruction algorithms are employed to create parallel axial slices from the cone beam dataset.

scanners have also been used for planning radiotherapy and most recently for dental applications. NewTom 9000 and 3G (QR), 3D Accuitomo (J Morita), CB MercuRay (Hitachi), and the i-CAT (Imaging Sciences International) are examples of CBCT scanners designed for dental and maxillofacial applications. Cone beam acquisition is very efficient and requires a lower radiation dose than a fan beam passing around the patient multiple times.

Advantages of CBCT

Most CBCT scanners are approximately the same size as a digital panoramic tomography machine, making them suitable for installation in a dental practice. Conventional MSCT scanners, in contrast, are lie-down machines that feature large gantries and are very costly to construct and maintain. Likewise, conventional CT scanners require heavy-duty engineering because the massive x-ray tube/detector assembly rotates around the patient at high speed (several rotations per second). CBCT scanners, by contrast, rotate about the patient once in approximately 20 seconds and are significantly smaller, lighter, and safer.

When patients lie down in a conventional CT scanner, the soft tissues tend to collapse. While not a diagnostic problem, accurate dental or surgical planning requires a precise assessment of the soft tissues in a natural sitting upright position. Most CBCT scanners are sit-up machines and therefore offer more accurate information. This is of particular importance when predicting the tissue changes likely to result from orthognathic surgery or orthodontic treatment, or for airway assessment.

In summary, CBCTs have the following advantages over the conventional MSCT:

- Convenience of having the machine in the dental office
- Modest cost
- Low radiation dose
- Patient sits up in a natural position for a shorter period

Table 2-2 Misch bone density classification*

Classification	Properties	Hounsfield unit (HU)
D1	Dense cortical bone	> 1,250
D2	Thick, dense to porous cortical bone on crest and coarse trabecular bone within	850–1,250
D3	Thin, porous cortical bone on crest and fine trabecular bone within	350–850
D4	Fine trabecular bone	150–350
D5	Immature, nonmineralized bone	< 150

*Reprinted with permission from Misch.[5]

CT Datasets

CT scanners build up 3D representations of the body from a series of thin cross-sectional slices. Because these images are most frequently taken transverse to the long axis of the patient, they are referred to as *transaxial* or *axial*.

At the completion of a CT examination, the operator will have a stack of axial slices stored in digital format. These slices can be represented by an array of gray-scale values called *pixels* (2D) and *voxels* (3D). Each voxel is characterized by a number of attributes, including its position within the 3D array, the size of the region it represents, and the x-ray attenuation measured by the CT scanner at the corresponding region within the patient's body.

The spatial resolution in an MSCT image is nonisotropic, which means that smaller objects can be better visualized within an axial slice (the X-Y plane) than between two slices (the Z direction). For dental CTs taken on an MSCT scanner, a voxel size of $0.25 \times 0.25 \times 0.50$ mm^3 is typical; in contrast, the resolution in CBCT images is isotropic, and a voxel size of $0.30 \times 0.30 \times 0.30$ mm^3 is typical.

Associated with each voxel is a number representing the average x-ray attenuation within the corresponding region of the patient's body. By convention, CT x-ray attenuation is expressed in Hounsfield units (HU) on a linear scale ranging from –1,000 (air) to 0 (water) and extending up to +3,000. Although there is no upper limit to the Hounsfield scale, for practical purposes many CT manufacturers set limits of –1,024 and +3,071. On the Hounsfield scale, fat is approximately –100, muscle is around 50, trabecular bone falls in the range of 150 to 850, and cortical bone extends above trabecular bone and continues to about 2,000. Dentin starts to appear at about 1,600 and enamel occurs in the range of 2,500 to 3,000.

Contrast resolution is the ability to distinguish between objects that are of similar radiographic density, such as neural tissue and fat. Objects differing by 5 HU or more are easily distinguished, so a rough estimate of the contrast resolution for CT is about 0.5%, or 10 times the sensitivity of radiographic film.

A mapping can be made between Hounsfield units and bone density on the Misch scale, as shown in Table 2-2.[5] According to this mapping, bone of type D4 lies between 150 and 350 HU, D3 lies between 350 and 850 HU, D2 lies between 850 and 1,250 HU, and D1 lies above 1250 HU. As a general rule, bone of quality 500 HU or more is usually adequate for placing implants.

The standard range of voxel values (–1,024 to +3,071) is too large to present subtle contrast differences to the human eye. A window/level transformation is applied to the voxel values before displaying them as gray-scale pixels on the computer screen in such a way as to maximize the contrast resolution for a specific tissue type. By interactively adjusting the controls while viewing the images, the operator can obtain views of either soft tissue or bone but not usually both in maximum detail at the same setting.

Random variations in gray scale from one voxel to another are called *noise*. The noise in a CT image depends primarily on how many x-ray photons pass through each voxel, which in turn depends on the exposure (x-ray tube current × scanning time) and the voxel size. For the same exposure, a smaller voxel size will result in a noisier image. The reconstruction algorithms and interpolation methods have an impact on the noise as well.[6] As a general rule, images with less noise require a higher radiation dose.

Structures in the image that have no counterpart in the object are termed *artifacts*. In CT images, streaking or starburst artifacts are commonly seen when dense objects such as dental restorations are encountered. Other types of artifacts are discussed in more detail later in this chapter.

Scout Views

The lateral scout view, sometimes called a *scan projection radiograph*, *localizer*, or *alignment image*, is obtained by putting the CT scanner into a special acquisition mode. The CT table and patient must be moved smoothly through the gantry while the x-ray tube and detectors remain fixed at the three o'clock or nine o'clock position. The resulting projected images, similar in appearance to conventional lateral skull radiographs, provide an overview of the patient's anatomic landmarks and precisely establish the region to be scanned. Scout views are used to ensure that (*a*) the patient is not rotated or misaligned laterally, (*b*) the scan plane is the one requested by the referring clinician, and (*c*) the volume to be scanned encompasses the required bony anatomy and radiologic scanning appliance with the minimum number of axial slices.

Because SimPlant (Materialise) and some of the other implant planning software packages incorporate the lateral scout view into the patient's dataset, the patient must not be moved between the time this view is obtained and when the diagnostic scans are taken.

Axial Views

Axial views are the original transaxial slices from which the panoramic, cross-sectional, and 3D images (but not the scout views) are reformatted using a dental software package. The axial slices are the gold standard used to identify anomalies such as tumors, osteomyelitis, extraction sockets, or retained root tips.

Reformatted CT Images

Some of the earliest dental CT scans were taken with the patient's head angled so that the slices were acquired in the coronal instead of the axial plane, but there are several drawbacks to this method. First, it is difficult to get patients to extend their neck sufficiently to obtain scans truly perpendicular to the alveolar ridge. Second, in the coronal plane, the x-ray beam traverses the crowns of the teeth and metal restorations, producing prominent streak artifacts that make it difficult or impossible to see the alveolar bone.[7] To avoid these problems, special computer software has been developed to produce virtual panoramic and cross-sectional images by reprocessing or reformatting a stack of CT slices acquired in the axial plane.

To reformat images using software tools, the operator draws a line following the entire midline of the bone (panoramic curve) on a representative axial slice. Once the central panoramic curve is established, the computer creates a family of panoramic curves equidistant from it. Then the computer searches through the stack of axial slices and finds all of the voxels along each panoramic curve, on each of the axial slices. These voxels are then organized into panoramic and cross-sectional images. Life-sized images can be printed for diagnosis and measurement (Fig 2-3).

SimPlant and similar software packages support 3D images as well as axial, panoramic, and cross-sectional views. Interactive computer tools make it possible to place "virtual" implants in optimal positions in alignment with predetermined tooth positions seen on the radiologic scanning appliance. Virtual implants and abutments depicting most manufacturers' platforms are available and can be placed and manipulated on the images at will. Other software packages such as coDiagnostiX (IVS Solutions), ImplantMaster (iDent Imaging), and implant3D (med3D) have broadly similar capabilities.

Panoramic views

Reformatted panoramic views are similar in some respects to conventional dental panoramic tomographs. The main differences are that the reformatted panoramic views are customized to follow the contours of an individual maxilla or mandible; there is no distortion or magnification in the image; and the image is a wafer-thin section, not a composite of the anatomy within a wide focal trough. Panoramic views can be printed at life size for taking direct measurement. Reformatted panoramic views are generated at right angles to the original axial slices and are especially useful for locating anatomic landmarks such as the inferior alveolar nerve canal, the incisive foramen and canal, and the maxillary sinuses. They are normally presented in multiple sections covering the full length, height, and thickness of the bone. About 10 to 15 panoramic views spaced 1 mm apart generated from a stack of closely spaced axial slices are sufficient to cover the entire jaw.

Cross-sectional views

Computer-generated cross-sectional views are reformatted in planes cutting across the maxillary or mandibular

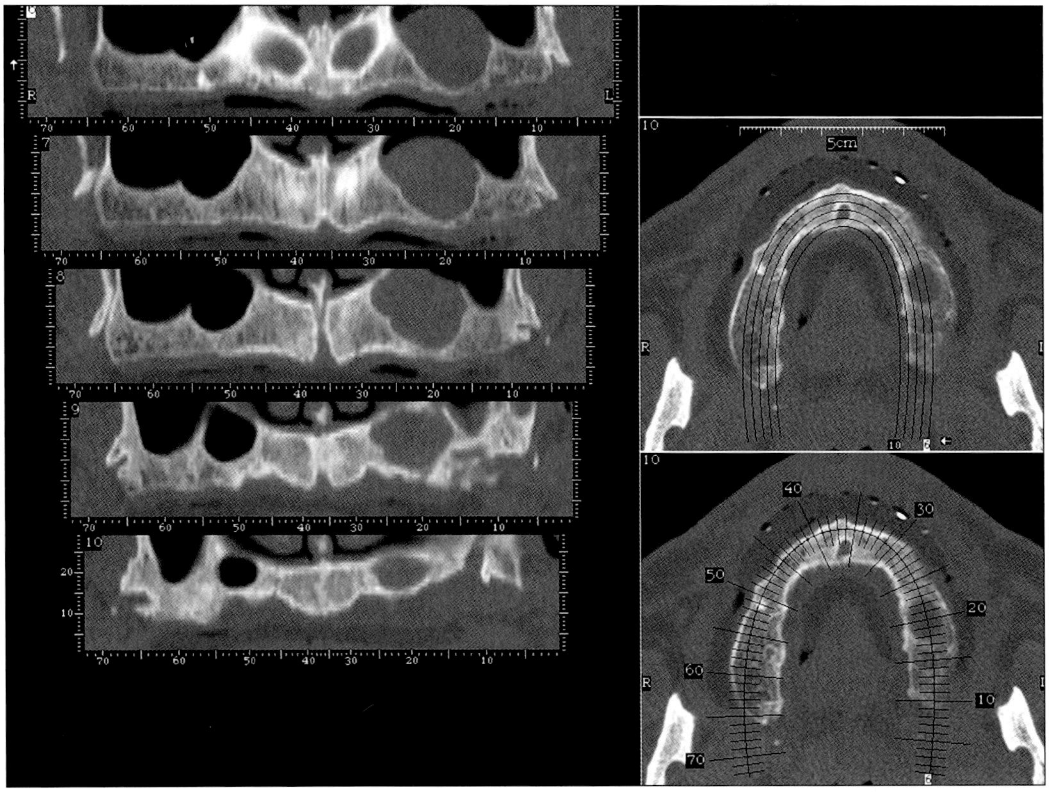

Fig 2-3 Life-sized images for direct measurement. The user traces a curve on a representative axial slice *(bottom right)*, and the computer calculates a family of equidistant curves *(top right)*. Then the computer creates a set of panoramic images, one for each curve *(left)*.

bone, at right angles to both the panoramic and original axial slices. Each cross-sectional view represents an image layer about 0.25 mm thick, commonly spaced 1 or 2 mm apart. The cross-sectional views may be the most important ones. It is from these images that observations of bone quality, implant size, and angulation are commonly made. By drawing a profile line across the cross-sectional image, the cortical plate thickness, cortical bone density, and trabecular bone density can all be estimated (Fig 2-4a).

When measuring distances from cross-sectional images, care must be taken to ensure that the cross-sectional slices are parallel to the direction in which the implants will be placed; otherwise, misleading information may result. This is especially important when working from hard copy such as film. The cross-sectional views are always generated at right angles to the axial slices, and this direction cannot be adjusted on hard copy.

In the posterior mandible, for example, one might think it is more logical to measure at right angles to the alveolar ridge; however, this is not necessarily the direction of the cross-sectional images (Fig 2-4b). In such cases it is important to take measurements from both the cross-sectional and panoramic views and, if necessary, make a mathematical correction for the oblique direction of the implant with respect to the reformatted planes. The CT images themselves are highly accurate, but failure to consider the direction of measurement or to use suitable planning software may lead to inaccurate results.

With some interactive software, the implants can be adjusted on the 3D view, and therefore the correct three-dimensional distance can always be obtained. Other software packages allow cross-sectional views to be generated in "double oblique" planes parallel to the implant direction, which is an alternative way of ensuring accurate 3D measurements.[8]

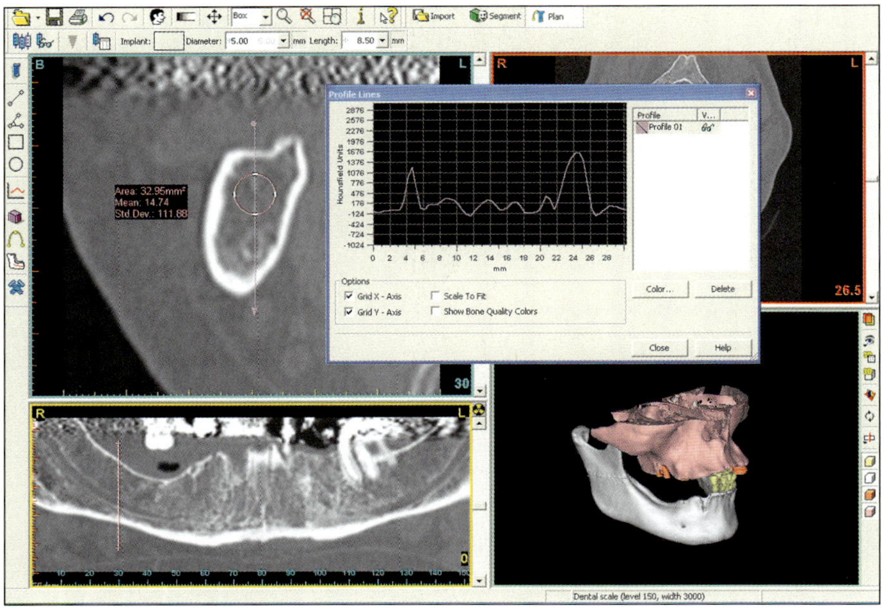

Fig 2-4a Cross-sectional image. Using the "Profile" and "Area" tools in SimPlant, a dense cortical plate is revealed. This posterior mandibular bone is type D4 at best.

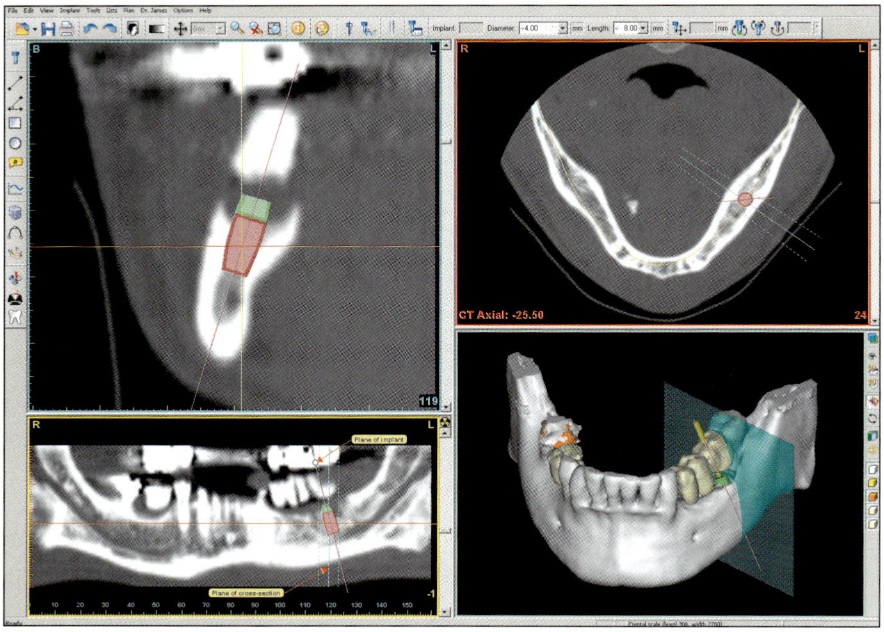

Fig 2-4b A cross-sectional image perpendicular to the axial slices, but not perpendicular to either the alveolar ridge or the lower border. When used on its own, such an image will not provide an accurate measurement of the available bone thickness. An accurate estimate of appropriate implant length may be obtained from the 3D view.

3D views

Computer-generated 3D views provide a superb overview of the bony architecture of the patient's mouth, the radiologic scanning appliance (representing desired tooth positions), and any remaining teeth. They can be very helpful in understanding structures that vary significantly in three dimensions, such as the floor of the maxillary sinuses.

By placing virtual implants on the 3D image, the clinician has an opportunity to determine the need for bone augmentation (such as grafting, ridge splitting, sinus lifting, etc) presurgically.

It is also possible to make the 3D image translucent and rotate it in all directions. While working in the 3D view, the clinician may plan to alter the angle of the implant preoperatively to avoid an important anatomic structure but retain the implant orientation in alignment with teeth depicted in the radiologic scanning appliance. An angulated abutment can then be placed to ensure the correct emergence angle.

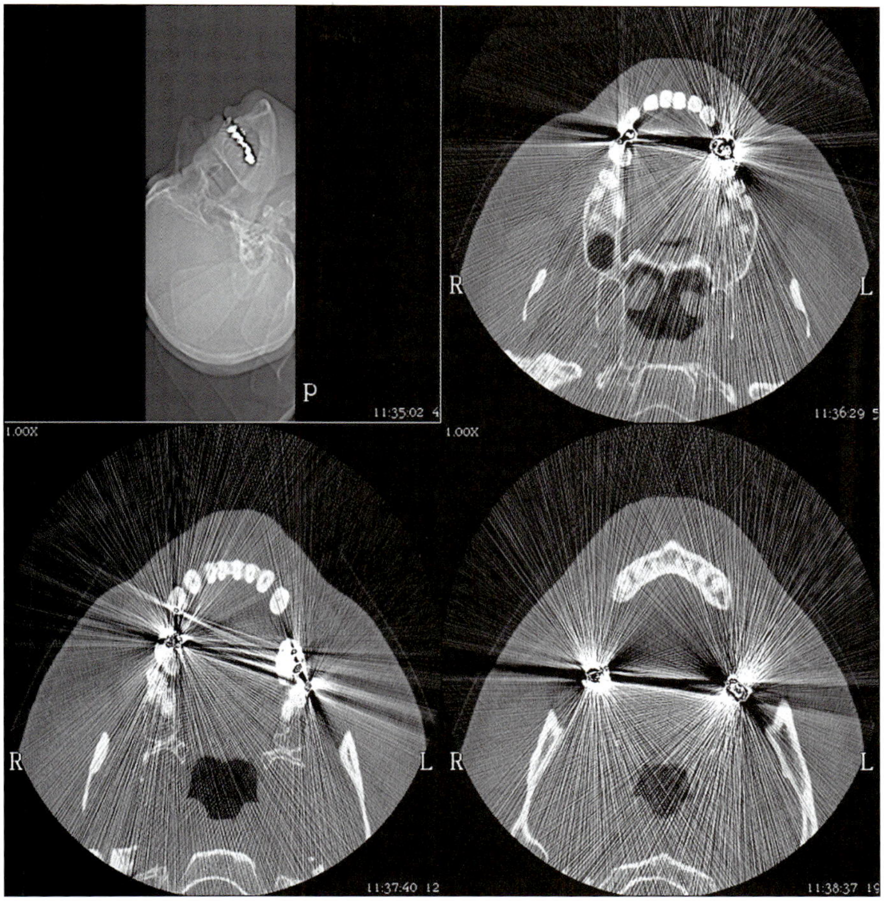

Fig 2-5 Starburst artifacts.

Artifacts in CT Images

Starburst

Starburst artifacts are produced by heavy metals, and they arise because of sampling limitations during scanning (Fig 2-5). The severity of the effect depends on the atomic number of the material; titanium causes little or no artifact, whereas gold causes a serious degradation of the image.

If the patient has been appropriately positioned, metal-ceramic restorations and large amalgam fillings may obscure detail at the occlusal plane level but rarely affect images apical to the alveolar crest. The primary exceptions are large gold or precious metal alloy posts extending down into the bone, which can cause loss of image detail at the bone crest or below.

Extensive artifacts produced by large posts in root canals or heavily restored teeth can render a CT unreadable. In such cases, either a compromise has to be made in the direction of scanning, or another method of examination (eg, complex motion tomography) must be chosen. Consideration should also be given to removing the metal before the scan. Starburst artifacts are always more pronounced on the axial slices. Reformatting the data into panoramic and cross-sectional views minimizes these artifacts. Datasets with severe artifacts in the axial slices still usually result in usable 3D, panoramic, and cross-sectional views.

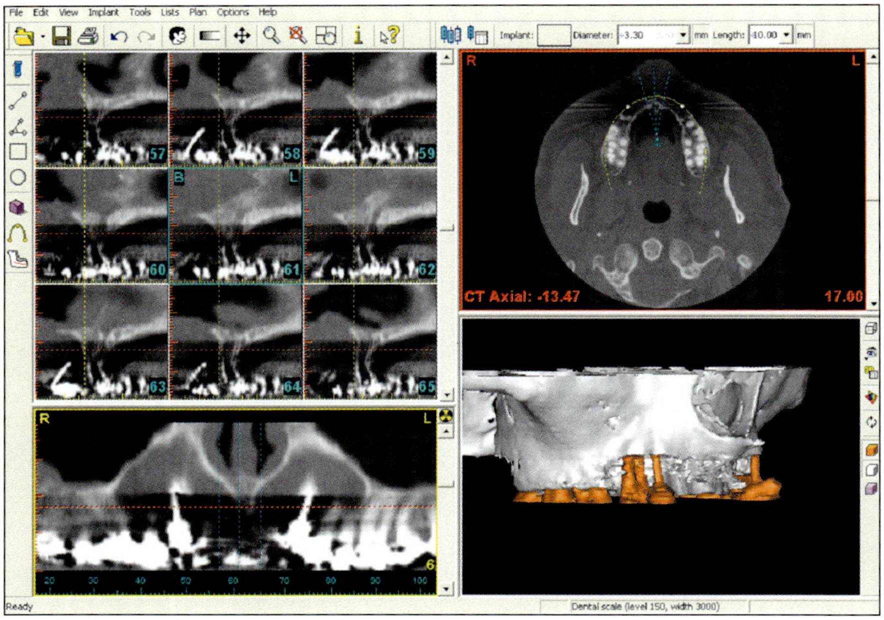

Fig 2-6 Beam-hardening artifacts.

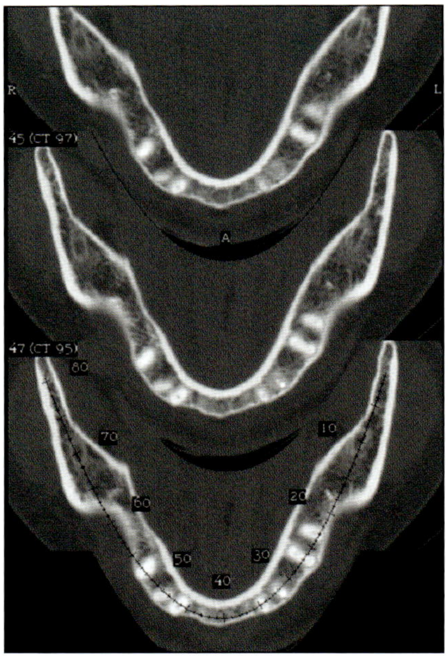

Fig 2-7 Helical artifact. The blurring arises from interpolation of the projection data at the time of scanning.

Beam hardening

Because x-ray tubes emit a spectrum of energies, low-energy photons are preferentially absorbed as the beam passes through metal. Consequently, the average energy increases while the Hounsfield number decreases. This artifact causes black streaks that connect objects with strong attenuation, such as metal pins (Fig 2-6). Beam-hardening artifacts are difficult to work around; the only alternatives may be to remove the offending metal before the CT scan or to use a different method of examination.

Compton scatter

The effect of Compton scatter is that not all photons follow a straight path. Some are deflected and continue at a lower energy and on a different path. In single-slice CT, the resulting image degradation is quite small, since photons that are scattered out of the slice are not collected. In multislice and CBCT, the effects are more significant because the wrong detector may collect the scattered photons. Compton scatter leads to loss of contrast and a background "fog" that is most noticeable in CBCT images.

Partial volume effect

The values of the individual voxels in a CT dataset are computed from photon intensity measurements that are averaged over the beam width or over the size of a detector element. Because the detector elements are not infinitely small, it is inevitable that, in some circumstances, air + soft tissue or soft tissue + bone may contribute to the same voxel value, resulting in distorted CT numbers. For example, very thin bone in the maxilla may be averaged with soft tissue and appear to have a lower density than it otherwise would have. The partial volume effect is reduced in MSCT scanners, which have multiple rows of very small detector elements.

Motion artifact

Patient movement during the data acquisition process results in blurring of the image. If the patient swallows, the trachea and esophagus may be blurred, but the bone and teeth may or may not be affected. However, if the teeth and bony structures are inconsistent from one slice to the next, then the patient will have to be rescanned.

Table 2-3 Choosing the scanning plane

Type of image	Indication	Advantages	Disadvantages
Axial slices parallel to occlusal plane	Maxilla, mandible, or both together	Minimal artifact from metal in occlusal surfaces of teeth Cross-sectional images are appropriate for planning implants vertical to the occlusal plane	
Axial slices parallel to lower border of mandible	Mandible only	Minimal number of slices required to cover the mandible Cross-sectional images are appropriate for planning implants vertical to the lower border	Images may be compromised by artifacts from metal restorations Position may be uncomfortable for the patient
Axial slices parallel to hard palate	Maxilla only	Minimal number of slices required to cover the sinuses Cross-sectional images are appropriate for planning implants vertical to the maxillary ridge	Images may be compromised by artifacts from metal restorations

Helical artifact

An artifact can occur on spiral or helical CT scanners because the individual axial slices are reconstructed from interpolated data. This artifact manifests itself as blurred regions in structures that change markedly from one slice to the next (Fig 2-7). The blurring is usually localized and does not affect the interpretation of the images.

Choosing the Scanning Plane

The optimal scanning plane depends on the architecture of the patient's mouth, the amount of metal in the remaining teeth, and the location and angulation of the desired implants. Since these are all clinical factors, the referring clinician is responsible for specifying the scanning plane. In an MSCT scanner, the patient should be positioned so that the scanning plane is vertical; in a CBCT scanner it should be horizontal. The correct CT scanning plane can help minimize the effects of artifacts from metallic restorations. It is always best to scan parallel to the metal to minimize the number of slices that are compromised by artifacts.

The reformatted panoramic and cross-sectional images are generated at right angles to the CT scanning plane. To ensure that these images have the same vertical orientation as the intended implant placements, choose the plane at right angles to the direction in which the implants will be placed (Table 2-3).

Occlusal plane

Advantages

- Scan the maxilla, mandible, or both together.
- Minimize the artifact from metal in occlusal surfaces of teeth.
- Cross-sectional images are appropriate for planning implants vertical to the occlusal plane.

Disadvantages

- None.

The occlusal plane is the arch-shaped area where the maxillary and mandibular teeth come into contact when the mouth is closed. If the patient's mouth is open, the occlusal plane can be taken as running from the tips of the anterior incisors and over the the occlusal surfaces of the posterior molars. The occlusal plane is generally curved, so it may be necessary to mentally "straighten out" the curve and scan parallel to the imaginary plane (Fig 2-8).

Sometimes, because of overeruption, the mandibular anterior teeth are much higher than the posterior teeth, especially when no opposing teeth are present. In such cases, it is best to ignore the anterior teeth and find the plane using only the posterior teeth. It is always best to have the chin up rather than down to ensure the entire jaw is scanned, without unnecessary slices. It is a common mistake to miss the bottom of the chin. By getting the chin up, this mistake is easily avoided and also allows for more of the ramus to be included.

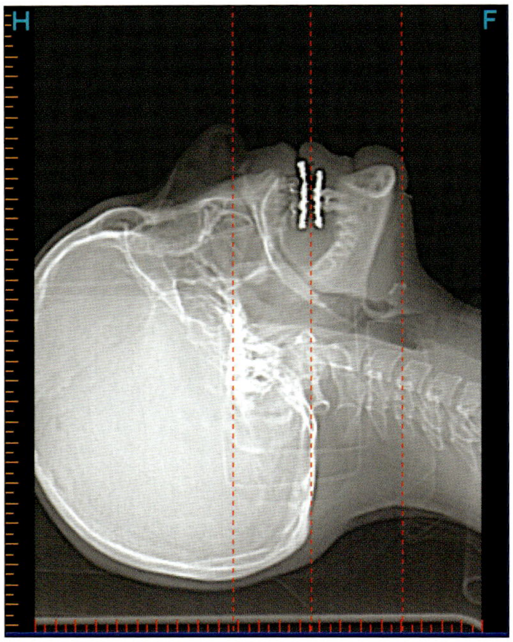

Fig 2-8 Scout view (alignment image) showing the patient correctly positioned for scanning parallel to the occlusal plane.

Lower border

Advantages

- Scan only the mandible.
- Minimal number of slices required covering the mandible.
- Cross-sectional images are appropriate for planning implants vertical to the lower border.

Disadvantages

- Images may be compromised by artifacts from metal restorations.
- Position is uncomfortable for the patient.

Scanning parallel to the lower border may be a good choice when implants are to be oriented vertical to the lower border (eg, in the mandibular molar and premolar regions). Scanning parallel to the lower border usually results in the minimum slices needed to cover the required anatomy.

When scanning parallel to the lower border, the effect of metal restorations should be carefully considered, since artifacts can seriously compromise the images. With a lie-down scanner it can be quite difficult for the patient to keep the lower border in a vertical direction. If both the mandible and the maxilla are to be scanned, the patient will need to be re-positioned after the mandibular scan is completed. Under no circumstances should the maxilla be scanned parallel to the lower border of the mandible, because the cross-sectional images will be seriously distorted.

Hard palate

Advantages

- Scan the maxilla only.
- Minimal number of slices required to cover the sinuses.
- Cross-sectional images are appropriate for planning implants vertical to the maxillary ridge.

Disadvantage

- Images may be compromised by artifact from metal restorations.

Some surgeons prefer scans taken parallel to the hard palate to assess the bony detail. This can be a useful option if the patient is edentulous and a radiologic template is not used.

Benefits and Risks of CT Scans

Most medical and dental procedures have associated risks as well as benefits, and radiologic imaging is no exception. The benefits of x-rays are obvious and the risks are small but should be addressed and placed into perspective.

Radiation dose

Every country has regulations and recommendations that provide an appropriate standard of radiation protection without limiting the beneficial use of x-rays. Although these regulations may vary, they are generally based on the work of the International Commission on Radiological Protection (ICRP), which emphasizes that "ionising radiation needs to be treated with care rather than fear and its risks should be kept in perspective with other risks."[9]

How should radiation doses be measured and expressed? Ionizing radiation, such as x-rays, interacts with living tissue by imparting energy. This absorbed energy may cause damage through chemical or molecular changes at the cellular level. Some of these changes may take a very long period of time (20 years or more) to become apparent.

The *absorbed dose* (expressed in milliGray [mGy]) represents the amount of radiation energy per unit mass received by the patient. However, this unit does not measure risk since it does not take into account the volume of tissue irradiated or whether this volume includes the more radiosensitive organs such as bone marrow, breast, colon, lung, or stomach.

Dental x-rays affect a relatively small portion of the body (just the head in most cases), whereas background radiation, to which we are all subjected, affects the whole body from head to toe. While the same amount of absorbed dose might be received in two different exposures, clearly it will do more damage if the whole body is affected since more radiosensitive organs will be involved.

The *effective dose* (expressed in milliSievert [mSv]) has been defined as "the dose that, if applied to the whole body, would involve the patient in the same degree of risk."[10] The effective dose is calculated using tissue-weighting factors to take into account the relative sensitivities of the different organs. In 2007, these tissue-weighting factors were revised by the ICRP,[10] which gave salivary glands a higher weighting.

The concept of effective dose allows comparisons to be made between one type of radiologic investigation and another and between the doses from medical and dental procedures and those from natural sources. The unit concept of background equivalent radiation time (BERT) is useful for explaining doses to patients.[11] BERT indicates the length of time it would take the patient to receive the same effective dose from naturally occurring background radiation, such as radon or isotopes in food and drink. In the United Kingdom, the average annual dose of background radiation acquired from natural sources (excluding medical and dental irradiation) is about 2.2 mSv, or about 6 μSv per day. A typical hospital CT scan of the maxilla (250 μSv) is therefore equivalent to 42 days of background radiation, while a typical cone beam CT scan of both jaws (68 μSv) is equivalent to 11 days of background radiation.

Radiation risks

Current medical statistics suggest that one in three people will develop some form of cancer resulting from the combined effects of genetics, environmental factors, background radiation, and medical and dental exposure. The additional risk from a dental imaging procedure is very low and needs to be viewed in the context of the risks posed by natural sources of radiation.

The two known types of adverse effect that can occur following exposure to ionizing radiation are deterministic and stochastic effects.

Deterministic effects

In this context, *deterministic* means that the severity of the effect is proportional to the dose received. The effect of skin erythema is a good example because the larger the dose, the more the skin becomes red. Another example is the formation of cataracts within the eye. Deterministic effects (including eye cataracts) do not occur below a threshold of about 1 Sv and should never be seen in dental imaging unless a bad mistake has been made. Therefore, we need not consider them further here.

Stochastic effects

Stochastic effects are based on a stochastic, or statistical model, in which the risk of a certain event occurring depends on the dose, but its severity does not. To understand this effect, consider the risk involved in crossing a busy street. The more times a person crosses the street, the more likely he or she is to be hit by a car. However, the *severity* of the accident does not depend on how many times the person has crossed the street before.

Stochastic effects include *genetic effects* (the possibility of the patient passing a defective gene on to a descendent) and *somatic effects* (the possibility of the patient developing a fatal cancer within the next 20 or so years following a dental imaging procedure). Genetic risks are extremely small in dental imaging, so we concentrate on somatic risks in this section.

The dose-dependent risks of radiation are very difficult to calculate. The best evidence shows a very small increase in cancer for doses of radiation of around 50 mSv or less.[12]

Table 2-4 Radiation doses from dental x-ray examinations (ICRP 1990 tissue weightings)*

X-ray mode	Technique	Typical effective dose (μSv)	Background equivalent radiation time	Theoretical cancer risk (per million exams)
Single periapical (PA) or bitewing[13]	Digital, rectangular collimation Digital, round collimation E-speed film, round collimation	1 2 4	4 hours 8 hours 16 hours	0.05 0.1 0.2
Lateral cephalogram[13]	Digital/film with rare earth screen	2	8 hours	0.1
Dental panoramic tomogram[14,15]	Digital/film with rare earth screen	20	3.5 days	1.0
Full-mouth set (20 PAs)	Digital, rectangular collimation Digital, round collimation E-speed film, round collimation	20 32 80	3.5 days 5.5 days 13.5 days	1.0 1.6 4.0
NewTom cone beam CT[16]	9000 series 3G	36 43	6 days 7 days	1.8 2.1
i-CAT cone beam CT[17]	20-second scan 40-second scan	29 68	5 days 11 days	1.5 3.4
Scanora[18]	1 cycle 6 cycles	65 390	11 days 65 days	3.3 19.5
Hospital CT[19]	Maxilla Mandible	250 480	42 days 80 days	12.5 24.0

*For comparison purposes: A 6-hour transatlantic flight delivers a typical effective dose of 24 μSv, with a background equivalent radiation time of 4 days and a theoretical cancer risk of 1.2 per million exams.[20]

Table 2-5 Recommended acquisition and reconstruction settings for two CT scanners

	GE LightSpeed 16	Siemens Sensation 16
Acquisition settings		
Gantry tilt	0 degrees	0 degrees
Tube potential	120 kVp	120 kVp
Tube current	80 mA	80 mA
Pitch	0.562	0.500
Table feed per rotation	5.62 mm	6.00 mm
Time per rotation	0.80 seconds	0.75 seconds
Collimation	16 × 0.625 mm	16 × 0.750 mm
Reconstruction settings		
Matrix	512 × 512	512 × 512
Field of view	150 mm	150 mm
Convolution kernel	Bone Plus	H60s
Slice thickness	0.625 mm	0.750 mm
Slice increment	0.5 mm	0.5 mm

However, there is clear evidence (mostly from atomic bomb survivors) that cancer has developed when doses of around 500 mSv or more have been involved. So the risk is calculated from these figures and then extrapolated back. The risk is usually expressed as 1 in 20,000 per mSv received. On this basis, a hospital CT scan of the maxilla (250 μSv) carries an additional risk of approximately 1 in 80,000 that the patient will develop a fatal cancer later in life (over and above the one in three risk that everyone bears). Put another way, one would expect to see 12.5 additional fatal cancers per 1 million hospital CT scans of the maxilla.

For perspective, here are some other activities that carry a 1 in 80,000 risk of a fatality:

- Smoking 10 cigarettes just once in your life
- Traveling 600 miles by car
- Working in a factory for 180 days
- Rock climbing for 25 minutes

A number of dental imaging examinations and the associated risks are shown in Table 2-4.

In 1990, the ICRP[9] issued a set of recommendations that have since been incorporated into European law. These recommendations were clarified in 2007[10] but the fundamental principles did not change. The ICRP's recommendations for medical and dental radiation exposures can be easily summarized: the benefit from each exposure to radiation must be greater than the risk, and radiation doses must be kept as low as reasonably achievable (abbreviated ALARA). Basically, if the slightly increased risk from radiation is outweighed by the greatly reduced risk of complications at the time of surgery, the CT scan is clearly justified.

The risk/benefit ratio is something that must be assessed individually for each patient. For example, if the patient has a medical condition that prevents him or her from remaining motionless during the CT scan, such a patient will not receive the full benefit of the CT study. It is unlikely that a CT scan could be justified in such a case. Once the CT scan has been justified, there is a responsibility to perform the CT scan using a radiation dose in keeping with the ALARA principle.

Because of the large natural contrast between bone and soft tissue, it is possible to perform dental CT scans using much lower exposure factors than those required for a diagnostic procedure such as a brain scan. Accurate patient positioning and strict adherence to a prescribed protocol are very important (Table 2-5). Minimizing the dose without considering image quality can lead to images that are not diagnostically useful.

The radiologist's responsibility is to provide the scout view and axial images of the region of interest. Radiation dose to the patient can be considerably reduced through the use of proper radiographic techniques, including:

- Avoiding rescans made necessary by patient movement
- Making sure the patient is properly prepared and instructed to remain motionless
- Scanning the minimum number of slices required
- Avoiding unnecessary slices under the chin (thyroid) or into the orbits (eyes)

Guidelines for the Referring Dentist

The importance of ensuring that a scan provides the most information at the lowest radiation dose cannot be overemphasized. The list below will help the referring clinician achieve these goals.

- Ensure that the patient is familiar with the procedures involved, and stress the importance of keeping completely still for the duration of the scan.
- Provide the patient with a radiologic scanning appliance containing radiopaque markers to indicate the ideal tooth positions and occlusal stops for keeping the jaws 1 to 2 mm apart.
- Make sure the patient knows how to insert and position the scanning appliance correctly.
- Instruct the patient to remove any removable metal dentures or other prostheses and all jewelry before the scan is taken.
- Consider removing any amalgam fillings and replacing them with composites, especially if the treatment plan calls for the tooth to be extracted.
- Provide clear and concise instructions to the radiologist or technician on a written referral form. This form should include the jaw(s) to be scanned, the intended use of a radiologic scanning appliance, the presence of removable dental prostheses, and the types of 3D masks required during processing of the CT scan. It is also important to provide instructions regarding the plane in which the axial views are to be taken.

Conclusion

Implantologists have many imaging modalities at their disposal; Table 2-1 summarizes the key properties of the ones most commonly used. Intraoral periapicals are useful in determining consistency at the time of surgery and osseointegration during follow-up. Dental panoramic tomograms provide an invaluable overview, which is often the start of the treatment planning process. However, only CT scanning can provide the clinician with the detailed images needed to plan implant placement to the required degree of accuracy.

The radiation dose from hospital-based CT scanners, while small, is a matter of concern. Care should be taken to keep the dose as low as reasonably achievable. Cone beam CT scanners, which deliver a considerably lower dose, will be important in implant planning in the future.

Distance measurements taken from correctly interpreted CT scans are extremely accurate, and CT is the only imaging modality to provide numerical values for bone density. However, CT is not suitable for patients who cannot remain immobile and/or have gold or heavy metal posts extending into the bone that cannot be removed.

References

1. Hounsfield GN. Computerized transverse axial scanning tomography: Part 1, description of the system. Br J Radiol 1973;46:1016–1022.
2. Herman GT, Naparstek A. Fast image reconstruction based on a Radon inversion formula appropriate for rapidly collected data. SIAM J Appl Math 1977;33:511–533.
3. McCollough CH, Zinc FE. Performance evaluation of a multi-slice CT system. Med Phys 1999;26:2223–2230.
4. Robb R, Hoffman E, Sinak LJ, Harris LD, Ritman EL. High-speed three-dimensional x-ray computed tomography: The dynamic spatial reconstructor. Proc IEEE 1983;71:308–319.
5. Misch CE. Bone density—A key determinant for success. In: Misch CE (ed). Contemporary Implant Dentistry, ed 2. St Louis: Mosby, 1999: 109–119.
6. Kalender WA. Computed Tomography. Munich: Publicis MCD Verlag, 2000:84–85.
7. Rothman SLG. Dental Applications of Computerized Tomography. Chicago: Quintessence, 1998:11–12.
8. Naitoh M, Katsumata A, Nohara E, Ohsaki C, Ariji E. Measurement accuracy of reconstructed 2-D images obtained by multi-slice helical computed tomography. Clin Oral Implants Res 2004;15:507–574.
9. 1990 Recommendations of the International Commission on Radiological Protection. ICRP Publication 60. Ann ICRP 1991;21:1–201.
10. 2007 Recommendations of the International Commission on Radiological Protection. ICRP Publication 103. Ann ICRP 2007;37:1–332.
11. Cameron JR. A radiation unit for the public. Physics Society 1991; 20:2.
12. Cardis E, Vrijheid M, Blettnet M, et al. Risk of cancer after low doses of ionising radiation: Retrospective cohort study in 15 countries. Br Med J 2005;10:1136.
13. Pendlebury ME, Horner K, Eaton KA (eds). Selection Criteria for Dental Radiography. London: Faculty of General Dental Practice (UK), Royal College of Surgeons of England, 2004.
14. Damforth RA, Clark DE. Effective dose from radiation absorbed during a panoramic examination with a new generation machine. Oral Surg Oral Med Oral Pathol Radiol Endod 2000;89:236–343.
15. Gijbels F, Jacobs R, Debaveye D, Bogaerts R, Verlinden S, Sanderink G. Dosimetry of digital panoramic imaging. Part 1: Patient exposure. Dentomaxillofac Radiol 2005;34:145–149.
16. Ludlow JB, Davies-Ludlow LE, Brooks SL. Dosimetry of two extraoral direct digital imaging devices: NewTom cone beam CT and Orthophos Plus DS panoramic unit. Dentomaxillofac Radiol 2003;32: 229–234.
17. Ludlow JB, Ivanovic M. Comparative dosimetry of dental CBCT devices and 64-slice CT for oral and maxillofacial radiology. Oral Surg Oral Med Oral Pathol Oral Radiol Endod 2008;106:106–114.
18. Dula K, Mini R, Lambrecht JT, et al. Hypothetical mortality risk associated with spiral tomography of the maxilla and mandible prior to endosseous implant treatment. Eur J Oral Sci 1997;105:123–129.
19. Dula K, Mini R, van der Stelt PF, Lambrecht JT, Schneeberger P, Buser D. Hypothetical mortality risk associated with spiral computed tomography of the maxilla and mandible. Eur J Oral Sci 1996;104: 503–510.
20. Hughes JS. Ionising Radiation Exposue of the UK Population: 1999 Review. Chilton: National Radiological Protection Board (NRPB-R311), 1999.

3

THE DYNAMIC NATURE OF SIMPLANT SOFTWARE

Alan L. Rosenfeld, DDS, FACD

The introduction of the modern dental implant by Per-Ingvar Brånemark initiated a paradigm shift in the treatment of the severely debilitated edentulous patient—the so-called oral invalid. The early prosthetic options for these patients were limited to the hybrid prosthesis, and implant placement was surgically driven. For treatment planning, a lateral cephalometric radiograph was used; this plain film radiograph provides a crude cross-sectional view of minimally sufficient accuracy and information about the atrophic jaw. Moreover, it is static, noninteractive, and does not allow the transfer of prosthetically relevant information for interpretation. Vital anatomic structures did not significantly influence treatment and posed relatively low risks to patients. Surgical decision making was performed intraoperatively rather than preoperatively.

Computed tomography (CT) was introduced to the dental profession in 1987 to facilitate radiographic examination of the jaws and implant treatment planning.[1,2] It allowed the dental profession for the first time to examine the anatomic structures of the maxilla and mandible in the form of accurate multiplanar, reformatted, contiguous images. Although analogue in nature, the reformatted images improved our ability to evaluate anatomic structures and the effects of postextraction resorptive patterns with submillimeter accuracy.[3,4] The technology also had significant limitations: there was no mechanism to interact with the CT data, transfer prosthetic outcome information into a CT dataset, or precisely transfer the CT plan back to the surgical setting.

Soon after, the concept of "optimal final tooth position" was introduced.[5–7] This concept was based in part on the ability to transfer patient-specific prosthetic information to the CT study via a scanning appliance.[8] In 1994, the computer-based interactive software SimPlant (Columbia Scientific) was introduced. Despite offering many advances, the SimPlant software did not allow treatment planning in 3D or the construction of accurate rapid prototype medical models and patient-specific surgical guides that could help ensure the preoperatively planned prosthetic outcome. These features were later incorporated into the real-time 2D-3D interactive imaging software developed in 1999 by Materialise, which at the same time introduced rapid prototype medical modeling to facilitate prosthetically guided surgical treatment.

Information Management

One of the most valuable functions of the SimPlant software is its capacity for information management. In a health care setting, information management involves collecting relevant clinical data that will be used to develop an accurate diagnosis and treatment plan. When accurate prosthetic information is incorporated into a CT study, parameters for effective collaboration can be established by the restorative dentist. Information management also serves as the driving force for collaboration and accountability on the part of all treatment participants.

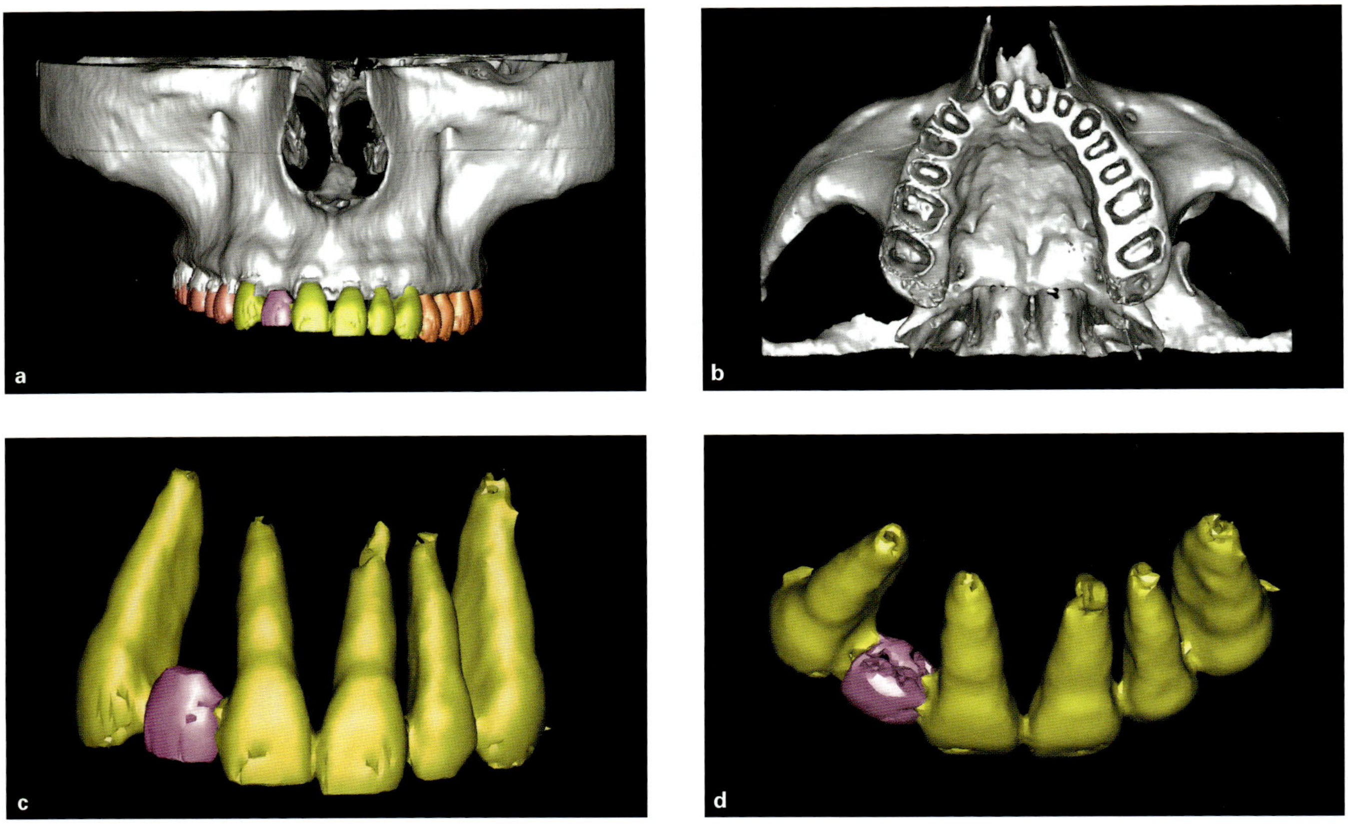

Fig 3-1 *(a)* 3D reconstruction of the maxilla and associated masks of the dentition. Each mask is represented by a different color that can be turned on or off to enhance viewing capabilities. *(b)* Occlusal view showing the socket of each tooth and allowing unimpeded examination of interradicular anatomy. *(c)* Anterior, and *(d)* superior views of the maxilla with the masks of the bone hidden.

Collaborative Accountability

The ability to manage information and develop a more precise diagnosis, in turn, helps to clarify the roles and responsibilities required of each participant for achieving a successful outcome. Such *collaborative accountability*,[9–11] as it has been called, represents a paradigm shift beyond interdisciplinary patient care, and it is one of the inherent benefits of using the SimPlant software. The restorative dentist assumes a leadership role by defining the prosthetic outcome, thereby establishing the surgical performance standards necessary to achieve the desired outcome before treatment has commenced. All treatment collaborators then have to determine whether the treatment plan is realistic, achievable, efficacious, and predictable. Preoperative rather than intraoperative planning drives treatment decisions.

The power of collaborative accountability lies in the shared knowledge that the patient, restorative dentist, implant surgeon, laboratory technician, and other dental and medical contributors can experience informed agreement in an atmosphere of disclosure and assume individual responsibility for achieving treatment objectives.

Accessing and Viewing CT Data in a 3D Environment

The ability to manage the complex array of treatment choices and optimize outcomes requires information management in a 3D environment based on a prosthetic outcome that is determined preoperatively. The true value of a CT study is that it contains relevant clinical information waiting to be accessed. Interactive CT software allows the clinician to formulate questions preoperatively and retrieve the data necessary to determine clinical performance standards. Not all of the software features must be mastered in order to realize this benefit. Users are motivated to learn the software in direct proportion to their desire to create an atmosphere of preoperative rather than intraoperative decision making.

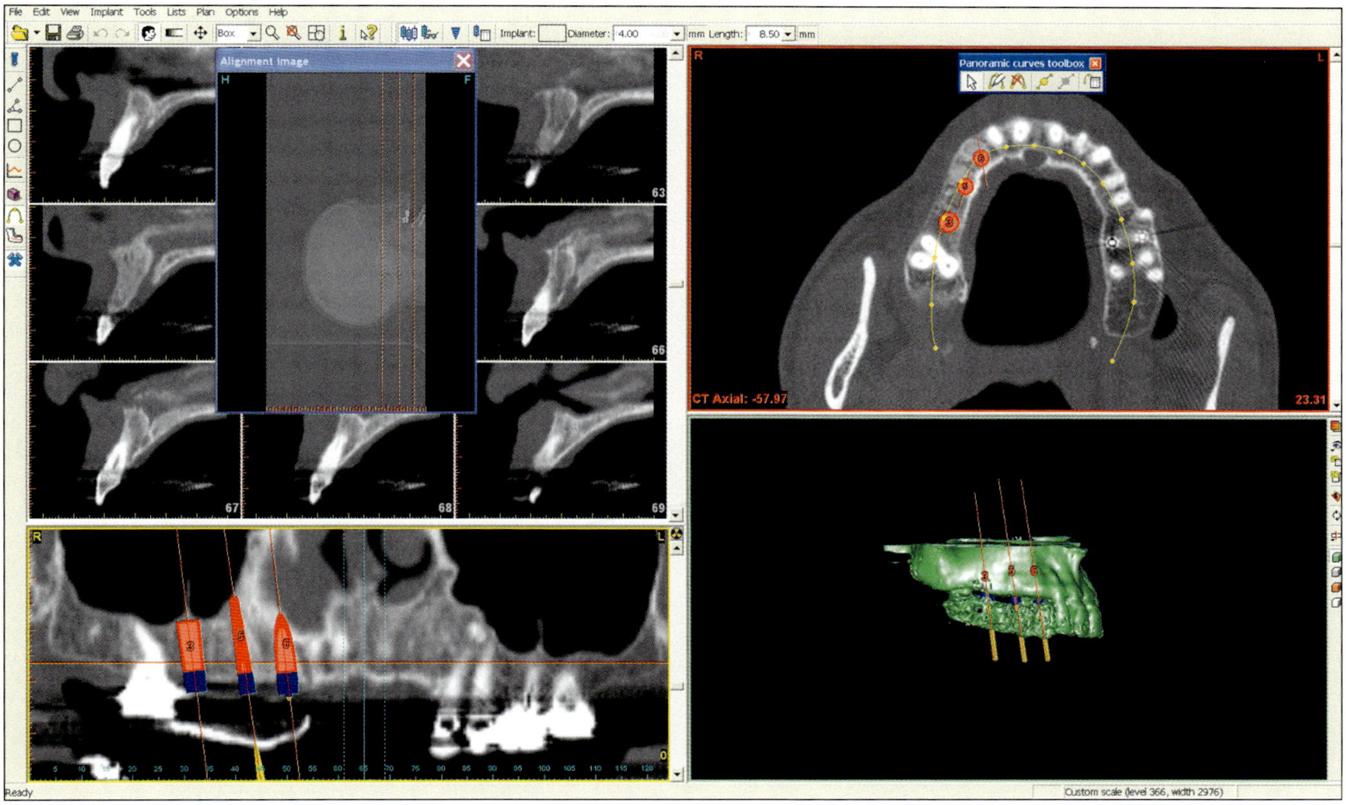

Fig 3-2 Four active work environments for SimPlant in the maxilla: cross-sectional, axial, panoramic, and 3D reconstruction. *Overlay, upper left:* The alignment image is used to confirm proper patient orientation at the time of CT imaging. *Overlay, upper right:* The panoramic curve modification tool is actively displayed.

The SimPlant software enables surgical treatment planning within the context of a prosthetically directed plan. Establishing a prosthetically driven treatment outcome leads to the fabrication of a patient-specific scanning appliance. The role of the scanning appliance is to transfer the prosthetic outcome to the CT dataset (see chapter 4).

All future surgical developments for the precise delivery of dental implants, either through the use of surgical guides or robotics, will be based on interpretation of CT images for each patient situation. The purpose of the SimPlant software is to facilitate a direct link between anatomic interpretation, treatment planning, and precise surgical execution. To allow for differential identification of tooth-related information in the CT study, all scanning appliances are made with barium sulfate. Within individual appliances, differential barium concentrations allow identification of tooth and soft tissue. Differential Hounsfield densities enable segmentation, isolation, and identification of influential regional anatomy.[12] Structures of different radiodensities are segmented so they can be isolated and viewed independently in the form of masks. This feature allows the user to disarticulate structures and view contiguous structures independently (Fig 3-1).

The Value of CT in Diagnosis and Treatment Planning

The brief examples that follow present various clinical situations in which patient treatment was influenced by preoperative discovery of influential regional anatomy. These examples demonstrate the different software features that are used to reveal relevant clinical information embedded within the CT dataset.

Upon opening a CT study, the user should perform the following three steps to confirm that it possesses the basic attributes necessary for interpretation:

1. Verify that the axial images are parallel to the occlusal plane, the scanning appliance was properly seated, and that the panoramic line was drawn properly, usually at the widest part of the jaw (Fig 3-2). Of the three attributes, only the panoramic line can be modified by the user.

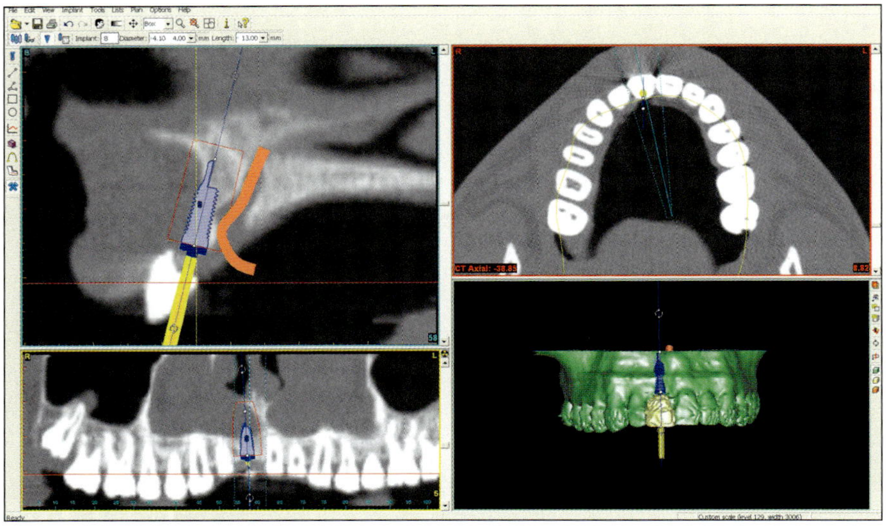

Fig 3-3a 2D and 3D maxillary views showing placement of a realistic implant in the anticipated optimal final tooth position. The available bone is insufficient to place an implant. In addition, the anatomy of the incisive canal, which will influence surgical treatment and informed consent, can be anticipated.

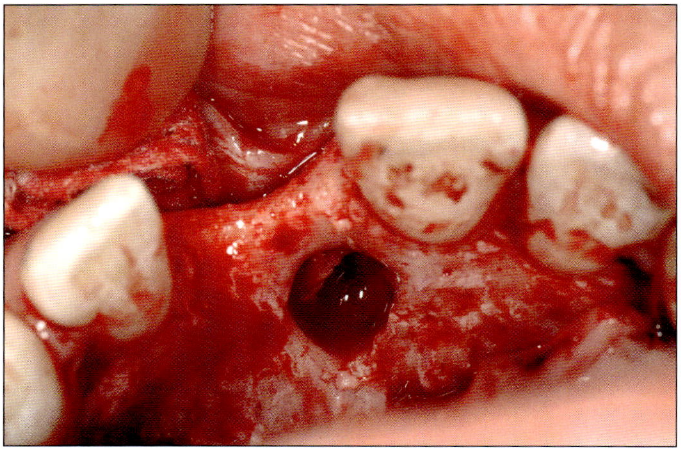

Fig 3-3b The clinical reality of the CT information is illustrated in this clinical view. The facial bone deficiency and the size of the incisive canal are problems that can be anticipated preoperatively.

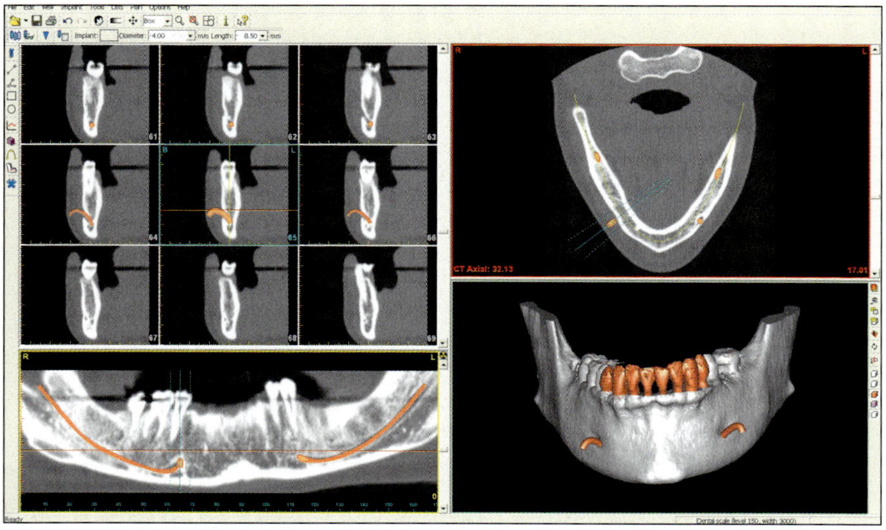

Fig 3-4 Four active work environments for SimPlant in the mandible: axial, panoramic, cross-sectional, and 3D reconstruction. The nerve drawing tool was used to highlight the anticipated position of the inferior alveolar nerve in all views. In addition, the 3D reconstruction has a mask of the dentition extending bilaterally from the first premolars.

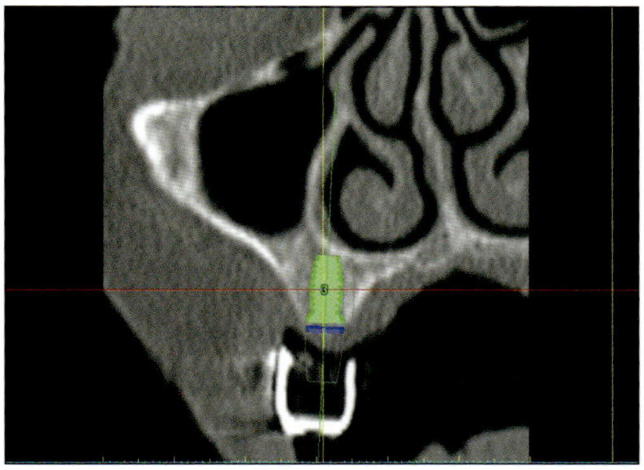

Fig 3-5a 2D cross-sectional view of the maxillary molar region. Note the size of the maxillary sinus and its medial and lateral walls; the osteomeatal complex; the nasal concha; the sinus floor; the bone inferior to the sinus; and the scanning appliance.

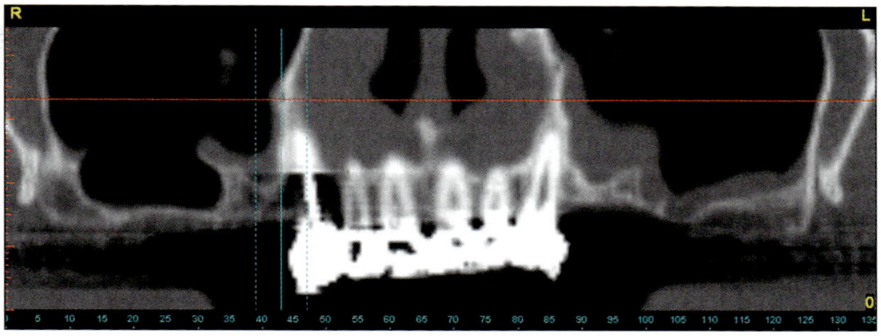

Fig 3-5b 2D panoramic view of the maxilla. Note thickening of the sinus membrane, irregular bony anatomy, and septa of the right and left sinuses.

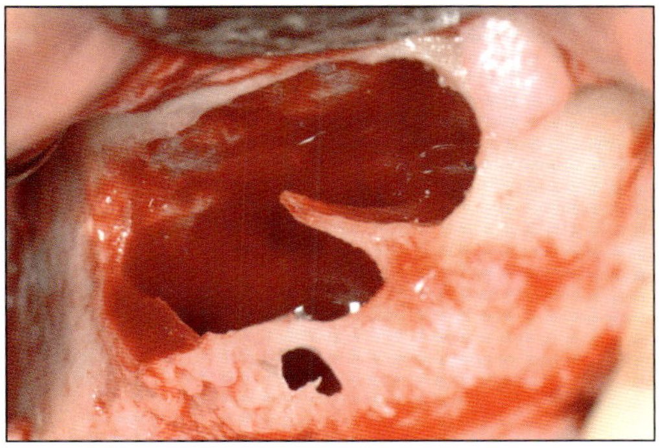

Fig 3-5c Clinical view of the regional anatomy shown in Figs 3-5a and 3-5b. Knowledge of the complex anatomy of the right sinus facilitated surgical management, which would not have been possible using any other radiographic modality. Note the bony fenestration of the sinus.

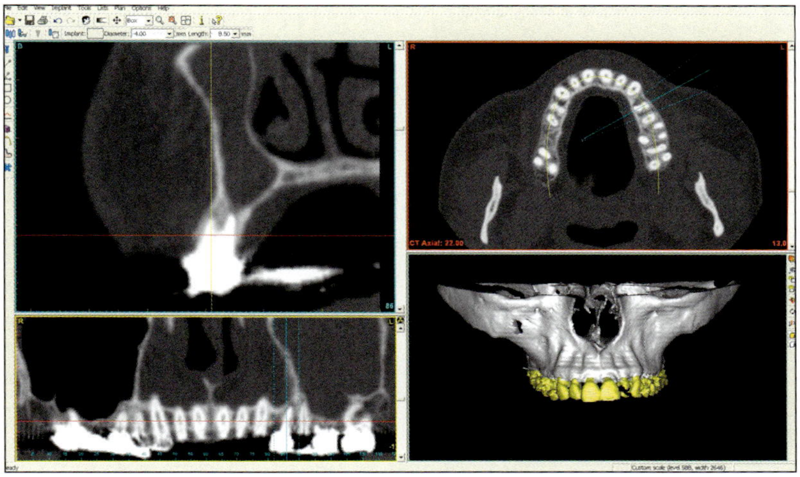

Fig 3-5d SimPlant presentation of maxillary left premolar periapical pathosis, revealing the perforation into the sinus. Such clear evidence of sinus disease requires critical decisions affecting patient treatment. It is important to view all of the images in order to appreciate the impact of the pathology.

2. Evaluate regional anatomy for vital structures and pathosis. Identification of neurovascular structures includes the nasopalatine foramen, mental foramina, and inferior alveolar canal (Figs 3-3 and 3-4). Regional anatomy can influence the location of implant placement. Evaluation of sinus pneumatization and the osteomeatal complex, linear circumference of the residual bone ridge, bone concavities, axial position of remaining teeth, periapical pathosis, and the relationship between bony resorption and anatomic structures influence the placement of dental implants (Figs 3-5 and 3-6).
3. Select a dental implant to be placed in the best prosthetically driven position dictated by the scanning appliance. Once an ideal implant position is determined, assessment of adequate bone volume and density can be completed (Fig 3-7). Implant selection can be generic or manufacturer specific. The software includes an implant library of realistic implants and abutments for each implant manufacturer. The need for site development can be determined and factored into the treatment plan (Fig 3-8).

In the CT study, the anterior maxilla and mandible appear as curvilinear structures, and each tooth represents a three-dimensional position within the jaw. By segmenting the bone from the teeth (Fig 3-9), SimPlant enables the user to view the teeth separately from the bone.

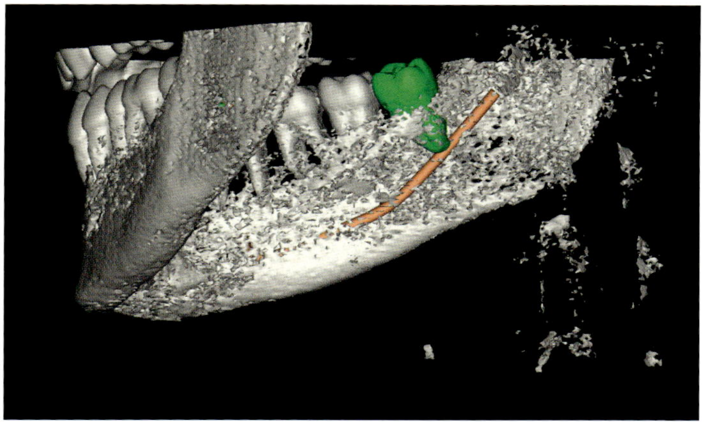

Fig 3-6a 3D reconstruction of the mandible created by adjusting the threshold values used to calculate the image. Once the best threshold value was determined, the software program created the reconstruction. A mask of the mandibular right third molar was created. The nerve drawing tool was used to display the relationship of this tooth to regional anatomy and vital structures.

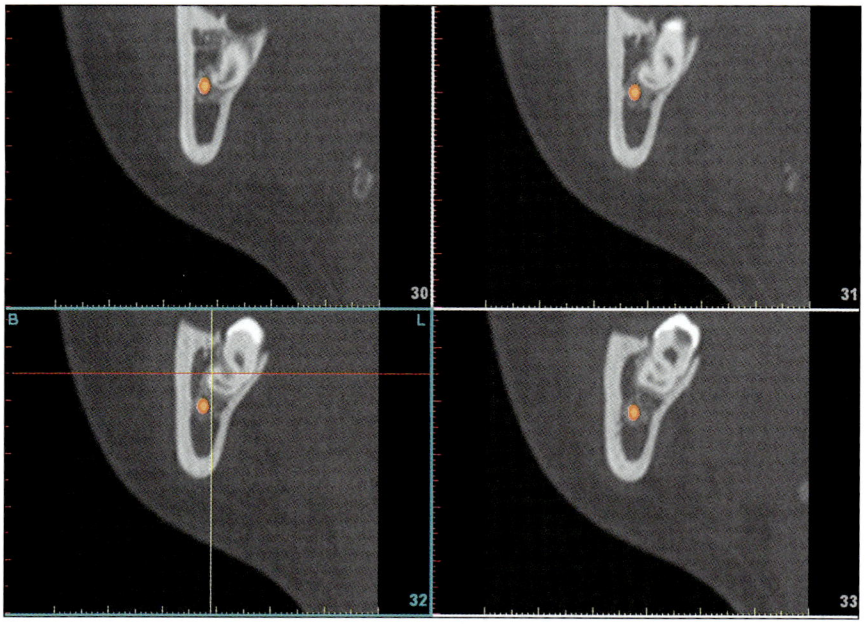

Fig 3-6b 2D cross-sectional view of impacted third molar and its relationship to the anticipated position of the inferior alveolar nerve.

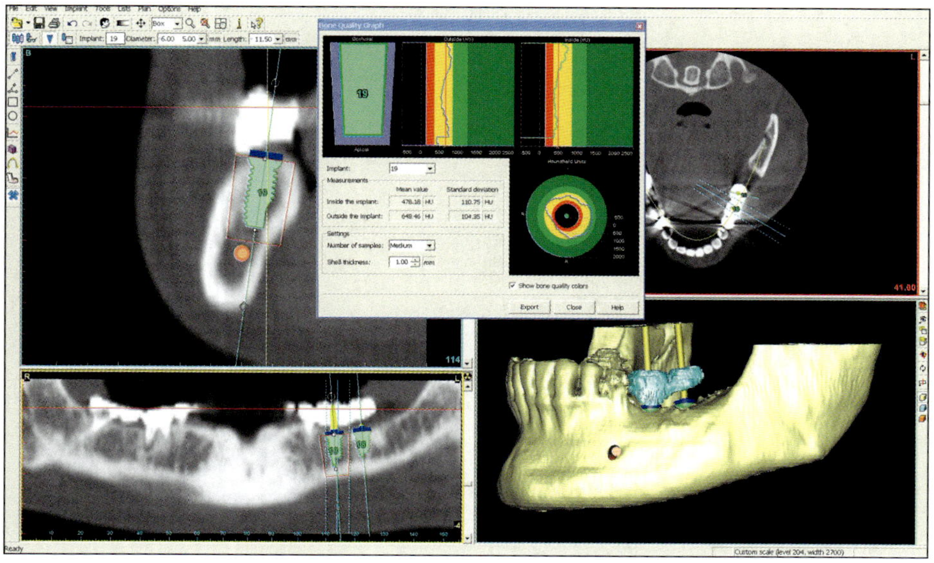

Fig 3-7 SimPlant presentation of the left posterior region of the mandible, scanning appliance, realistic implants, and bone density screen. This field summarizes the average Hounsfield values around the implant.

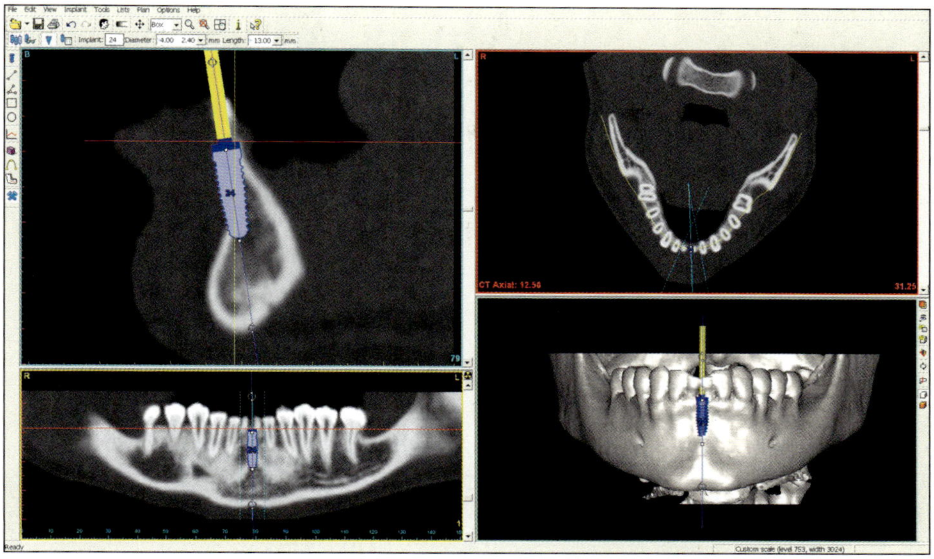

Fig 3-8 SimPlant presentation of 2D and 3D mandibular views. A realistic implant is placed in the anticipated optimal final tooth position; however, the available bone is insufficient to place the implant without bone grafting. Donor bone apical to the implant position can be used to augment the site.

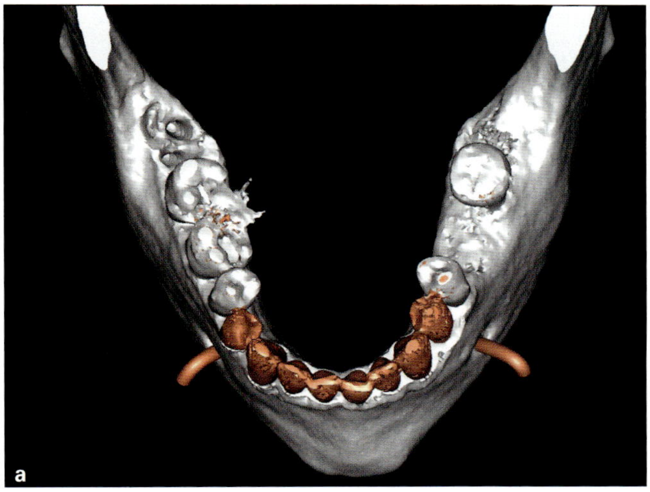

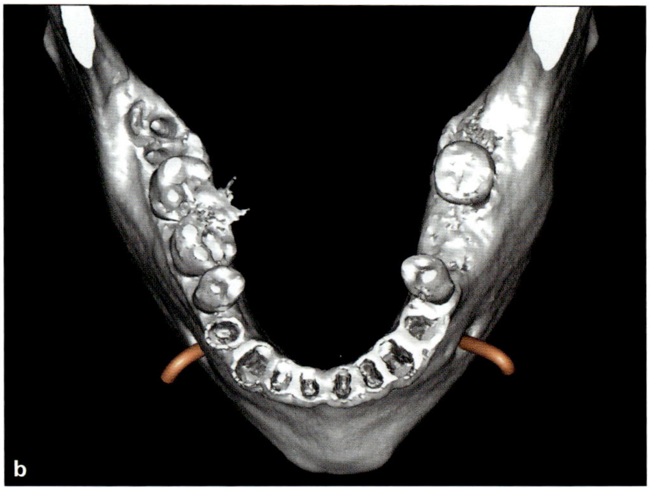

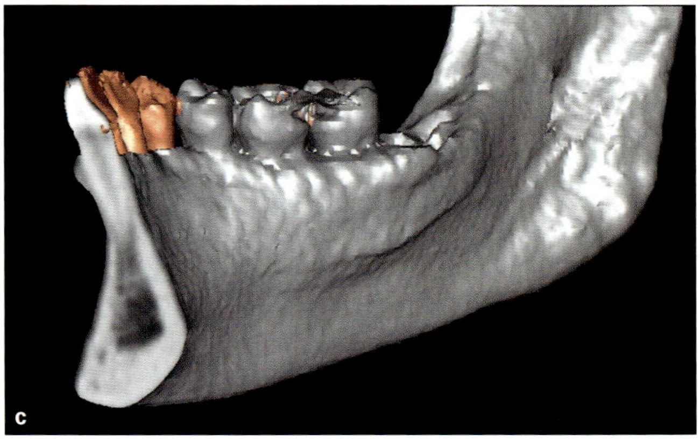

Fig 3-9 *(a)* Superior view of the mandible with a mask of the interforaminal dentition. Note the nerve tool illustration of the mental nerve as it emerges from the mental foramen. *(b)* The mask has been deactivated, revealing the underlying anatomy of the alveolar process. Note the divergent anatomy of the alveolar process and basal bone of the symphysis. *(c)* 2D cross-sectional view of a mandibular incisor that has been inserted into a 3D reconstruction of the mandible using the clip art software feature.

Clinical Examples

Congenitally missing maxillary lateral incisor

The patient is congenitally missing the maxillary right lateral incisor (Fig 3-10). At the end of orthodontic therapy, the roots lack parallelism and the apices of the teeth are convergent. Alveolar bone does not develop in the absence of tooth eruption, and the residual basal bone is palatal when compared to normal development. While the ridge width appears sufficient for implant placement, the interradicular spacing and root position of the adjacent teeth do not allow for simple implant placement.

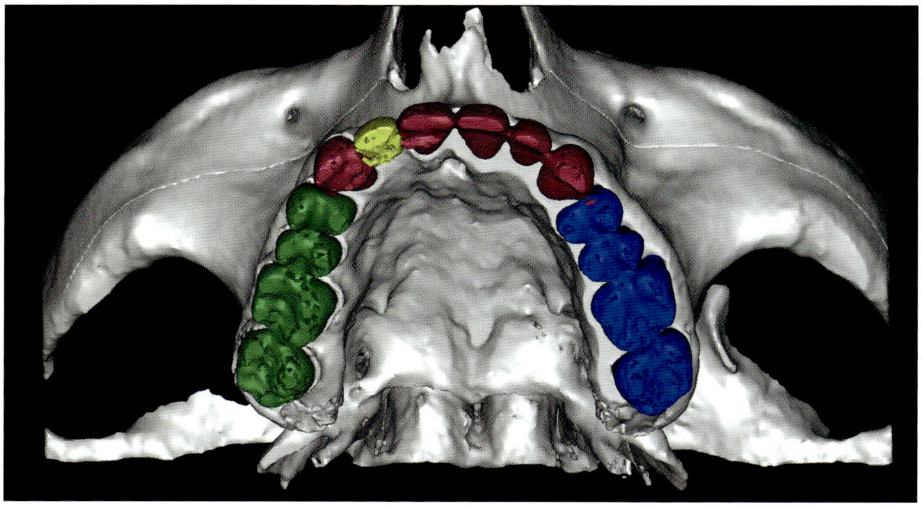

Fig 3-10a Masks for the anterior and posterior dentition. Each color represents a separate mask created to view each segment independently and assess regional anatomy.

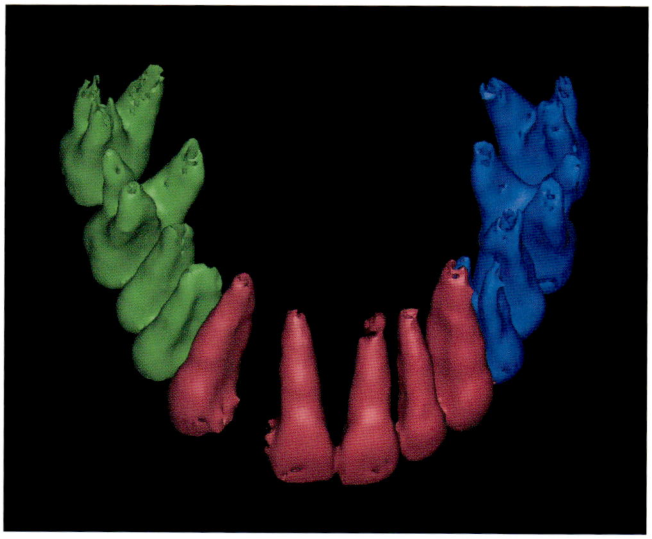

Fig 3-10b Isolation of the anterior dentition, revealing root convergence in the area of the congenitally missing right lateral incisor.

Clinical Examples Congenitally missing or impacted maxillary canine

A similar example is seen in a patient with a congenitally missing maxillary right canine (Figs 3-11a to 3-11c). A CT study allows for precise 3D determination of tooth position and its impact on adjacent structures. The dilaceration of the palatal root of the first premolar does not allow for implant placement without orthodontic correction. The impacted maxillary canine is not an uncommon developmental abnormality. This information facilitates an assessment of the risks associated with its removal (Figs 3-11d to 3-11g).

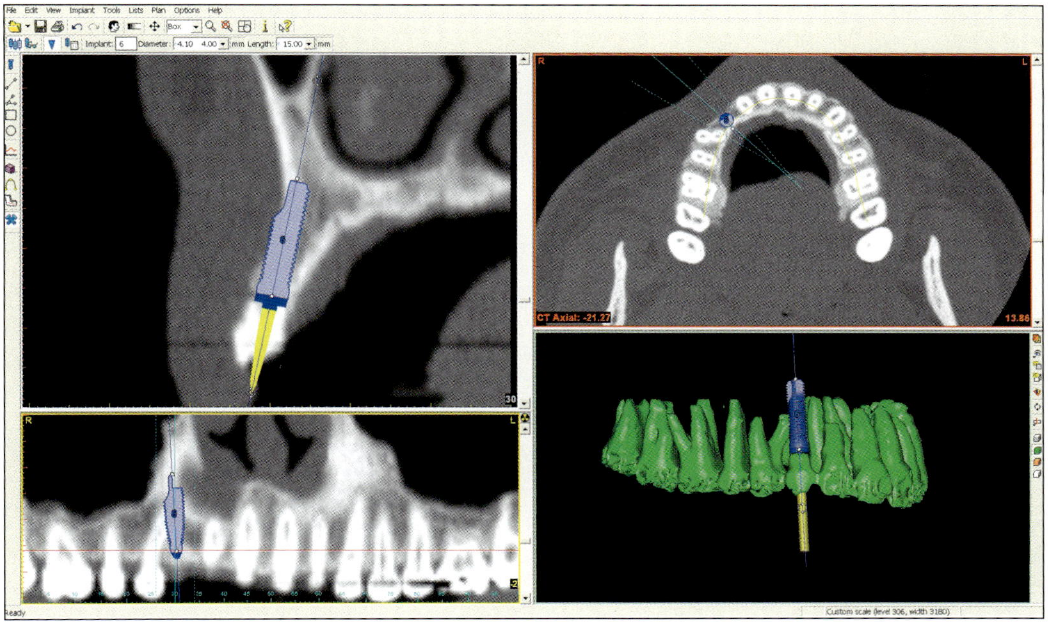

Fig 3-11a SimPlant presentation of 2D and 3D maxillary views illustrates the primary canine. The mask of the maxillary dentition (green) provides a unique opportunity to view the teeth.

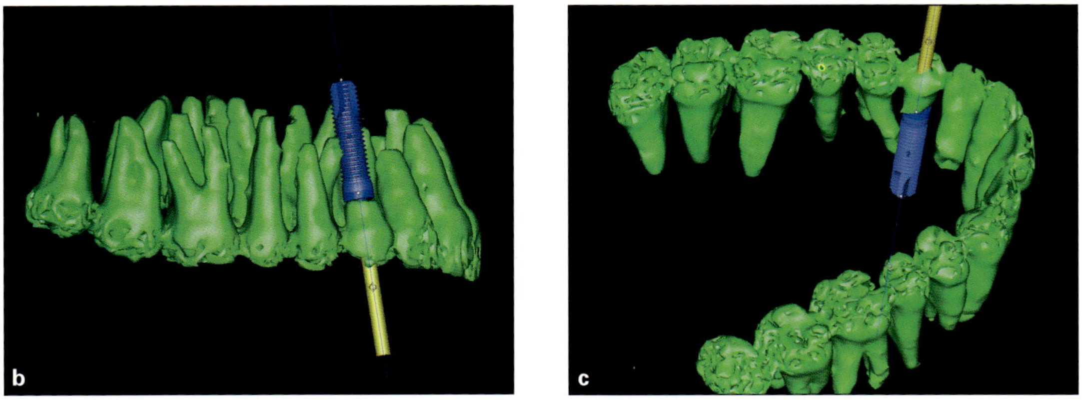

Figs 3-11b and 3-11c Enlarged 3D views of the dentition masks reveal a severe dilaceration of the palatal root of the maxillary right first premolar. No other imaging modality could have identified this clinically important anatomic abnormality.

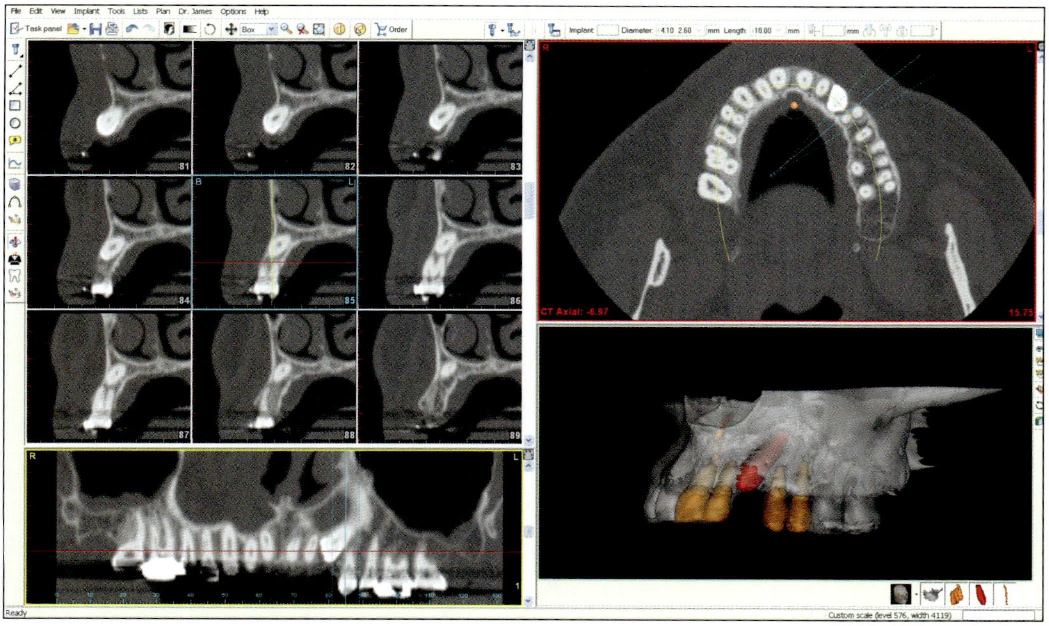

Fig 3-11d Neighborhood view revealing ankylosed and impacted maxillary left canine and its relationship to adjacent teeth. Note the 3D transparency and associated masks.

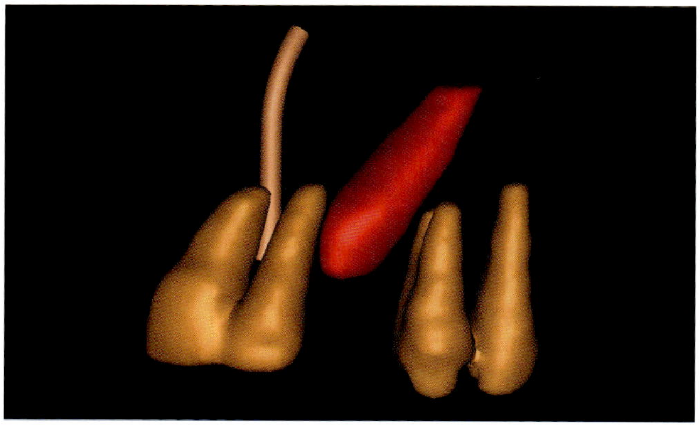

Fig 3-11e The mask of the maxillary bone has been removed, isolating the adjacent dentition and the impacted canine. Note the graphic representation of the incisive nerve.

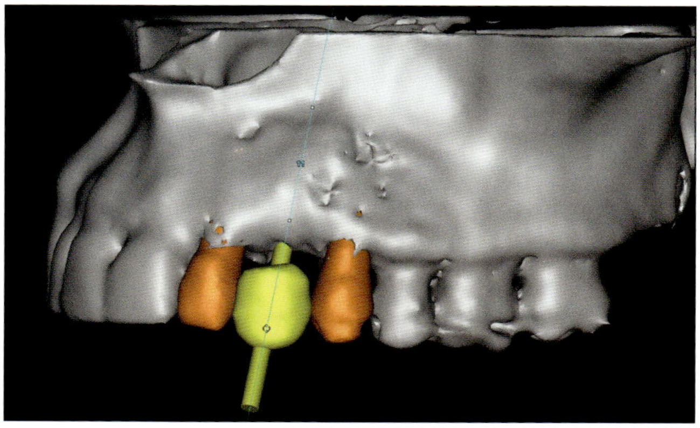

Fig 3-11f Postoperative extraction with site development outcome in the canine position. Note the mask of the adjacent teeth and scanning appliance.

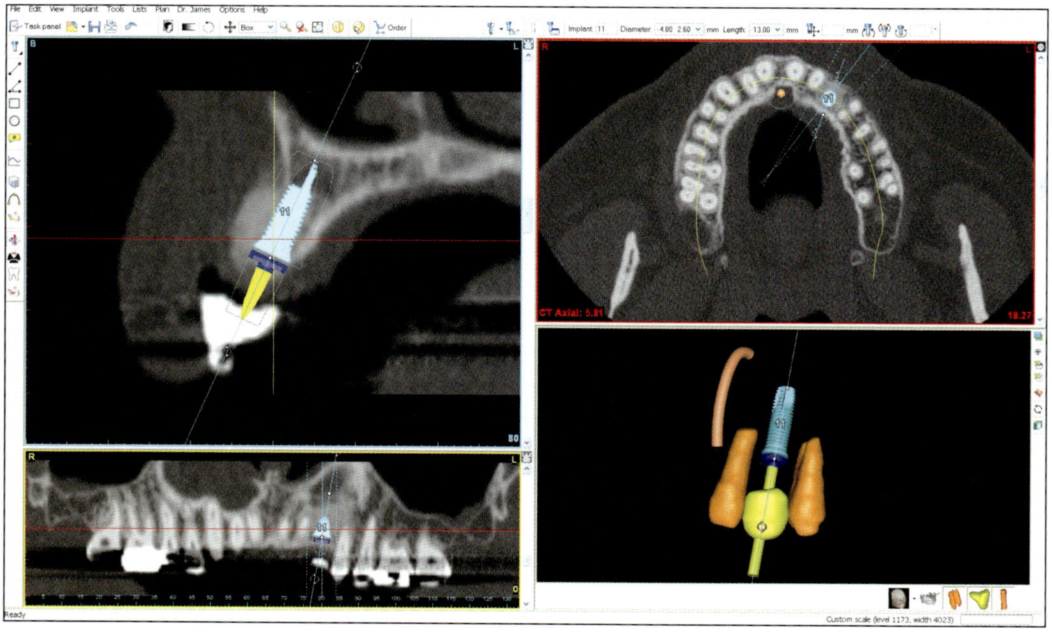

Fig 3-11g Neighborhood view of final treatment plan using several software features for analysis.

Clinical Examples

Root fracture

A common discovery is that a patient's clinical presentation is frequently misleading. A patient presented with a root fracture of the maxillary right lateral incisor. The anterior clinical photograph suggests a rather straightforward and uncomplicated situation (Fig 3-12a). The CT study, however, reveals several clinical issues that significantly altered treatment, including adjacent tooth rotation, convergent roots of the right lateral and central incisors, and a severe disturbance of tooth position and underlying basal bone (Figs 3-12b to 3-12h). This information influenced the sequence and nature of treatment.

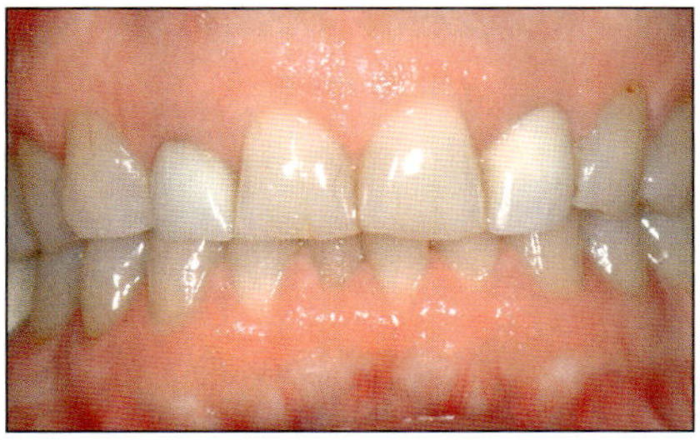

Fig 3-12a Clinical anterior view of the retracted dentition. Note the relative thickness of the soft and hard tissues, which differs from the CT assessment.

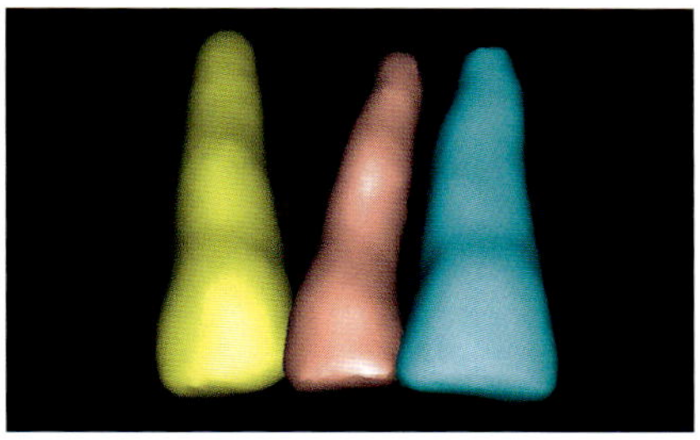

Fig 3-12b 3D frontal reconstruction. Note that a mask has been created for each of the right anterior teeth.

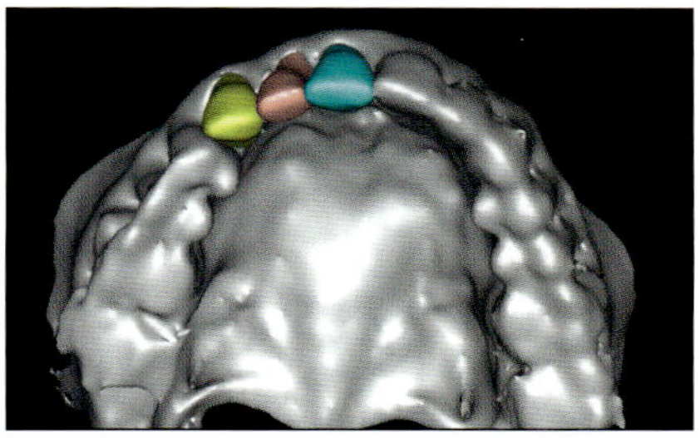

Fig 3-12c 3D reconstruction from an occlusal view. Note the masks of the right anterior teeth and maxilla.

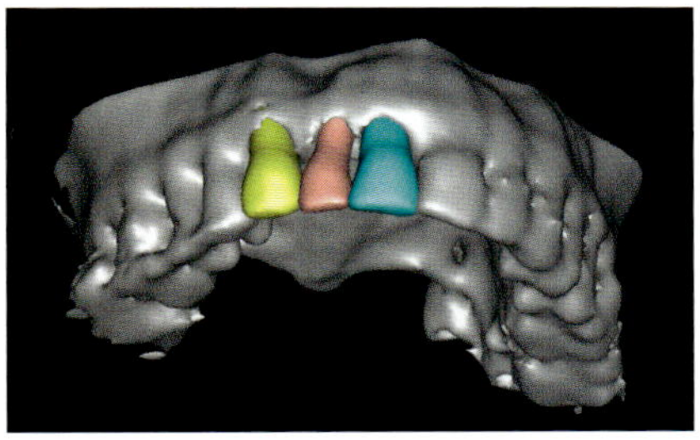

Fig 3-12d 3D reconstruction from an anterior oblique view. Note the masks of the right anterior teeth and maxilla.

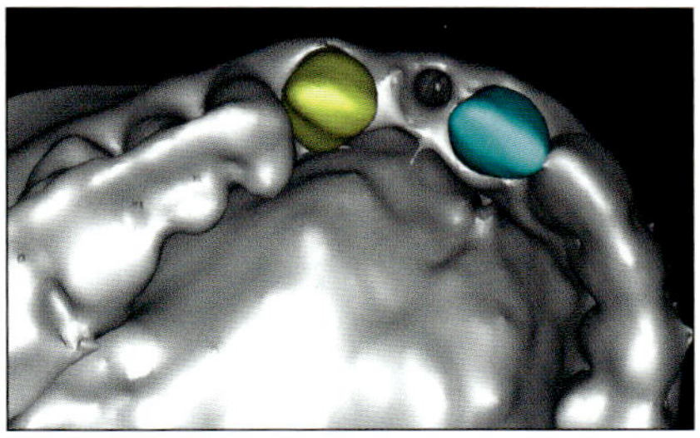

Fig 3-12e 3D reconstruction from an occlusal view. The masking feature allows for selective removal and viewing of each tooth independently.

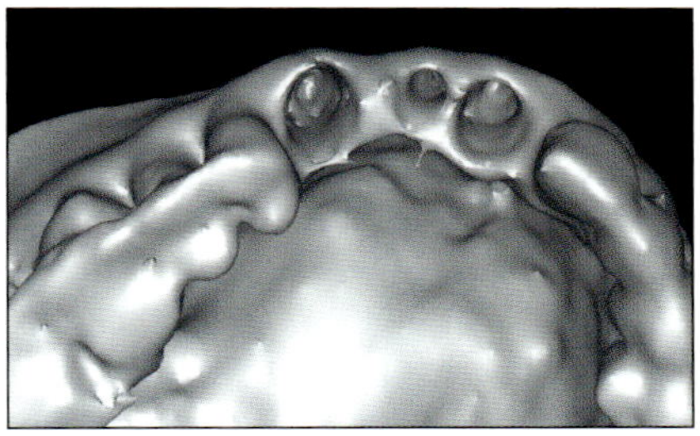

Fig 3-12f 3D reconstruction from an occlusal view with all teeth removed to allow a better view of the local alveolar anatomy of the sockets.

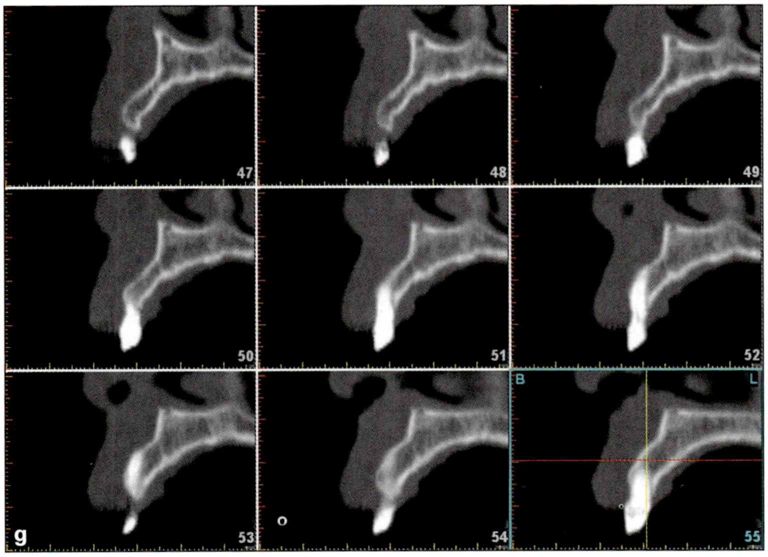

Fig 3-12g 3D cross-sectional view of the maxillary right lateral incisor. Note the axial divergence between the tooth position and alveolar process. This clinical information has considerable impact on the patient's treatment plan.

Fig 3-12h 3D reconstruction illustrating the use of clip art to isolate 2D cross-sectional anatomy in the 3D reconstruction.

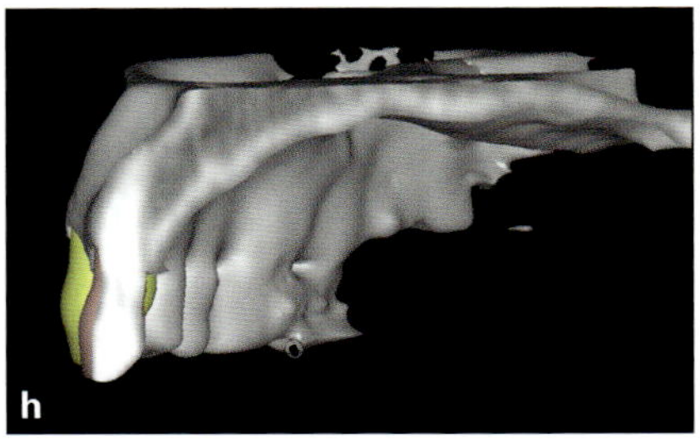

Clinical Examples

Skeletal abnormality

Preoperative recognition of clinical problems dramatically influences the patient's treatment strategy. A young adult female with congenitally missing maxillary canines had completed orthodontic treatment to correct a Class II malocclusion. The periapical radiographs suggest sufficient interradicular space for the placement of dental implants (Figs 3-13a and 3-13b); however, they offer no information about the final prosthetic outcome. At first glance, the cross-sectional images do not appear particularly unusual. Yet, the scanning appliance for both canines, as shown in the cross-sectional images, reveals clinical crown length deficiencies and abnormal relationships between the proposed final tooth position and the underlying bone. The orthodontic treatment positioned the teeth into a Class I tooth relationship but had no influence on the underlying Class II skeletal abnormality (Figs 3-13c and 3-13d).

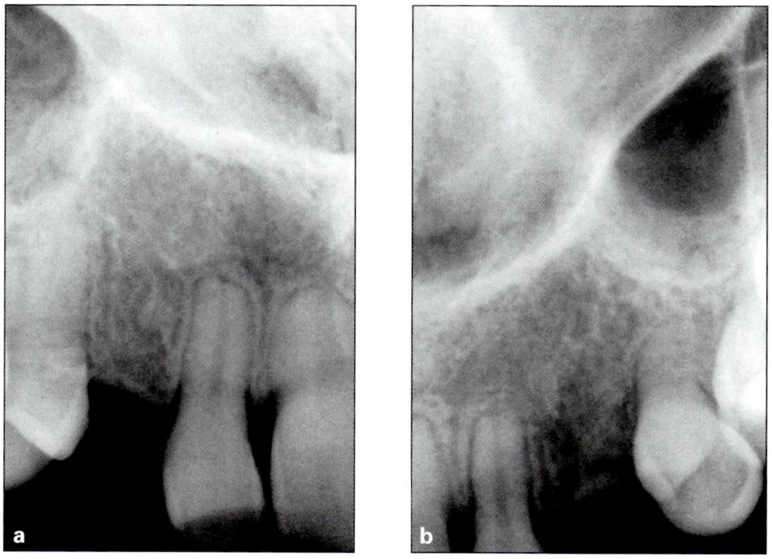

Figs 3-13a and 3-13b Postorthodontic periapical radiographs of the maxillary right *(a)* and left *(b)* canine sites in a 20-year-old female.

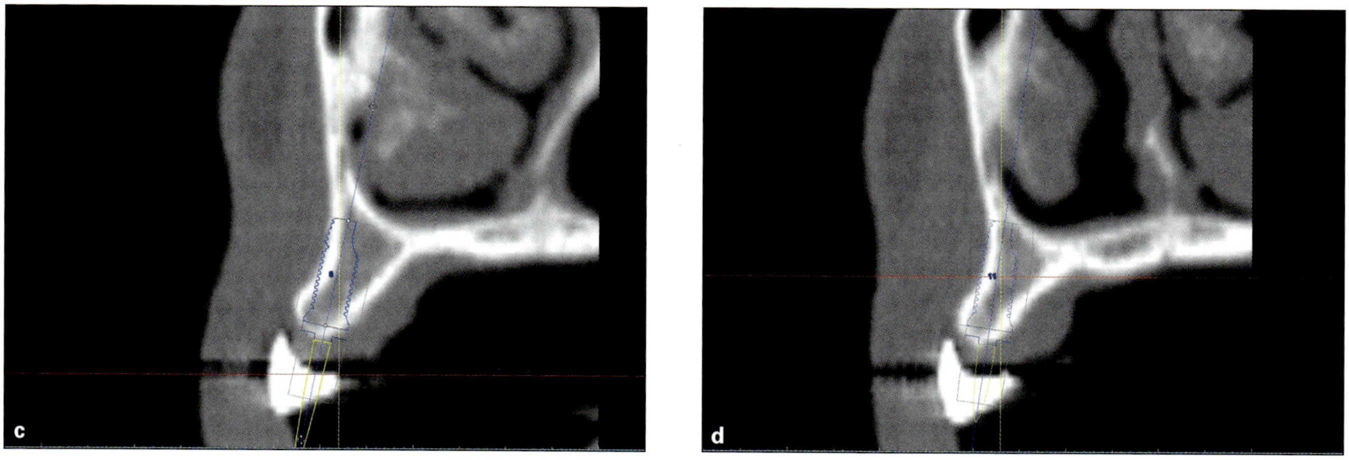

Figs 3-13c and 3-13d 2D cross-sectional views of the right *(c)* and left *(d)* canine sites with the scanning appliance clearly visible. Note the Class II skeletal pattern of the bone and the Class I tooth position represented by the scanning appliance. The teeth represented by the scanning appliance appear short due to a discrepancy between alveolar bone and tooth positions, reducing the vertical restorative space.

Clinical Examples Influential developmental abnormality with insufficient bone

The treatment dynamics in the care of this patient were best served by preoperative planning and meaningful informed consent. The patient's treatment plan was based on a prosthetically directed outcome. The CT study revealed a developmental abnormality of the alveolar process and an enlarged nasopalatine canal (Figs 3-14a and 3-14b). The nerve drawing tool was used to highlight the expected position of this vital structure. The SimPlant collision-detection feature automatically activated to warn of close proximity to the nasopalatine nerve. After thorough analysis of the anatomic situation, it was determined that treatment would include guided bone regeneration to increase facial bone width and a neurectomy to increase palatal bone volume (Figs 3-14c and 3-14d).

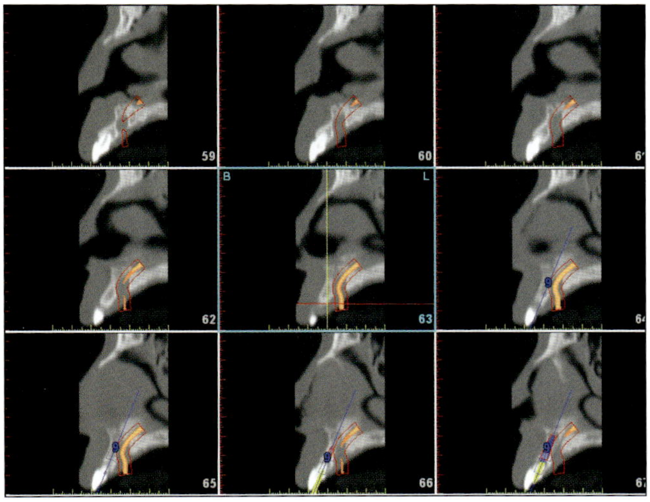

Fig 3-14a Series of cross-sectional views of the maxillary central incisors. Note the developmental abnormalities of the alveolar process and nasopalatine canal.

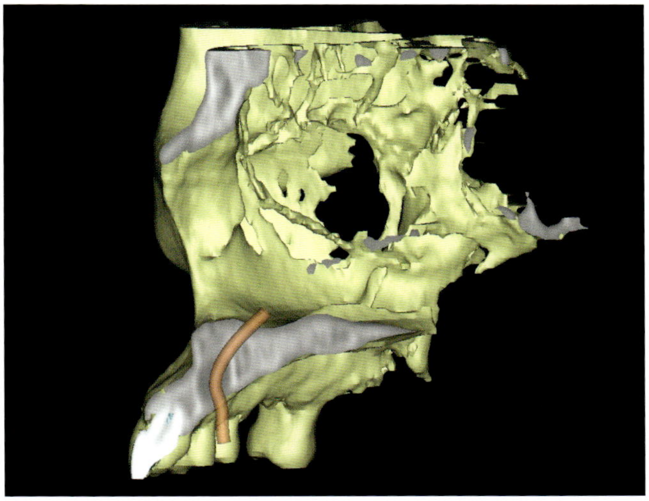

Fig 3-14b 3D view obtained using axial clip art to insert cross-sectional 2D image into the 3D reconstruction.

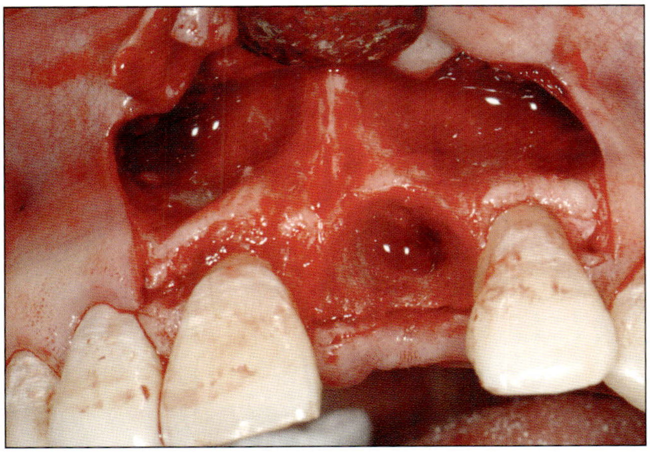

Fig 3-14c Facial view of surgical exposure and extraction of the maxillary left central incisor.

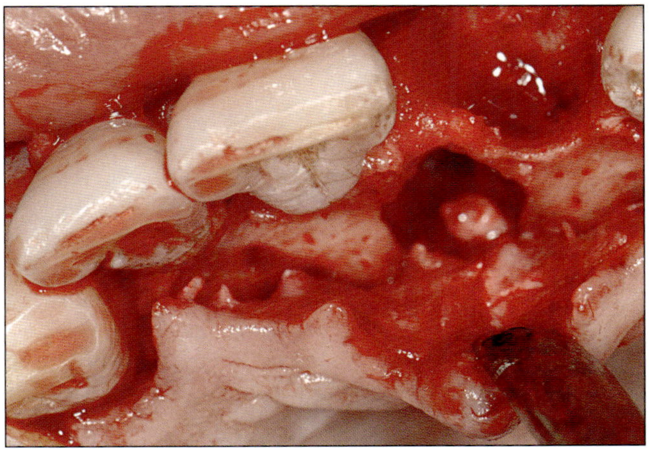

Fig 3-14d Palatal view of surgical exposure and completion of incisive nerve neurectomy.

Clinical Examples

Donor site evaluation

One interesting feature of the anterior mandible is the divergence between the alveolar process and underlying residual ridge (Figs 3-15a and 3-15b). This feature of normal anatomy can be more clearly understood by disarticulating teeth and bone anatomy through use of masks. The cross-sectional view of a mandibular central incisor can be simultaneously examined by using the clip art feature (Fig 3-15c). This feature allows the user to view the cross-sectional image superimposed on the 3D reconstruction. Use of the mandibular symphysis as a donor site for guided bone regeneration can be evaluated using these same features. Its application in the treatment of a patient with congenitally missing mandibular central incisors showed that insufficient bone was available for the placement of a single implant at the midline. The cross-sectional image revealed sufficient bone to obtain a corticocancellous block bone graft for site development apical to the future implant site (Fig 3-15d). A single-tooth implant-supported restoration was accomplished.

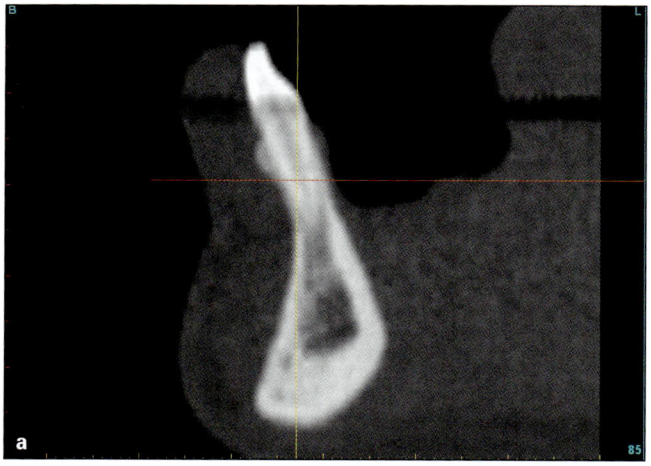

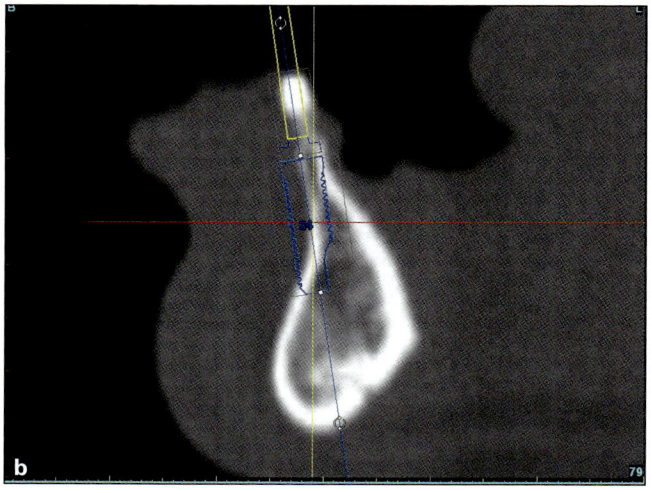

Figs 3-15a and 3-15b 2D cross-sectional view of a mandibular incisor, clearly illustrating the divergence between the axial inclination of the tooth–alveolar bone complex and the underlying basal bone of the chin.

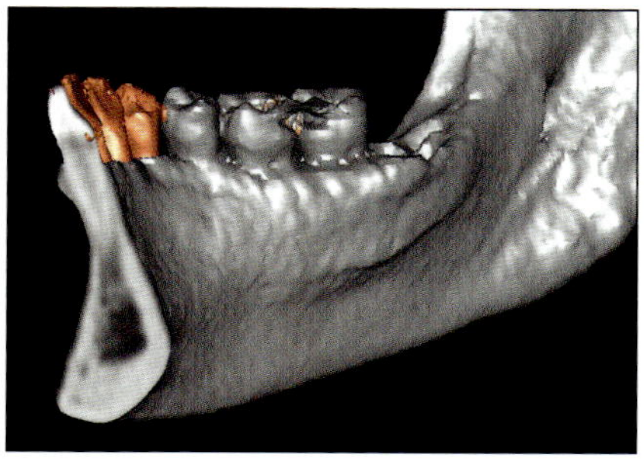

Fig 3-15c 2D cross-sectional view of a mandibular central incisor region, which has been inserted into a 3D reconstruction of the mandible using the clip art software feature.

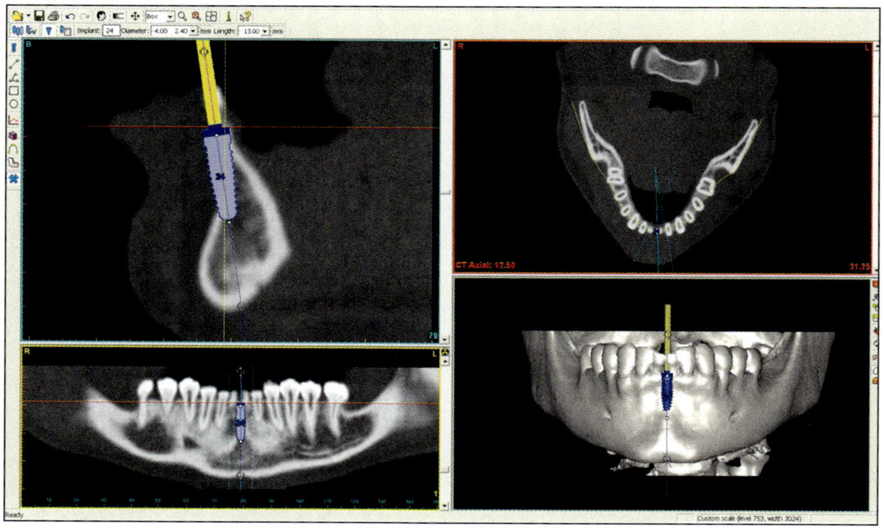

Fig 3-15d SimPlant presentation showing multiple views of the mandibular anterior region. Sufficient bone apical to the anticipated implant position is available to harvest a corticocancellous block bone graft for augmentation of the region.

Clinical Examples — Complexity of maxillary and mandibular posterior regional anatomy

The posterior maxilla and mandible have important anatomic characteristics that influence implant treatment. In the posterior maxilla, the maxillary sinus often exhibits complex anatomic characteristics and disease, which affect patient treatment (Figs 3-16a to 3-16c). Periapical pathosis is often not visible on analog dental radiographs. Sinus disease can be the direct result of periapical pathosis, which can cause bony perforations in the floor of the maxillary sinus (Fig 3-16d). The success of sinus bone grafting is directly related to absence of active disease (Figs 3-16e and 3-16f). When planning sinus bone augmentation, a volumetric tool can be used to evaluate the volume of bone grafting material required for treatment. In the posterior mandible, anatomic characteristics present unique challenges. Bone density, concavities, and location of neurovascular structures influence treatment decisions. By locating the inferior alveolar nerve canal, the nerve drawing tool can be used to highlight its anticipated entry, traverse, and exit through the mandible. The impacted mandibular third molar and its relationship to the inferior alveolar nerve are important considerations that require informed consent because of the potential for nerve injury. By accessing multi-dimensional information, a more effective surgical extraction strategy can be facilitated to minimize surgical morbidity (Figs 3-16g and 3-16h).

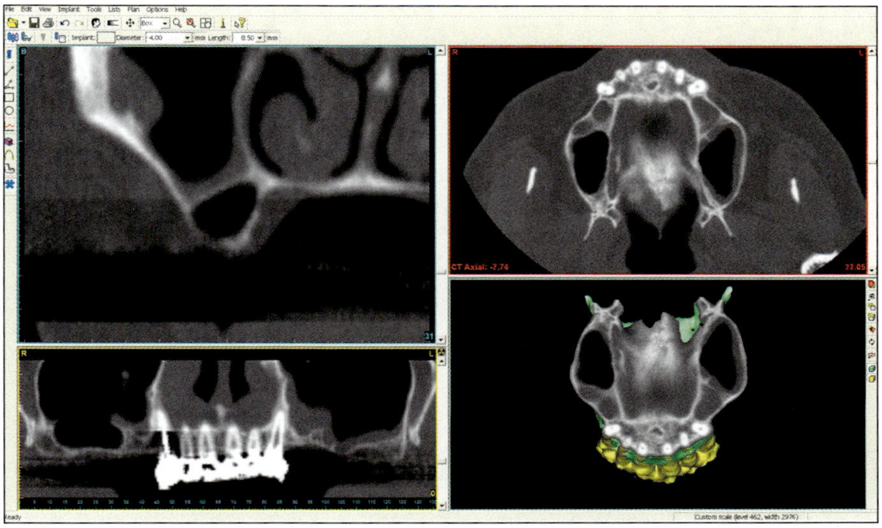

Fig 3-16a SimPlant presentation of the maxilla. Note the insertion of a 2D axial view in the 3D reconstruction using the clip art feature. From a superior perspective, many important anatomic features can be seen.

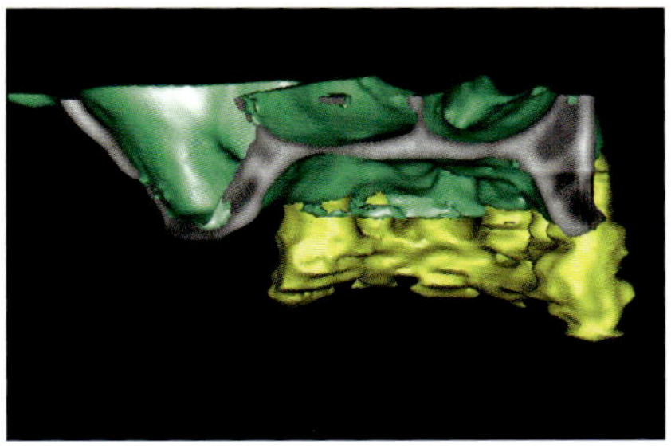

Fig 3-16b 3D reconstruction of the maxilla viewed from the posteroanterior perspective. A cross-sectional image was inserted to capture the mediolateral plane. The floor of the nose, hard palate, sinus, mask of the anterior teeth, and residual jaw are all illustrated in this single view.

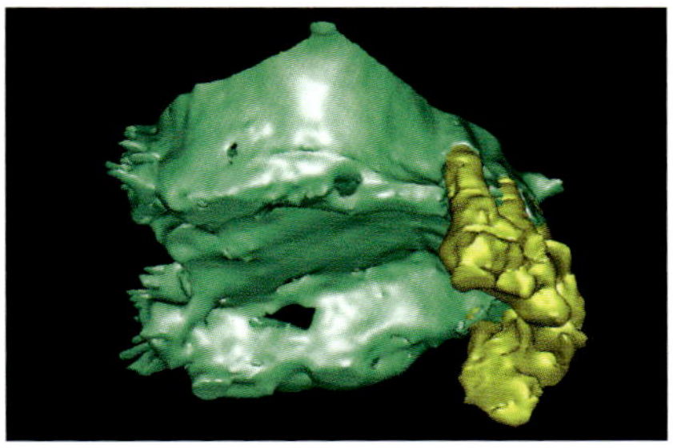

Fig 3-16c 3D reconstruction of the maxilla, reoriented to view the right maxilla, mask of the anterior teeth, and fenestration of the sinus.

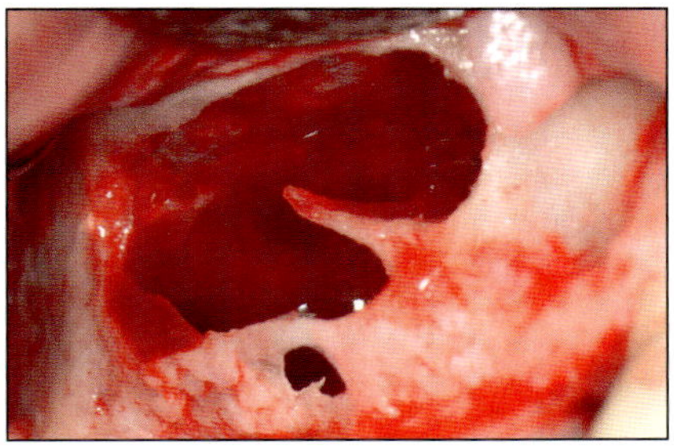

Fig 3-16d Clinical view of the regional anatomy shown in Fig 3-16c. Knowledge of the complex anatomy of the right sinus facilitated surgical management and could not have been obtained using any other radiographic modality. Note the bony fenestration of the sinus.

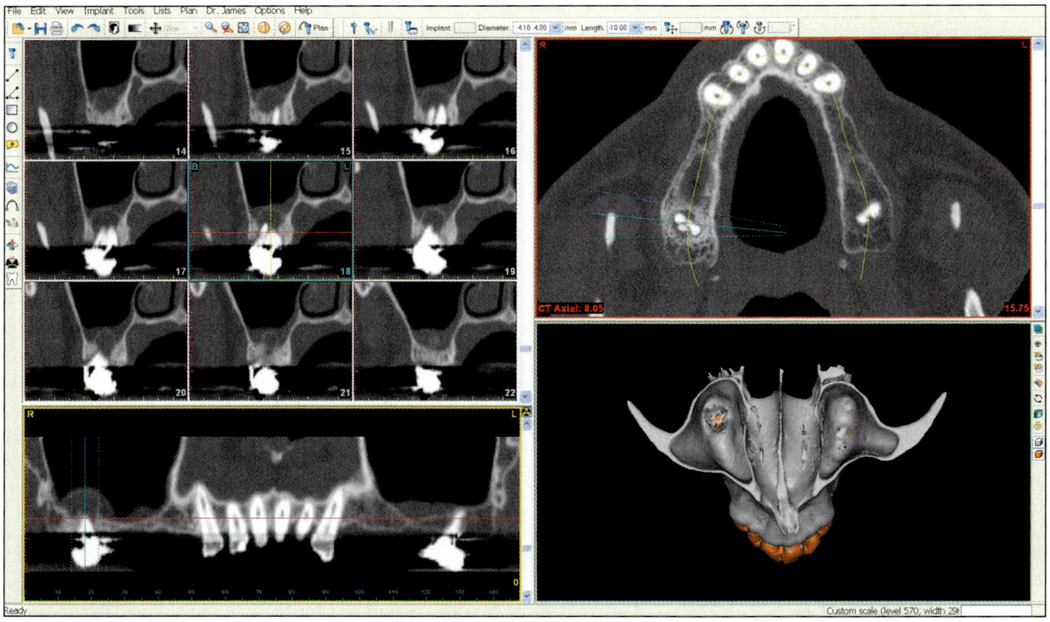

Fig 3-16e SimPlant presentation of sinus disease related to the periapical pathosis of the maxillary right third molar. All views illustrate the relative risk associated with sinus augmentation.

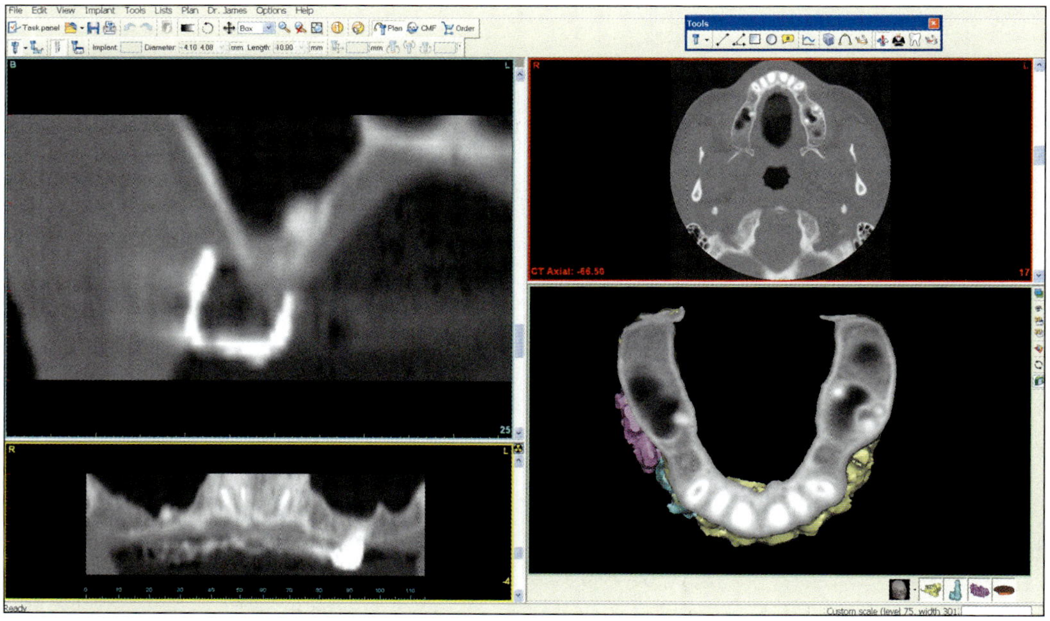

Fig 3-16f SimPlant presentation of retained palatal root tip associated with the medial wall of the sinus. This unanticipated finding influenced the nature of the sinus grafting surgery, which would likely lead to a more successful outcome.

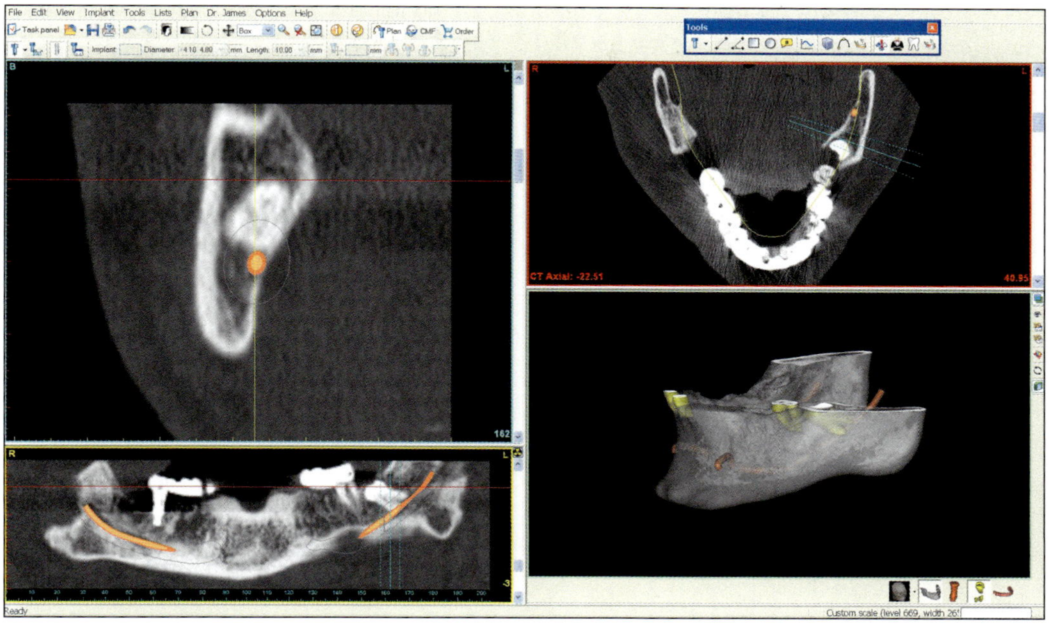

Fig 3-16g The entire anticipated course of the inferior alveolar nerve can be illustrated with the nerve drawing tool. Each of the SimPlant presentation windows can be manipulated to provide the best view of the impacted mandibular left third molar.

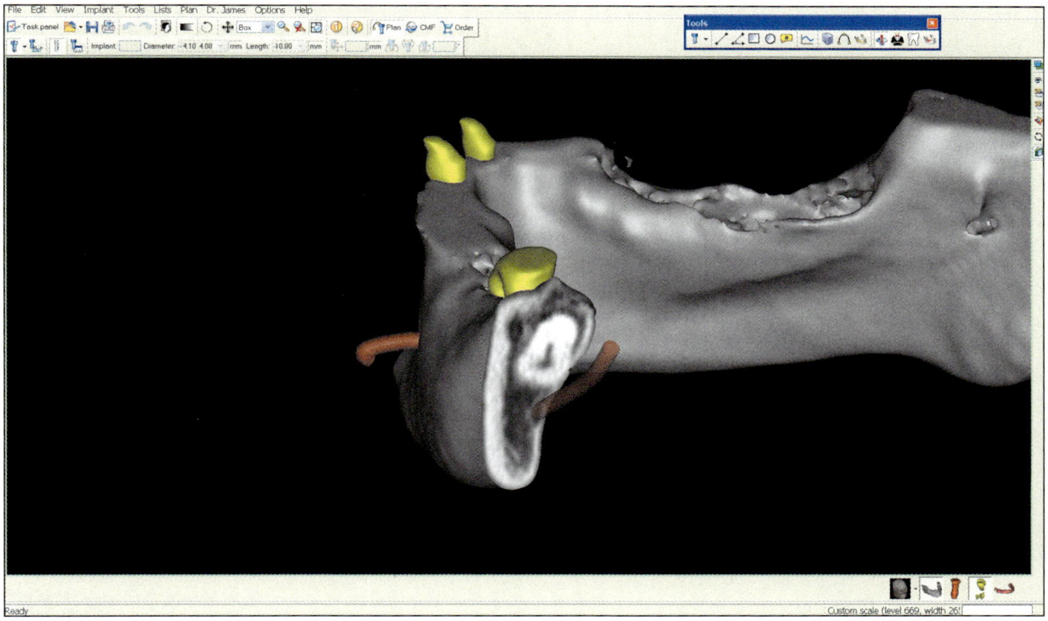

Fig 3-16h Use of the cross-sectional clip art feature allows in-depth assessment of the impacted third molar shown in Fig 3-16g.

Clinical Cases

Use of SimPlant in the posterior maxilla

The anatomy of the posterior maxilla often presents a challenge to the implant team. In this particular case, sinus pneumatization robbed the posterior maxilla of sufficient bone for the placement of dental implants. The left sinus was grafted 8 months before via a lateral antroscopy approach. A prosthetically directed scanning appliance was fabricated, and a CT study was obtained (Fig 3-17a). From the implant library, four manufacturer-specific realistic implants were placed in the left posterior sextant in alignment with the collaboratively generated scanning appliance. Careful attention to implant-tooth and interimplant positions was observed. The collision-detection feature warned of insufficient distance between premolar implants (Fig 3-17b). Four masks were created to isolate and better visualize anatomic features critical to determining the most favorable implant positions. Masks of the maxilla, sinus graft, adjacent canine, and scanning appliance were created by the radiology technician. These masks were independently manipulated to offer treatment-planning insight otherwise unavailable (Figs 3-17c to 3-17f). The most notable feature of the CT study was the anteroposterior limitation of the sinus graft. The defined posterior limitation could be visualized in both the 2D and 3D images.

The principles of information management and collaborative accountability defined the position of the most posterior implant. Without this information, the risk of placing the terminal implant outside the boundaries of the sinus graft was significant. After careful review and modification, a final treatment plan was developed (Figs 3-17g to 3-17j), and this was uploaded to Materialise for fabrication of a tooth- and mucosa-supported SurgiGuide for osteotomy preparation and implant placement without bone exposure (Figs 3-17k and 3-17l). Osteotomy sites were prepared using the surgical guides that were matched to accommodate the step-wise drill diameters used to prepare the osteotomy sites. The implants were then placed into the prepared osteotomy sites (Fig 3-17m). Treatment was completed as a single-stage surgery, thus avoiding an additional surgical procedure to expose the implants. Soft tissue autogenous grafting was completed on the buccal aspect to create a more favorable environment for hygiene and restoration (Fig 3-17n). The definitive prosthesis consisted of four porcelain-fused-to-metal single-tooth restorations (Figs 3-17o and 3-17p).

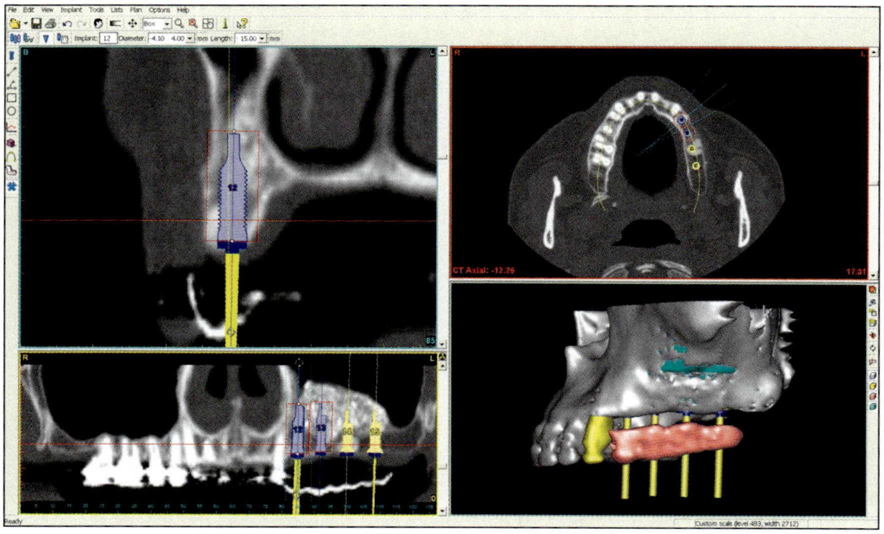

Fig 3-17a SimPlant presentation of the left region of the posterior maxilla following sinus grafting, showing realistic implants, a mask of the maxillary left canine, the scanning appliance, and the sinus graft. The collision-detection feature warns that the proposed interimplant distance is less than the parameter set by the user. This safety feature is a 3D calculation transferred to the 2D reconstruction, thus ensuring that limitations of 2D interpretation do not compromise treatment plan safety.

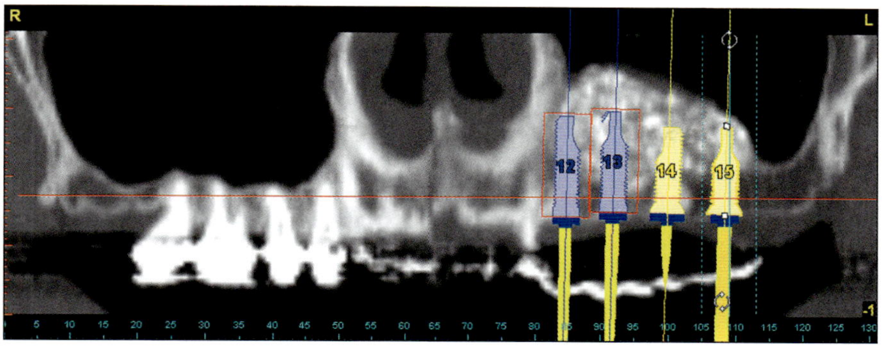

Fig 3-17b Enlarged panoramic view.

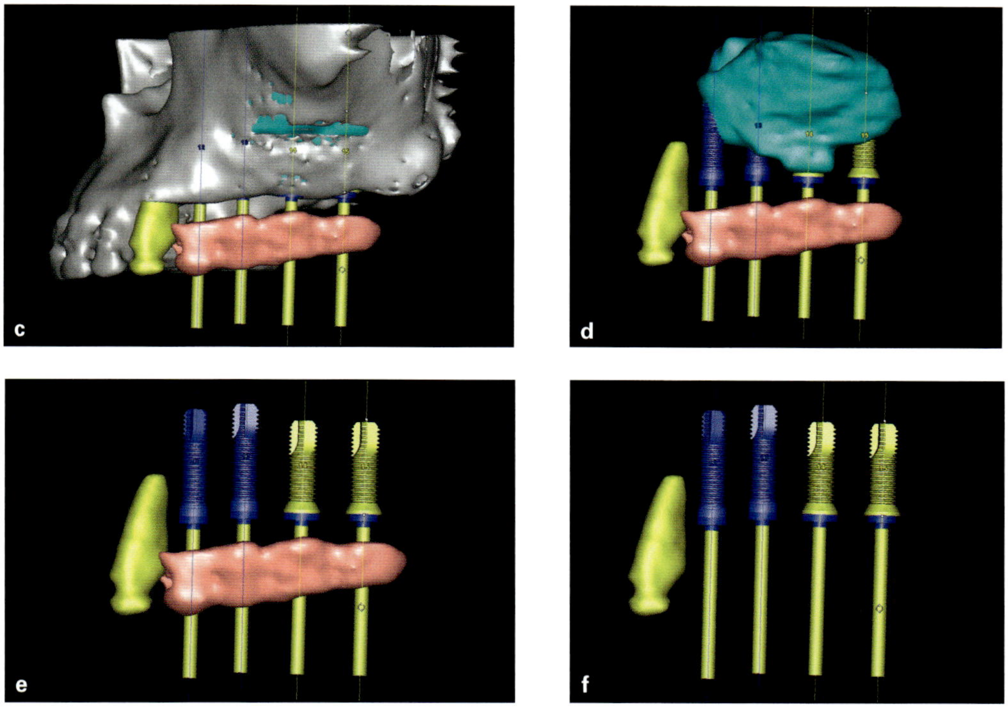

Figs 3-17c to 3-17f *(c)* 3D reconstruction of the maxilla, left lateral view, showing masks of the left canine, scanning appliance, implants, sinus graft, and maxilla. *(d)* When the mask of the maxillary bone is removed, there is a visual opportunity to examine the relationship between the natural tooth, implants, and maxillary sinus bone graft within the context of the proposed final tooth position created by the scanning appliance. *(e)* Removal of the sinus graft allows a view of the realistic implants. *(f)* Removal of the scanning appliance further enhances implant assessment.

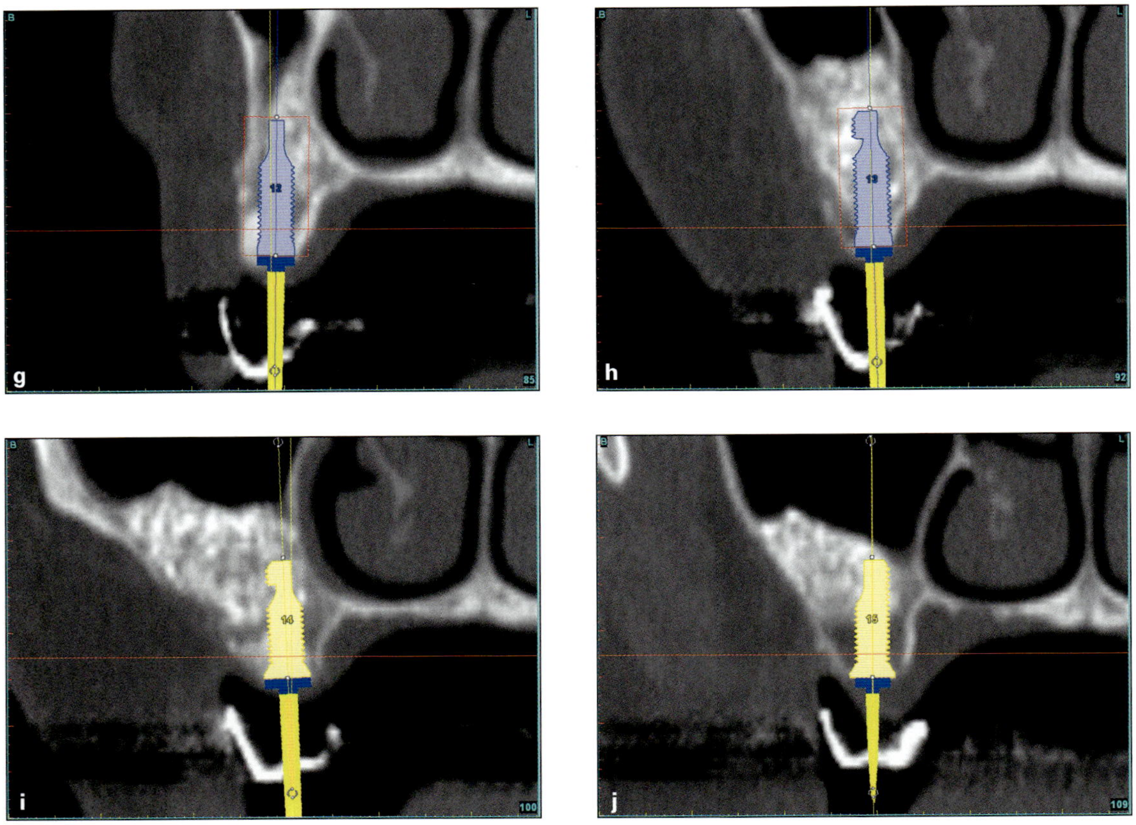

Figs 3-17g to 3-17j 2D cross-sectional views illustrating the relationship between the realistic implants, native bone, sinus graft, medial wall of the sinus, and scanning appliance. It is important to note that the collision-detection feature became activated, reminding the user to assess the implants in the proposed premolar sites.

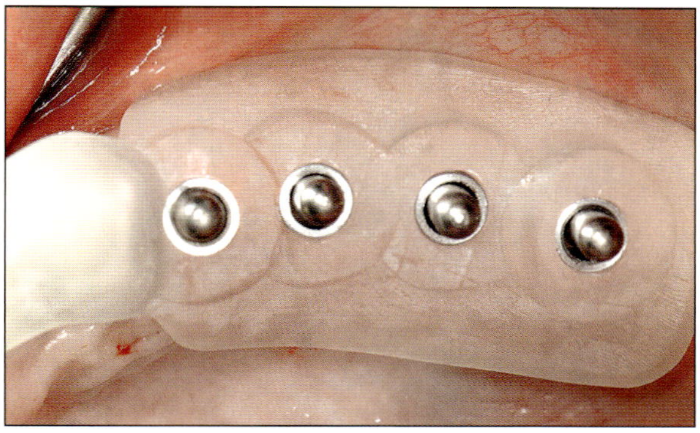

Fig 3-17k The treatment plan established using these features resulted in the fabrication of a SurgiGuide and an opportunity to place implants without bone exposure. After the preparation of 2-mm osteotomy sites, guide pins were inserted into the prepared sites. The guide was then replaced to photographically verify the favorable outcome of osteotomy preparation.

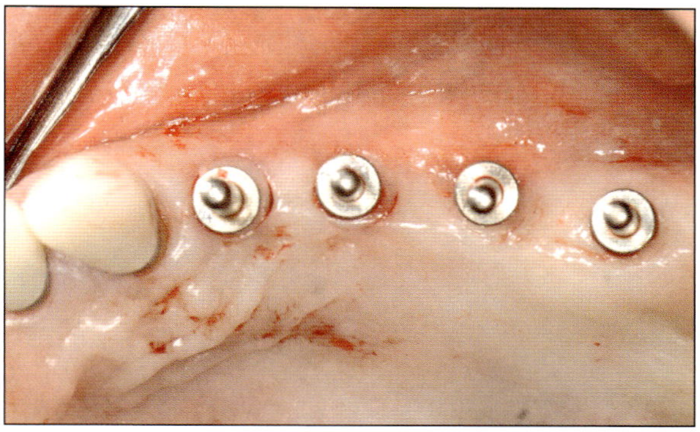

Fig 3-17l Position of the guide pins after SurgiGuide-directed 3-mm osteotomy preparation following removal of the guide. Note the minimally invasive nature of osteotomy site preparation.

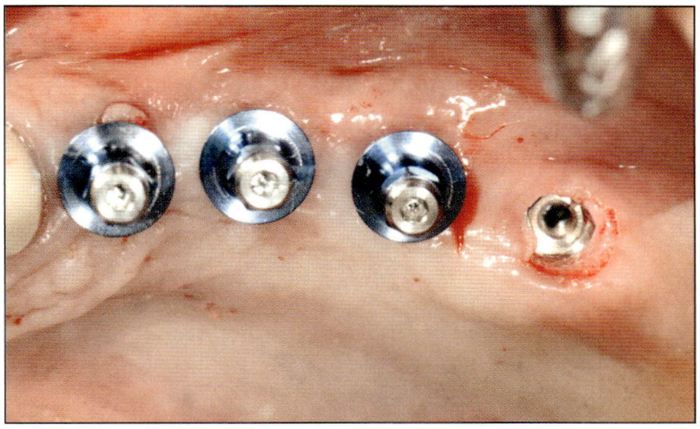

Fig 3-17m Manual implant placement completed. The implant mount on the most distal implant was removed to illustrate the relationship of the platform to the soft tissue. Treatment was completed as a single-stage surgical procedure.

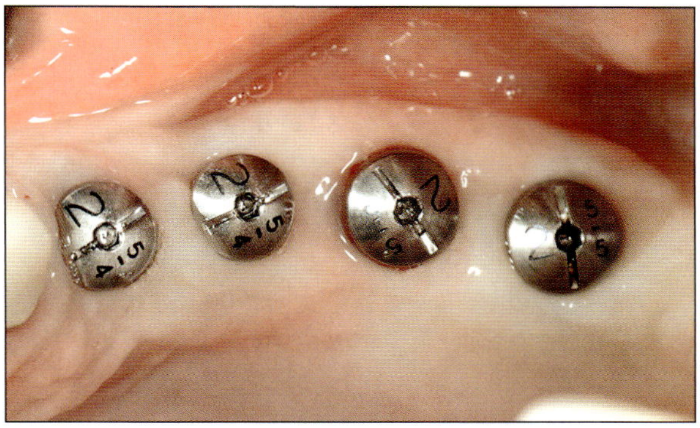

Fig 3-17n Soft tissue grafting was completed to create a more favorable environment for hygiene and restorative emergence in the final prosthetic restoration. Healing abutments were placed at the time of implant placement.

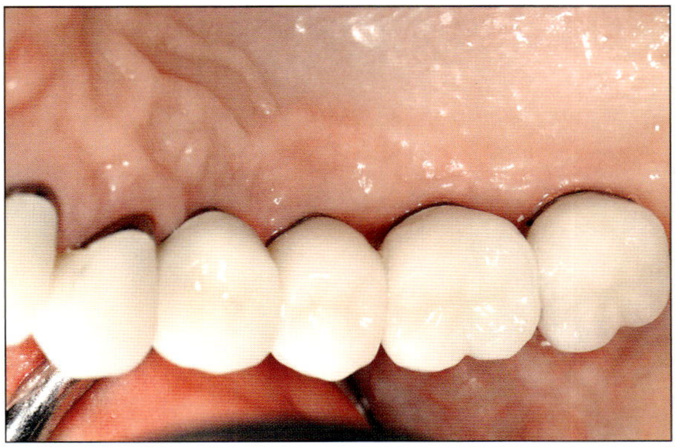

Fig 3-17o Final prosthetic outcome.

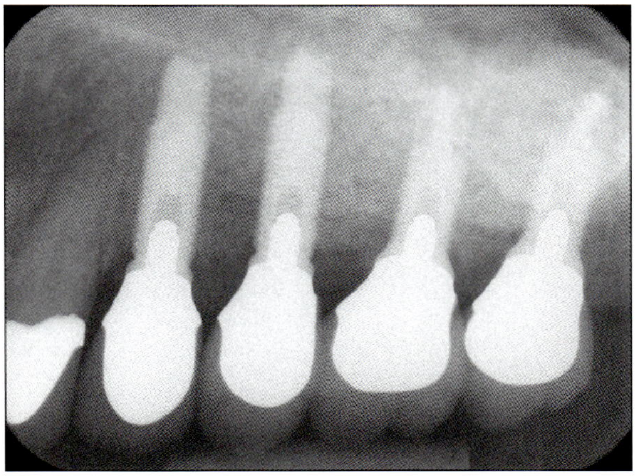

Fig 3-17p Periapical radiograph of the definitive prosthesis.

Clinical Cases

Use of SimPlant in the mandible

SimPlant can facilitate the principle of collaborative accountability used to coordinate more complex treatment strategies in the mandible. Perhaps one of the most exciting uses of the SimPlant software is to plan immediate-load prosthesis therapy. For example, in the edentulous mandible the use of a differential barium gradient scanning appliance can identify soft tissue, bony anatomy, and optimal final tooth positions (Figs 3-18a and 3-18b). A decision about whether implant placement can be accomplished with or without bone exposure can be made.

This patient lost teeth due to advanced periodontal disease. The patient was fitted with immediate maxillary and mandibular dentures following tooth extraction. After 6 months, new dentures were fabricated, and they established the esthetic, phonetic, and esthetic requirements at an acceptable physiologic vertical dimension. A duplicate was made of the mandibular denture, and differential concentrations of barium were incorporated into the denture base and teeth (Figs 3-18c to 3-18f). The barium-impregnated denture base helped delineate the mucosa overlying the bone. Under suitable conditions, this can enable the fabrication of mucosa-supported surgical guides. The CT study revealed a knife-edge ridge, which required approximately 10 mm of vertical bone reduction to create sufficient ridge width for implant placement (Figs 3-18g and 3-18h). The cross-sectional and axial clip art features enabled the treatment collaborators to determine the precise amount of vertical bone reduction necessary to achieve sufficient bone width for the placement of five dental implants (Figs 3-18i and 3-18j). A bone density analysis was performed at the level of the anticipated implant position. A treatment plan was developed that took into consideration the amount of vertical bone reduction required to obtain sufficient width for implant placement. A bone reduction guide was manufactured to precisely guide the amount of vertical ostectomy required for the placement of five dental implants (Figs 3-18k to 3-18m). The extension of distal cantilevers bilaterally was determined by incorporating the position of the mental foramina and their influence on the anteroposterior spread (Figs 3-18n and 3-18o). A bone-supported surgical guide was manufactured to fit the bone at the preoperatively determined reduction level. The implants were placed in the prepared osteotomy sites.

The surgical guides used during the actual surgery were first used for a surgical dress rehearsal on the stereolithographic bone model. Implant analogs were then placed in osteotomy sites prepared on the bone model to simulate final implant position. In addition, a stereolithographic mucosa model with prepared osteotomy sites was fabricated. The patient's existing denture was seated, articulated, and prepared on the model. At the time of surgery, the denture would be luted to cylinders that were attached to the implant abutments (Figs 3-18p to 3-18r). The combined surgical and prosthetic procedure was successfully accomplished as a direct result of collaborative accountability. The roles and responsibilities of the dentist, implant surgeon, laboratory technician, and patient were clearly defined preoperatively.

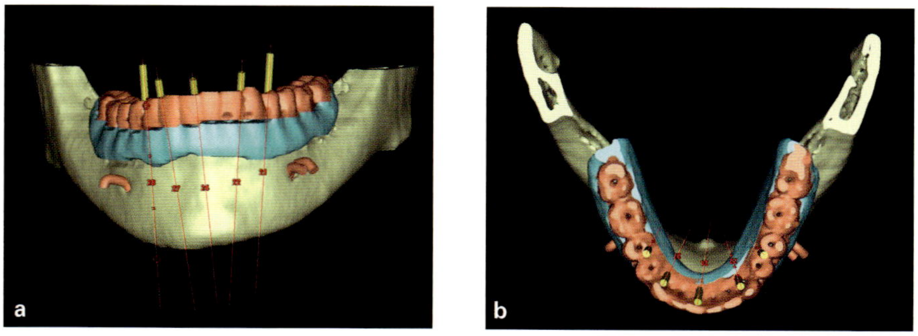

Figs 3-18a and 3-18b 3D view of mandibular ScannoGuide with holes fully penetrating into the central fossae of posterior teeth and the cingula of anterior teeth.

Figs 3-18c and 3-18d 2D cross-sectional clip art image of the scanning appliance, realistic implant with abutment, and anterior mandible. *(c)* Note the thin crestal bone, requiring the placement of the implant platform approximately 8 to 10 mm below the crest. *(d)* Axial clip art was used to determine the approximate amount of vertical ostectomy required to achieve sufficient bone width for implant installation.

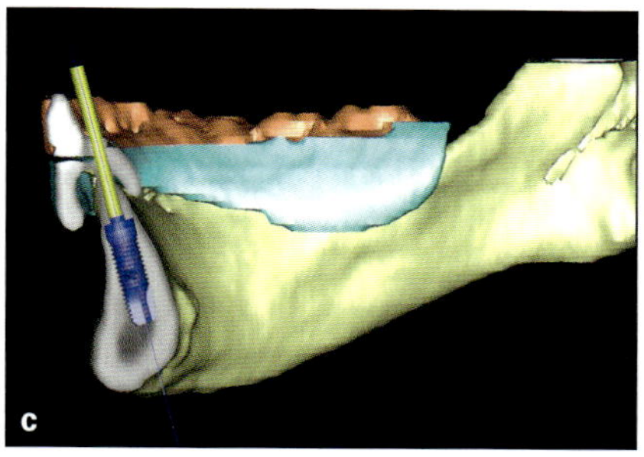

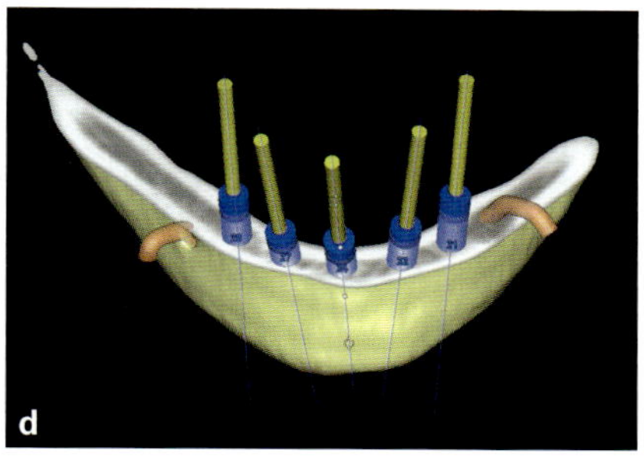

Fig 3-18e Dual-density mucosa-supported scanning appliance (30% barium for teeth and 10% barium for denture base) used for the CT scans shown in Figs 3-18c and 3-18d.

Fig 3-18f 2D cross-sectional view of scanning appliance relative to native bone and proposed implant site.

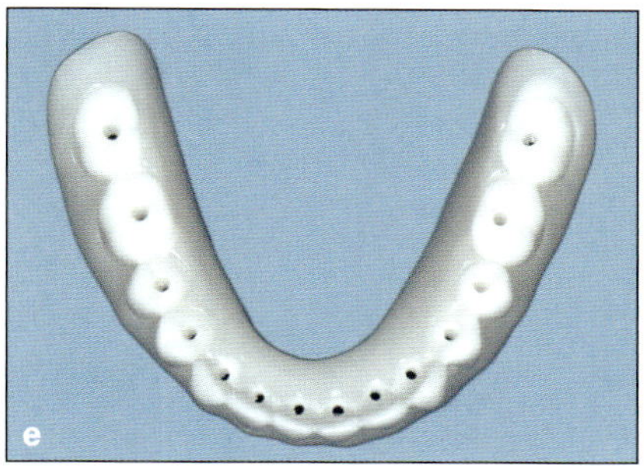

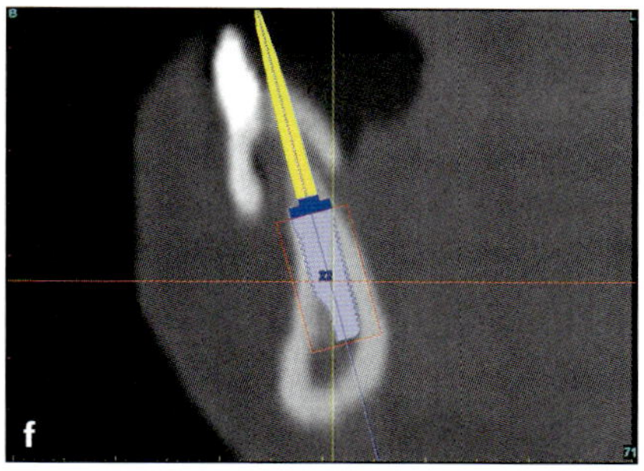

Figs 3-18g and 3-18h Facial and occlusal clinical photographs confirm the very thin crestal bone. This anatomic deformity was discovered in the CT study and its management determined preoperatively. Note the bone reduction guide, which was fabricated presurgically to establish the vertical bone reduction level necessary to establish the correct position of the implant platforms.

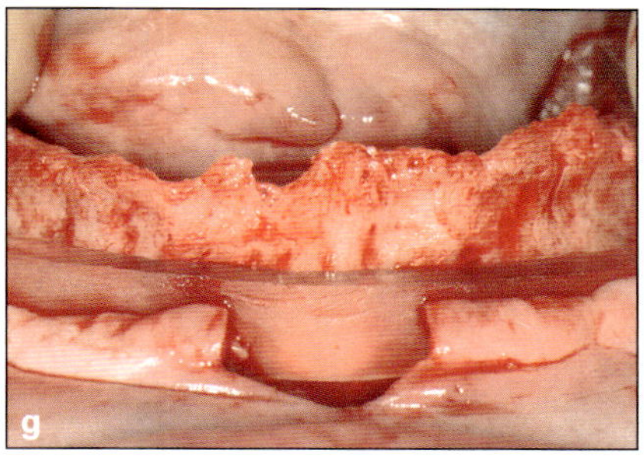

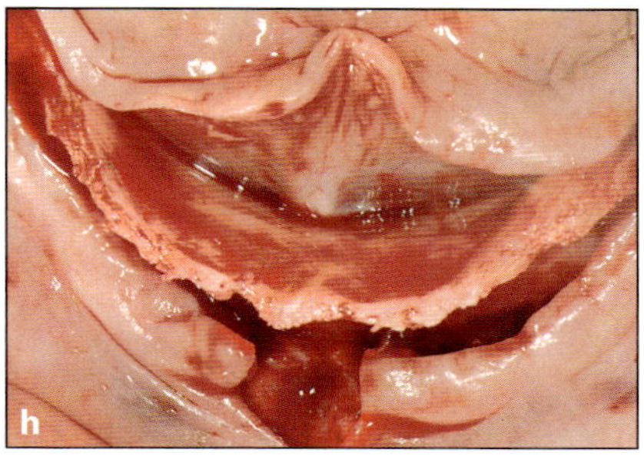

Figs 3-18i and 3-18j Facial and occlusal clinical views of the completed vertical bone reduction. A bone-supported SurgiGuide was fabricated to fit at the level of reduced bone to facilitate osteotomy preparation.

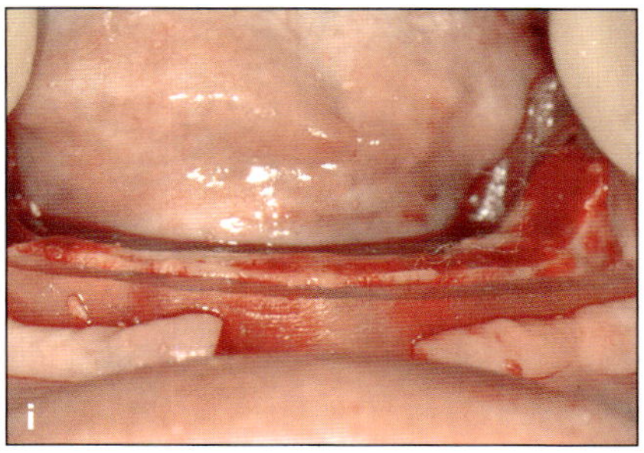

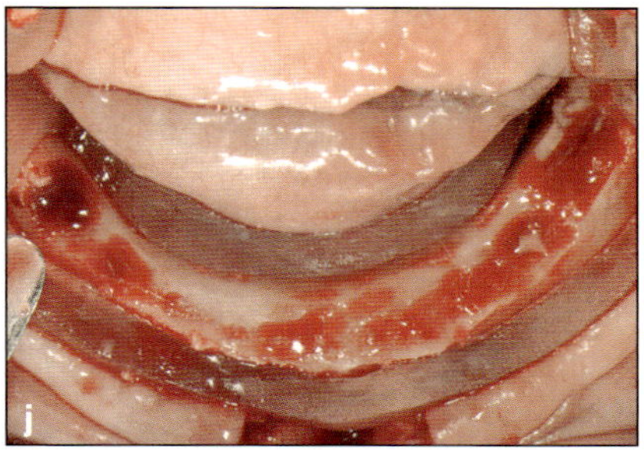

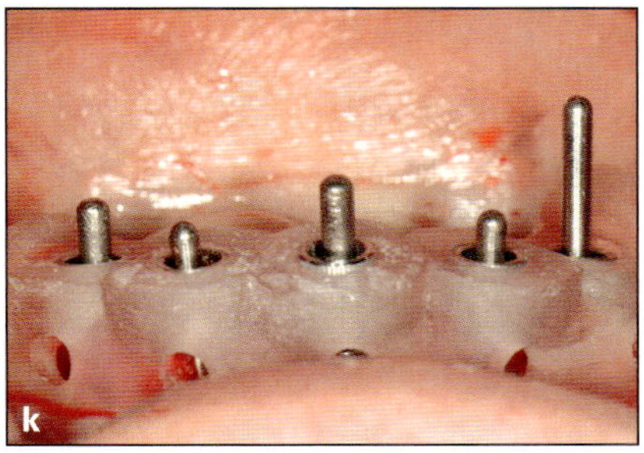

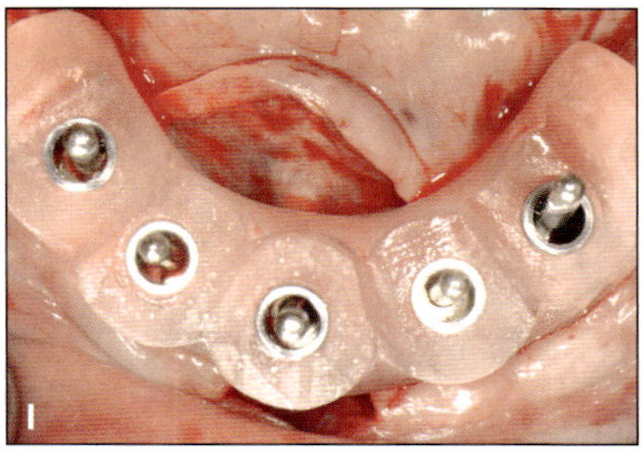

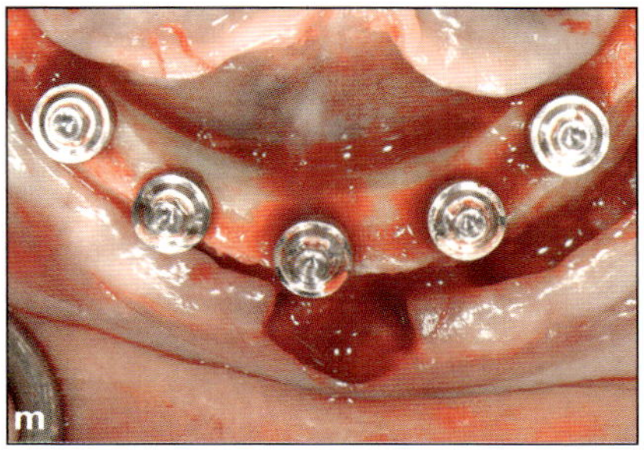

Figs 3-18k and 3-18l Facial and occlusal clinical views of the SurgiGuide used for osteotomy preparation. In these views, the guide pins have been inserted into the osteotomy preparations and the SurgiGuide replaced. Note the guidance accuracy.

Fig 3-18m Occlusal clinical view of the implants and abutments.

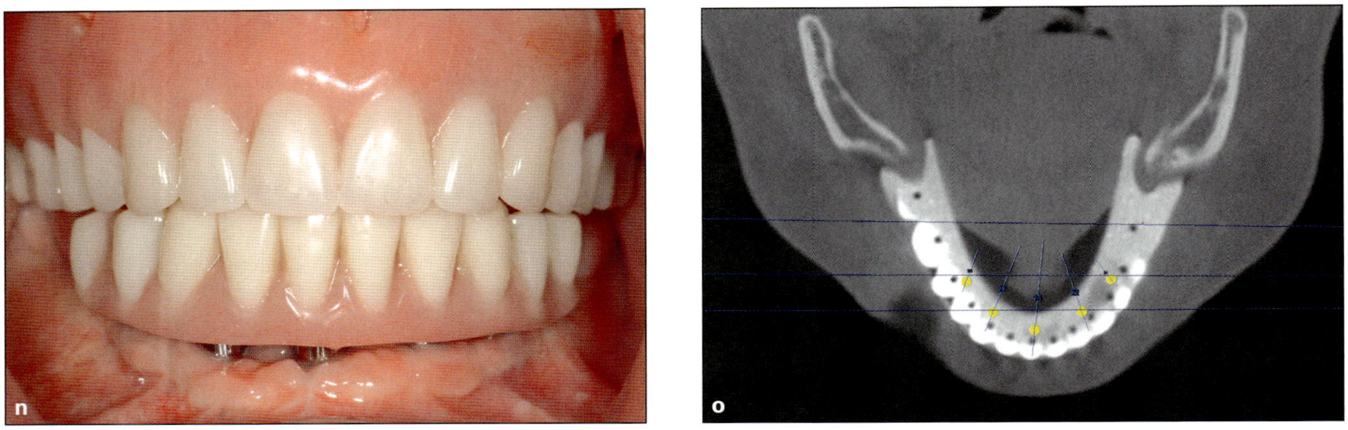

Figs 3-18n and 3-18o *(n)* A 24-hour postoperative view of the maxillary complete denture and implant-supported immediate-load mandibular denture. *(o)* The axial CT image shows the scanning appliance used to plan the patient's treatment and the anteroposterior spread to determine the distal cantilever extension.

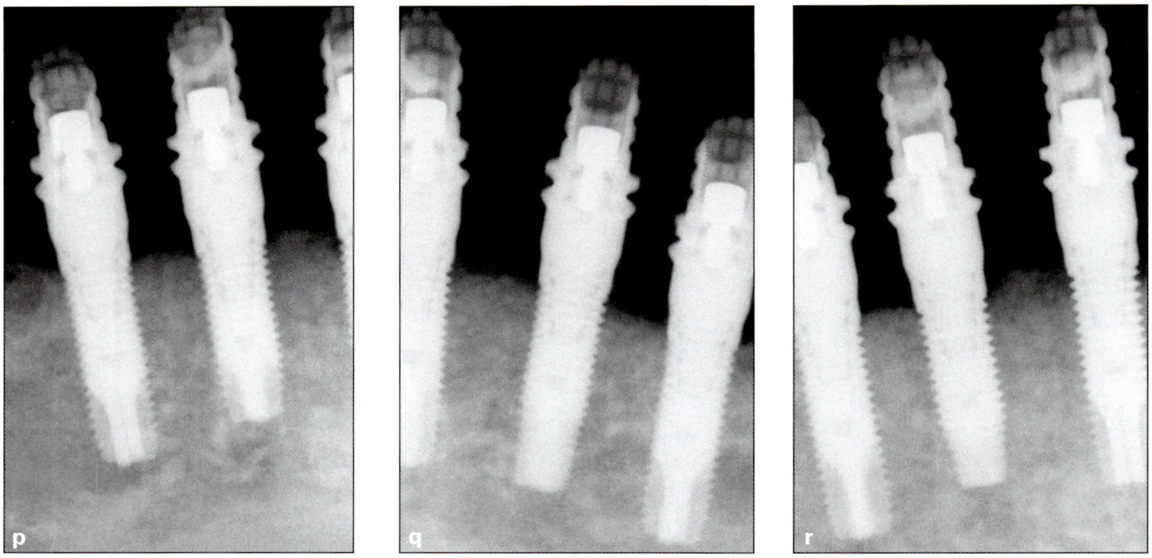

Figs 3-18p to 3-18r Postoperative periapical radiographs taken 4 months after the completion of the surgical treatment. Note the stability of crestal bone levels and uniformity of bone density.

Conclusion

The use of SimPlant software features discussed in this chapter can facilitate preoperative planning and surgical execution. The reader should understand that interpretation of CT data is directly related to familiarity and experience. The biggest challenge lies in the interpretation and correlation between the CT images and clinical reality. With increased experience and confidence, the value of preoperative inquiry becomes increasingly important. The SimPlant software has many additional features not covered in this section. The need to learn advanced software features will be directly related to the perceived value of preoperative planning and collaboration.

References

1. Schwarz M, Rothman S, Chafetz N, Rhodes M. Computer tomography. Part II. Preoperative assessment of the maxilla for endosseous implant surgery. Int J Oral Maxillofac Implants 1987;2:133–148.
2. Schwarz M, Rothman S, Chafetz N, Rhodes M. Computed tomography. Part I. Preoperative assessment of the mandible for endosseous implant surgery. Int J Oral Maxillofac Implants 1987;2:137–141.
3. Sonick M, Abrahams J, Faiella R. A comparison of the accuracy of periapical, panoramic and computerized tomographic radiograph in locating the mandibular canal. Int J Oral Maxillofac Implants 1994;9:455–460.
4. Gher M, Richardson A. The accuracy of dental radiographic techniques used for evaluation of implant fixture placement. Int J Periodontics Restorative Dent 1995;15:268–283.
5. Mecall R, Rosenfeld A. Influence of residual ridge resorption patterns on implant fixture placement and tooth position. Part I. Int J Periodontics Restorative Dent 1991;11:8–23.
6. Mecall R, Rosenfeld A. The influence of residual ridge resorption patterns on implant fixture placement and tooth position. Part II. Presurgical determination of prosthesis type and design. Int J Periodontics Restorative Dent 1992;12:32–51.
7. Mecall R, Rosenfeld A. Influence of residual ridge resorption patterns on fixture placement and tooth position, Part III: Presurgical assessment of ridge augmentation requirements. Int J Periodontics Restorative Dent 1996;16:322–337.
8. Israelson H, Plemons J, Watkins P, Sory C. Barium-coated surgical stents and computer-assisted tomography in the preoperative assessment of dental implant patients. Int J Periodontics Restorative Dent 1992;12:52–61.
9. Rosenfeld L, Mandelaris GA, Tardieu PB.Prosthetically directed implant placement using computer software to insure precise placement and predictable prosthetic outcomes. Part I. Diagnostics, imaging and collaborative accountability. Int J Periodontics Restorative Dent 2006;26:215–221.
10. Rosenfeld L, Mandelaris GA, Tardieu PB. Prosthetically directed implant placement using computer software to insure precise placement and predictable prosthetic outcomes. Part II. Rapid prototype medical modeling and stereolithographic drilling guides requiring bone exposure. Int J Periodontics Restorative Dent 2006;26: 347–353.
11. Rosenfeld L, Mandelaris GA, Tardieu PB. Prosthetically directed implant placement using computer software to insure precise placement and predictable prosthetic outcomes. Part III. Stereolithographic drilling guides that do not require bone exposure and the immediate delivery of teeth. Int J Periodontics Restorative Dent 2006;26: 493–499.
12. Borrow J, Smith J. Stent marker materials for computerized tomography-assisted implant planning. Int J Periodontics Restorative Dent 1996:16:61–67.

4

SCANNING APPLIANCES AND VIRTUAL TEETH

Philippe B. Tardieu, DDS

Prosthetically Driven Implant Selection and Placement

Because early implant placement was surgically and not prosthetically driven, there were major discrepancies between the anticipated and actual outcomes. We now know it is necessary to include meaningful prosthetic information in the computed tomography (CT) dataset to obtain the best prosthetic and esthetic results. The following case illustrates a variety of implant strategies based on different prosthetic objectives that are influenced by patient anatomy. Each option influences the design of the scanning appliance. This case represents a common clinical situation: three teeth missing between a mandibular canine and a mesially inclined second molar (Fig 4-1a).

Option 1: The obvious solution would be to replace the missing teeth with a three-unit implant-supported prosthesis. However, closer examination reveals that the mesiodistal prosthetic space is limited, so the restorations would be quite small and unesthetic and there would be limited access for proper hygiene (Fig 4-1b).

Option 2: Another option (Fig 4-1c) would be to reduce the number of implants while keeping the same number of teeth. The middle implant would be removed, but the position of the two remaining implants would remain unchanged. This option offers better access for hygiene but does not address the issue of tooth size.

Option 3: The third option replaces the three missing teeth with only two teeth. This results in a normal-sized premolar and an anatomically incorrect first molar (Fig 4-1d). In this scenario, the mesial implant remains the same, but the position and size of the distal implant are changed. It is possible that esthetics, the volume and density of the bone, and the regional anatomy could make this an undesirable choice.

Option 4: The fourth option also involves replacing the three missing teeth with two implants except it is based on a two-molar diagnostic waxup (Fig 4-1e). The position and size of both implants have been changed accordingly. This option may be more acceptable with regard to the size and position of the implants, but it is esthetically unacceptable.

Option 5: Here, the mesial aspect of the inclined molar is reduced to allow for the placement of a third more anatomically correct implant-supported prosthesis (Fig 4-1f). While the prosthetic outcome appears more esthetically pleasing, little improvement is gained in hygiene accessibility.

Option 6: With this option, the middle implant is removed to improve accessibility for hygiene (Fig 4-1g). While resolving the hygiene situation, the tooth size problem is not addressed. A variation of this option would be to increase the diameter of the distal implant to better accommodate the available space.

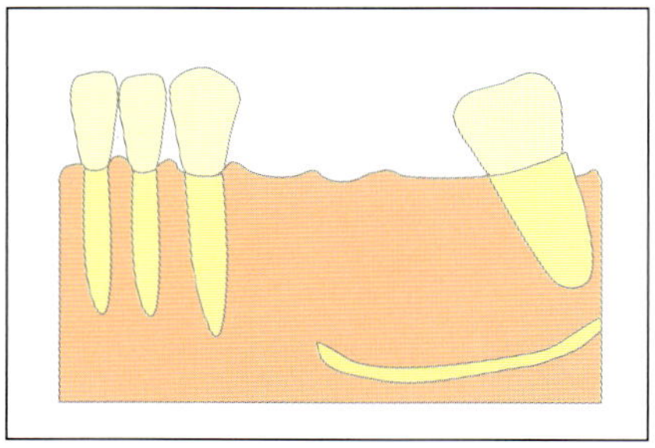

Fig 4-1a Schematic representation of the partially edentulous area: three teeth missing between a mandibular canine and a mesially inclined second molar.

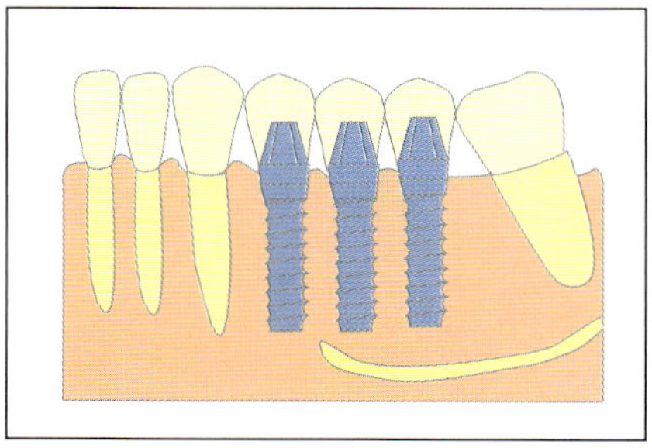

Fig 4-1b Option 1: Replacement of three teeth with a limited volume on three standard implants.

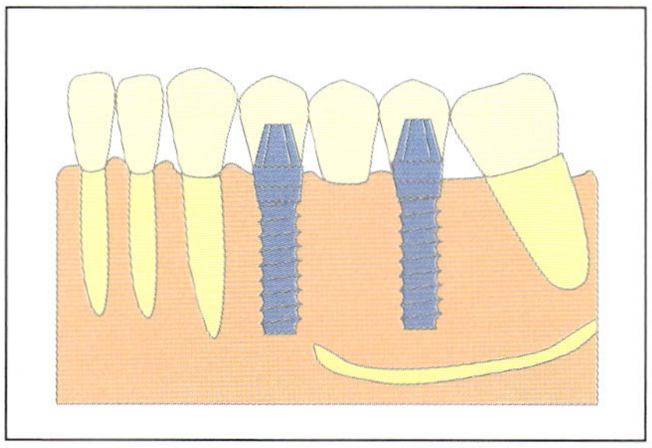

Fig 4-1c Option 2: The middle implant has been removed and the position of the two remaining implants is unchanged.

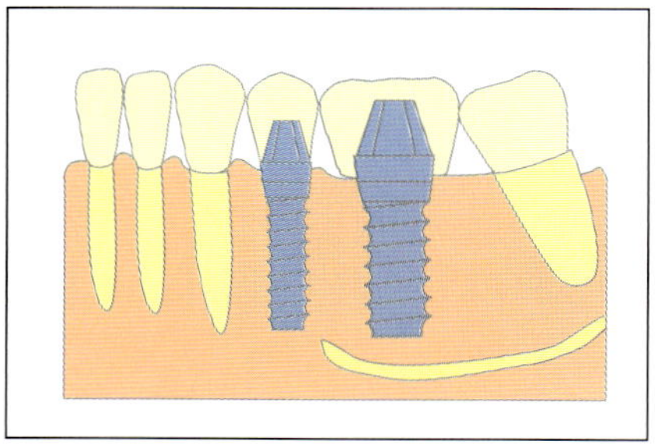

Fig 4-1d Option 3: The replacement of the three missing teeth with two teeth supported on implants.

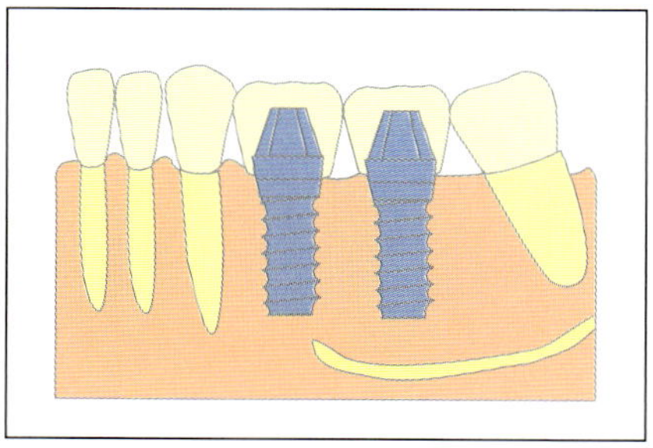

Fig 4-1e Option 4: Replacement of three teeth using two implants based on a two-molar diagnostic waxup.

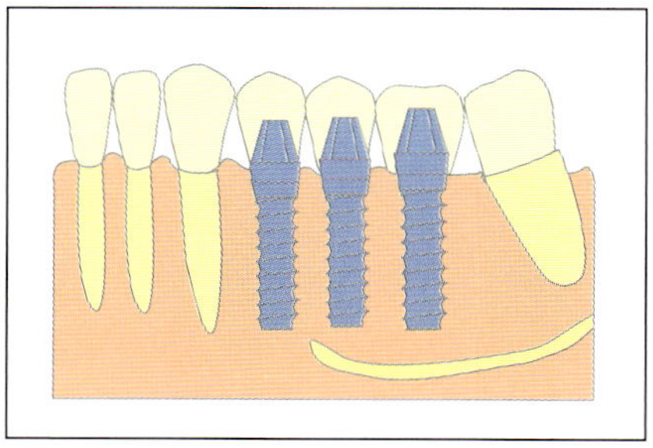

Fig 4-1f Option 5: The mesial aspect of the inclined molar has been modified to allow for the placement of a more anatomically correct implant-supported tooth.

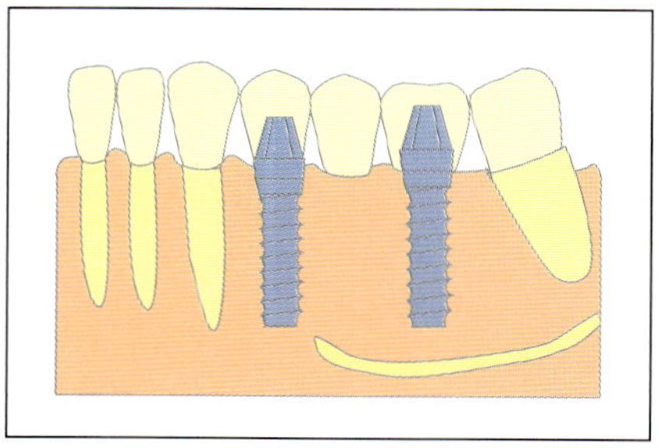

Fig 4-1g Option 6: Removal of the middle implant to improve accessibility for hygiene.

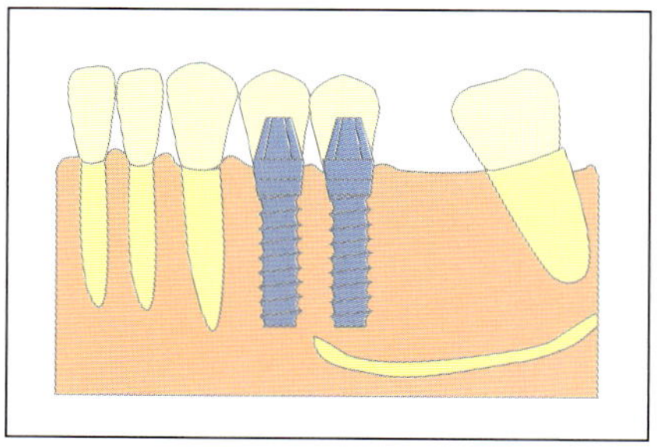

Fig 4-1h Option 7: Replacement of the two premolars only.

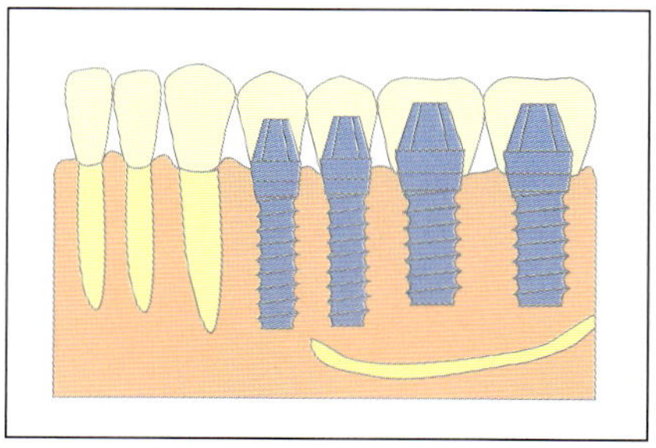

Fig 4-1i Option 8: Extraction of the inclined molar and placement of four implants.

Option 7: This option calls for replacing only the premolars (Fig 4-1h). Should the second molar require extraction later, additional implants could be placed in more appropriate positions.

Option 8: The second molar is extracted to facilitate the placement of four implants in this option (Fig 4-1i). Now the implant size and position closely resemble the natural tooth configuration, leaving the patient with more pleasing esthetics and access for oral hygiene.

These treatment options demonstrate the importance of evaluating final tooth position and size before determining the type and number of implants needed to achieve the prosthetic outcome. For the prosthetic outcome to drive the implant treatment plan, the final position, size, and number of teeth must be determined and then integrated into a scanning appliance worn by the patient during the CT scan. The resulting images provide a blueprint for treatment.

Scanning Appliance

A scanning appliance, sometimes referred to as a *scan prosthesis*, *radiologic template*, or *CT appliance*, is a radiopaque duplicate of the planned provisional tooth arrangement. The appliance is worn by the patient during the scanning process, and the radiopaque images of the planned tooth arrangement are visible in the CT data. Having this information incorporated into the same images as the patient's anatomic data enhances the clinician's ability to plan treatment, since both clinical and esthetic considerations are integrated. The main objective of a scanning appliance is to visualize the diagnostic tooth arrangement in CT images. A properly designed appliance enables visualization not only of the soft tissue but also of underlying ridge defects, which often are not observed clinically.

ScannoGuide

The author has developed a protocol for fabrication of a scanning appliance, called a *ScannoGuide*, that greatly facilitates the entire treatment planning process. The ScannoGuide offers several important advantages for both the clinician and the patient:

1. The ScannoGuide stabilizes, correctly positions, and maintains the jaws during CT scanning so that the radiologist can assess proper patient orientation using the scout view.
2. During the implant planning phase, the ScannoGuide allows visualization of the teeth to be replaced, determines the longitudinal axis of teeth, and relates teeth to surrounding anatomic structures. This allows assessment of ridge defects at the level of tooth emergence, provides information about the relationship between soft tissue and bone crest, and facilitates segmentation of teeth, soft tissue, and regional anatomy in three-dimensional (3D) reconstructions.
3. In edentulous patients, the ScannoGuide allows for the precise outline of the soft tissue surface. This unique imaging of the soft tissue enables fabrication of a surgical guide supported by mucosa. The same principles can be applied in the partially edentulous patient.
4. Since the ScannoGuide provides all of the relevant clinical information to restore function and esthetics, it can, with some modification, be used as a provisional immediate prosthesis. The patient's original prosthesis remains intact instead of being modified to fabricate an immediate temporary bridge. In the event of an unfavorable surgical outcome, the patient's original denture can be used as a back-up prosthesis.
5. The ScannoGuide provides a preoperative assessment of the need for facial support. In many cases, a prosthetic flange is required to meet the esthetic needs of the patient.
6. The ScannoGuide allows the patient to experience a prosthesis similar to the final outcome.
7. Perhaps the most underappreciated value of the ScannoGuide is that it enables the doctor and patient to participate in an atmosphere of informed consent and complete disclosure.

Fabrication of Scanning Appliance

The procedure for the fabrication of scanning appliances is different for edentulous and partially edentulous cases. The reason is that the design of a purely soft tissue–supported surgical guide (only possible in edentulous cases) and a combined tooth and soft tissue–supported surgical guide (in partially edentulous cases) is different. Soft tissue surface is needed to fabricate a surgical guide lying on the mucosa. Since the soft tissue is not visible on a CT scan, a method for visualizing the soft tissue surface was developed as part of the scanning appliance. The underlying surface of the base of the scanning appliance represents the outer surface of the soft tissue. In the combined tooth and soft tissue–supported surgical guide, the surface of the mucosa comes from the plaster cast of the jaw, and not from the CT scan image. This is a mere technical consideration that is explained in more detail in the chapter on surgical guides.

Edentulous patients

If the patient's current denture meets the physiologic requirements necessary to provide esthetics, phonetics, lip support, vertical dimension, and proper occlusion, an impression of the denture is made. If the existing denture does not meet these criteria, a new trial tooth setup is necessary. In some instances, it may be necessary to fabricate a new denture. If the existing denture is unstable, a hard reline is mandatory before duplication.

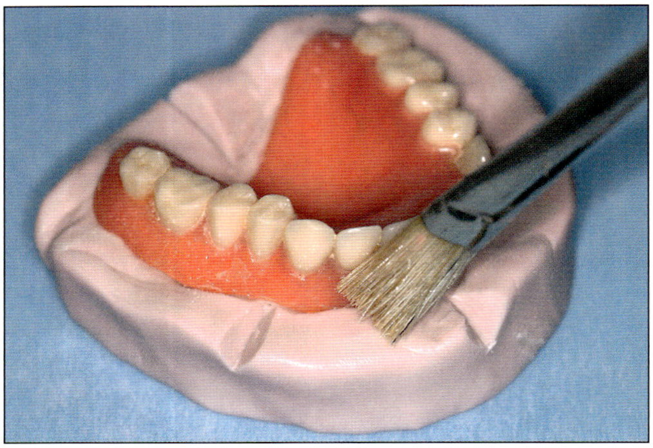

Fig 4-2 Small notches have been placed around the cast, which is being brushed with lubricant.

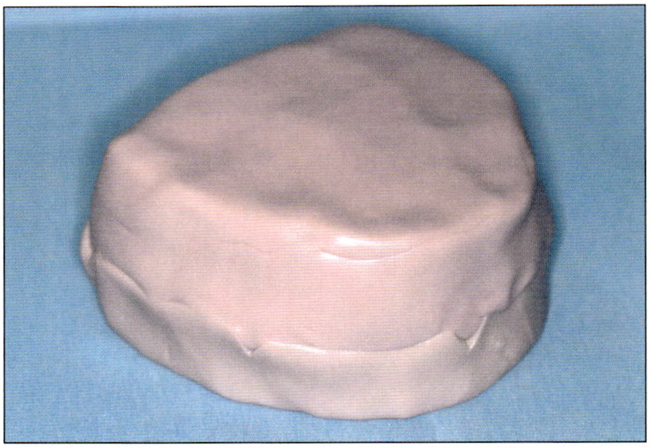

Fig 4-3a Upper part of the impression.

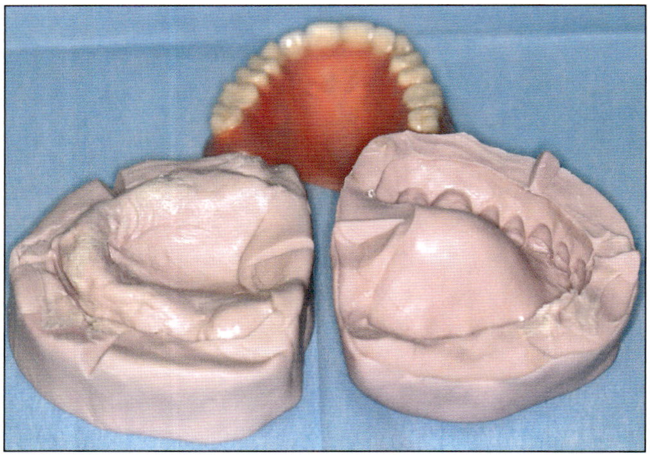

Fig 4-3b After setting, the molds and the denture can easily be separated.

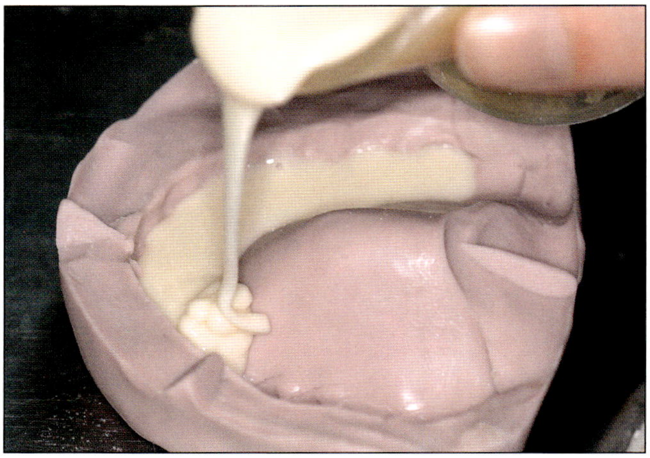

Fig 4-4 Filling of the impression.

Obtaining an impression

While there are a number of methods for denture duplication, the use of a silicone impression material is most common. To construct the scanning appliance, an impression of the underlying tissue surface is made in silicone. The impression material must be firmly adapted to ensure the absence of voids on the tissue surface of the denture and confined to the tissue-bearing surface of the denture.

A scalpel is used to make reference notches in the maxillary and mandibular molds for proper alignment, and a separating lubricant is applied (Fig 4-2). Once the material has set, the molds and the denture are separated (Figs 4-3a and 4-3b).

A barium sulfate mixture ($BaSO_4$) is incorporated into the appliance to create radiopaque CT images of the prosthesis. The $BaSO_4$ powder is mixed with resin powder in two specific ratios by weight: a 30% $BaSO_4$ and resin powder mixture for the teeth, and a 10% $BaSO_4$ and resin powder mixture for the denture base. This gradient radiopacity differentiates the teeth from the denture base. The mixture must be homogeneous to avoid dense spots caused by excessively high concentrations of $BaSO_4$ in the appliance, which will cause unwanted artifacts to appear in the images.

A monomer is then added to the powders to obtain a sufficiently low viscosity. It is important to minimize the air bubbles in the mixtures so that the entire volume is homogeneous.

If two different cold-polymerizing resins (tooth- and tissue-colored) are incorporated in the $BaSO_4$ mixtures to produce a lifelike appliance, the resulting appliance can be used as an implant-supported provisional prosthesis. Use of a single-colored resin does not diminish the diagnostic value of the appliance, although it does limit its use as a prosthesis.

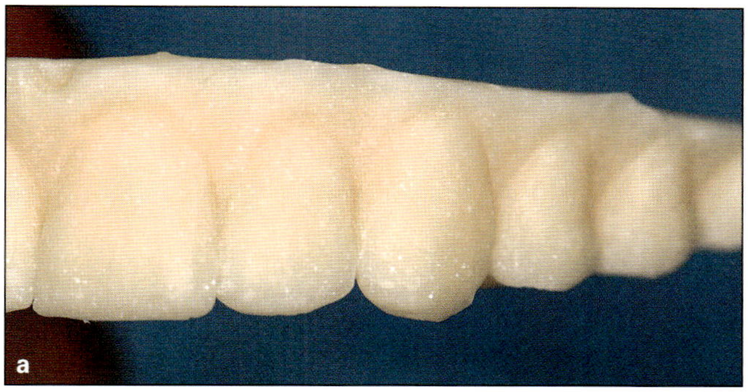
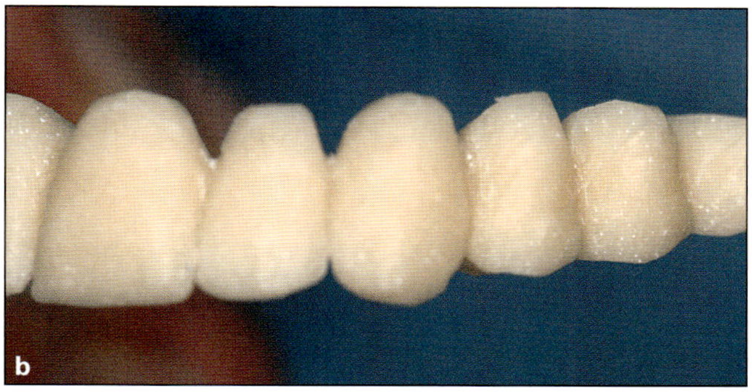

Fig 4-5 *(a,b)* Excess acrylic is removed to define the cervical tooth contour.

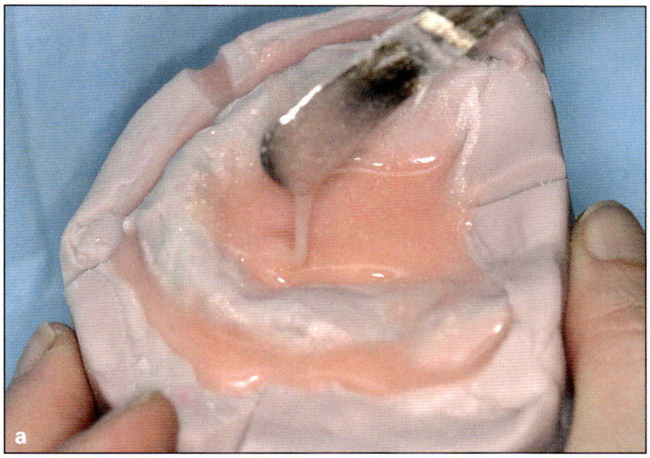
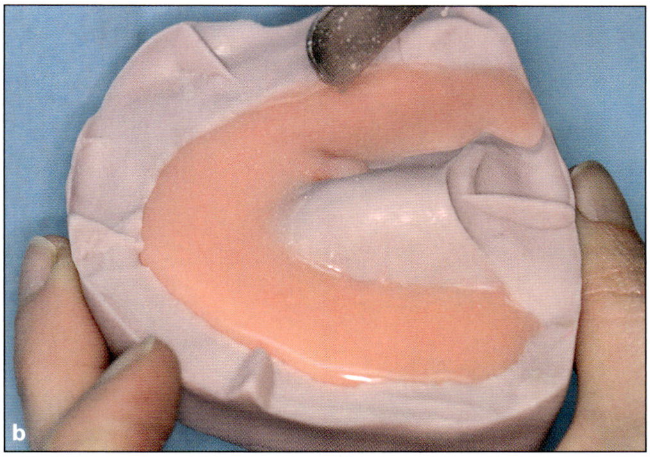

Fig 4-6 *(a)* The tissue portion of the mold is filled. *(b)* The mold containing teeth is filled.

Fabrication

The 30% $BaSO_4$-resin mixture is placed into the tooth portion of the mold (Fig 4-4) and allowed to harden in a pressure cooker with hot water. When the resin is completely hardened, the excess resin should be trimmed before removing it from the mold (Figs 4-5a and 4-5b). The maxillary and mandibular tooth molds should be aligned using the reference notches.

To create the denture base, the 10% $BaSO_4$-resin mixture is placed into the denture base mold and any excess resin removed. To limit the introduction of bubbles, the molds are filled separately (Figs 4-6a and 4-6b) and manually pressed together. The molds are then hardened in a pressure cooker. When the resin has set, any excess resin is trimmed off, and the appliance is separated from the mold.

To ensure that the center of each tooth will be visible on the CT images, a hole (0.5 to 1 mm in diameter) is drilled in the occlusal center of the posterior teeth and the cingulum of the anterior teeth, following the long axis of each tooth until the denture base is penetrated (Fig 4-7).

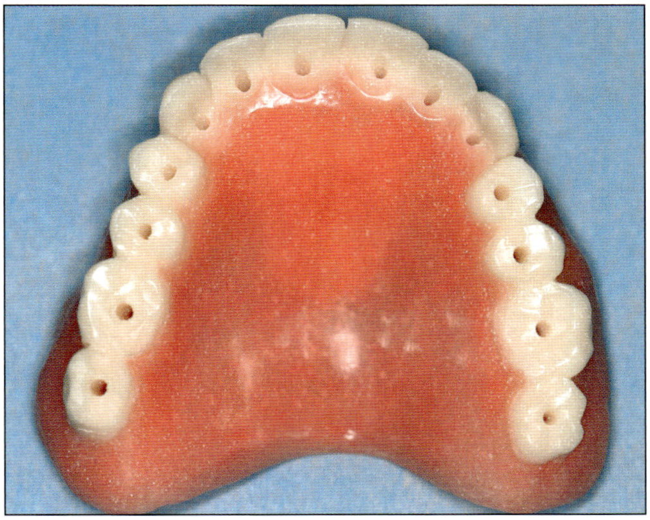

Fig 4-7 The completed scanning appliance with drill holes representing the center of each tooth.

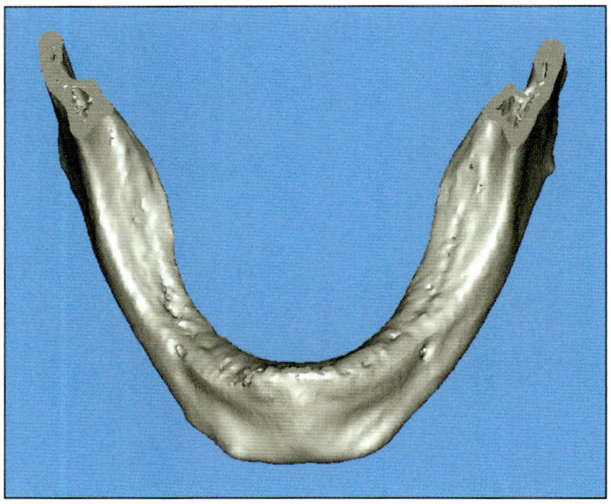

Fig 4-8a 3D image of the bone only.

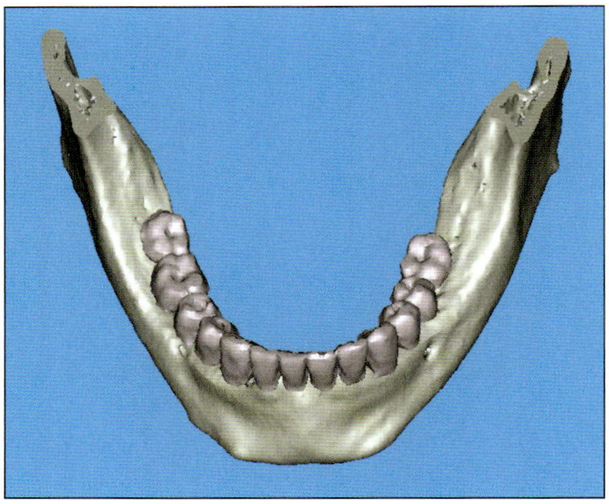

Fig 4-8b Bone and teeth of the ScannoGuide.

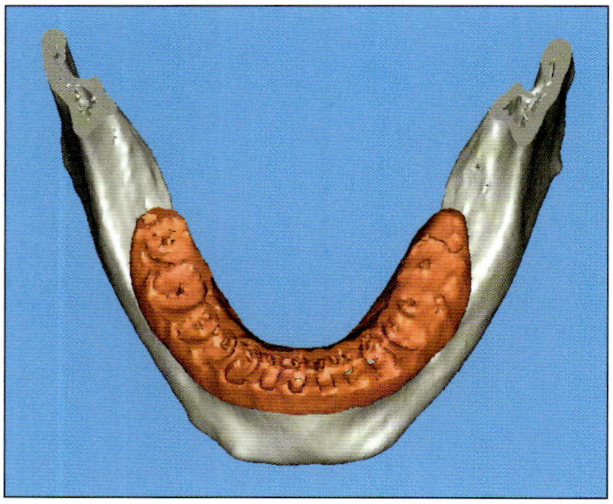

Fig 4-8c Bone and base plate of the ScannoGuide.

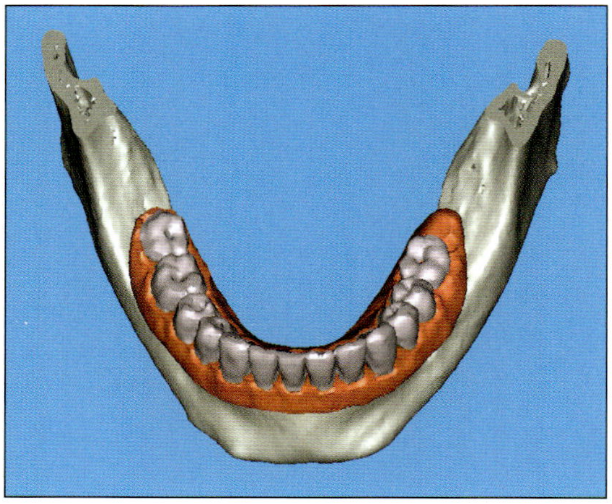

Fig 4-8d Bone and ScannoGuide.

If the holes are not accurately placed, they can be filled with the appropriate $BaSO_4$-acrylic mixture and new holes drilled. Gutta-percha should not be used because it will introduce a radiographic artifact that will interfere with CT interpretation.

Positioning the appliance for scanning

The appliance should fit comfortably and securely in the patient's mouth. To stabilize the appliance, cotton rolls should be placed between the maxilla and mandible with the patient biting down firmly. Any adjustment can be done as a chairside reline using the same mixture used for the denture base.

Imaging the appliance

All of the clinical information is now embedded in the CT study. The software allows the user to manipulate the 3D information and evaluate the characteristics necessary to design the definitive prosthesis, such as choosing the type of implants and abutments and determining whether a bar-supported removable or fixed denture is most appropriate.

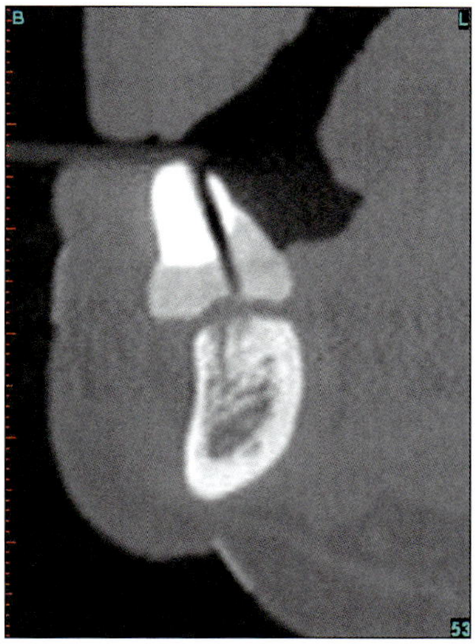

Fig 4-8e Drill hole appears black on 2D cross sections.

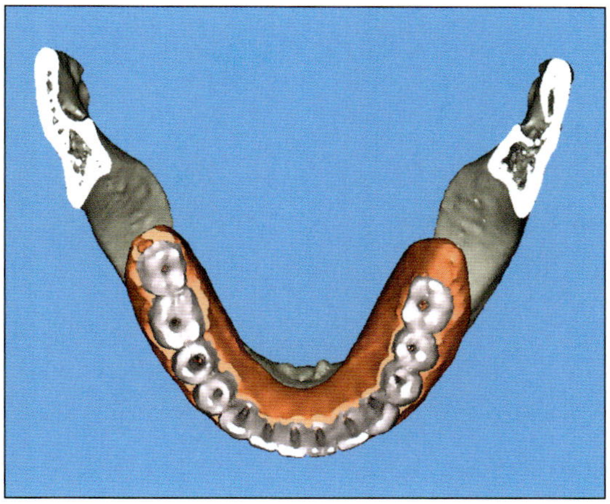

Fig 4-8f Drill holes visible in the 3D representation of the ScannoGuide.

The appliance can be viewed in all CT images and, because of the differences in radiopacities, the teeth and denture base can be viewed separately from the bone anatomy in the 3D reconstruction (Figs 4-8a to 4-8f). Furthermore, the software allows the user to activate or deactivate selected images, making it possible to evaluate bone anatomy independently or in combination with the prosthetic information.

Partially edentulous patients

Most of the characteristics of the ScannoGuide can be used to design a scanning appliance for the partially edentulous patient. First, a diagnostic waxup representing the planned final restorative outcome (ie, information to be transferred to the CT scans) should be completed on properly mounted study casts. Be aware that denture teeth may not accurately represent the natural dentition anatomy and that commercially available radiopaque denture teeth do not exhibit the barium concentration necessary for proper imaging. Each case requires special attention during the diagnostic waxup, which influences the relationship between the implant and the restoration. For example, in some cases there may not be adequate space to replace all of the missing teeth, making it necessary to modify the tooth size to accommodate both implant placement and tooth position. In the case illustrated in Fig 4-9, the normal appearance of the lateral incisor and the premolar was maximized, and the residual space was used for the canine (Fig 4-9a). The mesial aspect of the canine was left intact and the distal aspect reduced to give the impression that the canine had full volume. If implants were placed without preoperatively establishing this situation, it would not be possible to create the illusion of three natural-looking teeth.

Teeth fabrication

An impression of the waxup is made (Fig 4-9b) and the wax completely removed from the plaster cast. A separating lubricant is applied over the edentulous area and adjacent teeth. Then the same basic procedures used to create a fully edentulous scanning appliance are followed: The entire tooth volume is filled with the 30% barium concentrate mixture (Fig 4-9c); the impression is placed over a plaster cast and secured with rubber bands (Fig 4-9d); and the entire mold is placed in a pressure cooker with hot water. When the teeth are removed from the mold, excess resin is trimmed away, leaving the underlying surface undisturbed. This is important since this surface represents the outer aspect of the soft tissue (Fig 4-9e). As with fully edentulous cases, holes are drilled completely through the teeth to allow precise location of the centers of the teeth (Fig 4-9f).

The acrylic teeth are firmly attached to the plaster cast with adhesive (Fig 4-9g). A radiolucent thermoplastic plate is heated and compressed over the cast using a vacuum system (Fig 4-9h). The thermoplastic plate, which now incorporates the teeth, is removed from the cast and then trimmed to remove those undercut areas that would restrict passive fit of the appliance in the patient's mouth (Fig 4-9i).

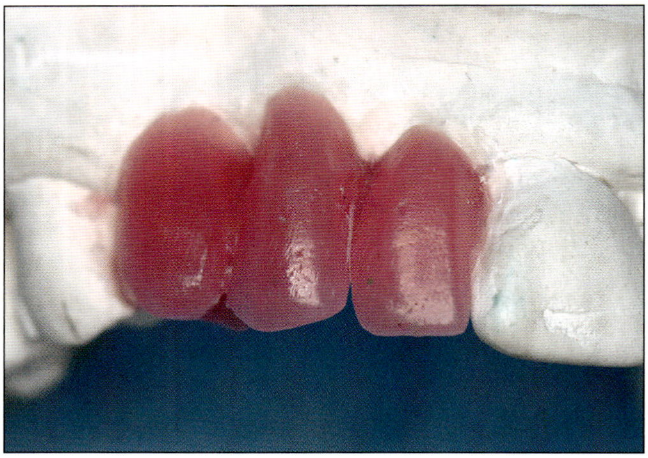

Fig 4-9a Waxup of the teeth to be replaced.

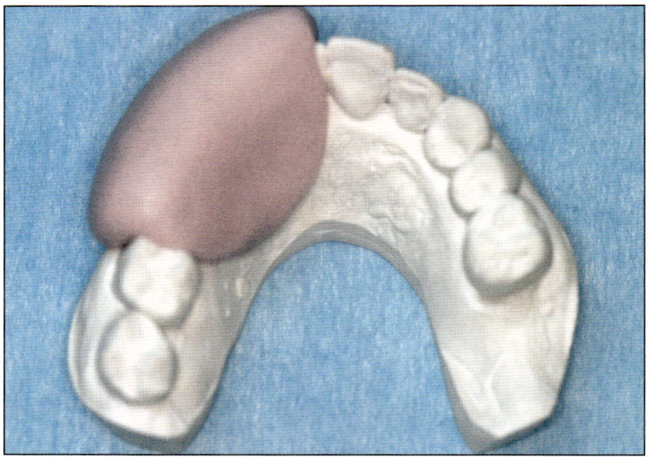

Fig 4-9b Impression of the waxup, occlusal view.

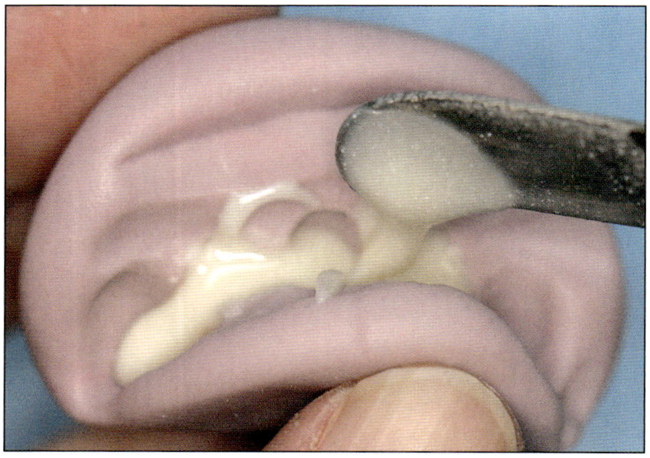

Fig 4-9c The entire teeth volume is filled with the mixture.

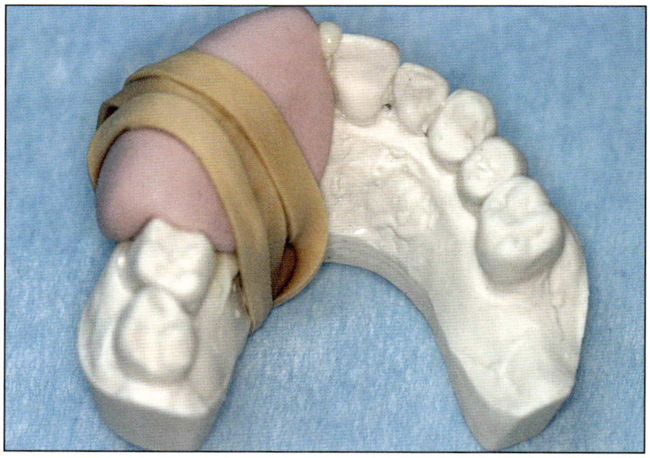

Fig 4-9d The mold containing the resin mixture is secured with rubber bands.

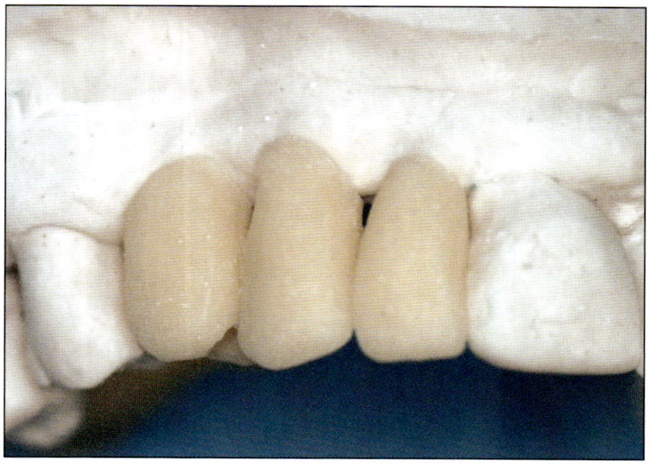

Fig 4-9e Excess resin is removed.

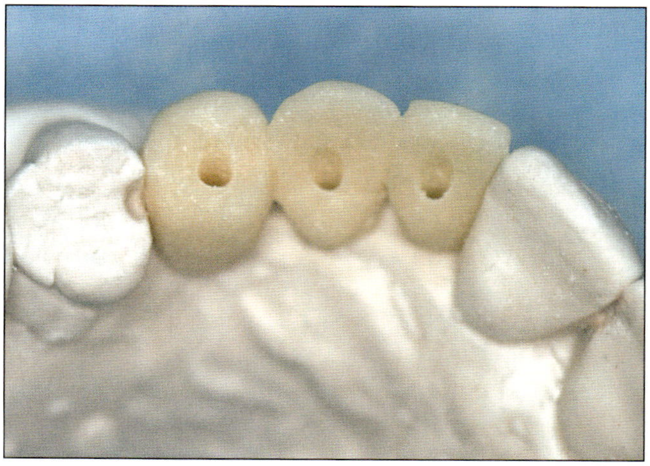

Fig 4-9f Holes are drilled through the teeth.

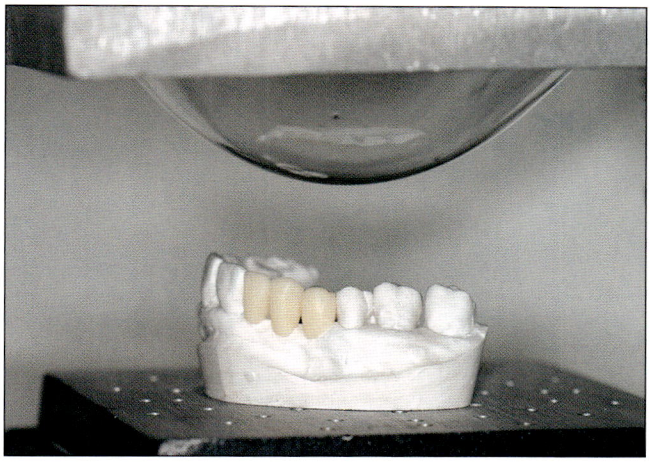

Fig 4-9g Thermoplastic plate that has been heated in the vacuum machine.

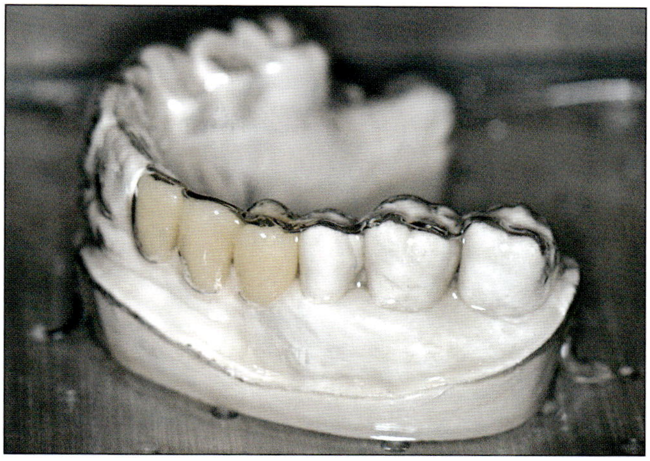

Fig 4-9h Thermoplastic plate, adapted over the plaster cast.

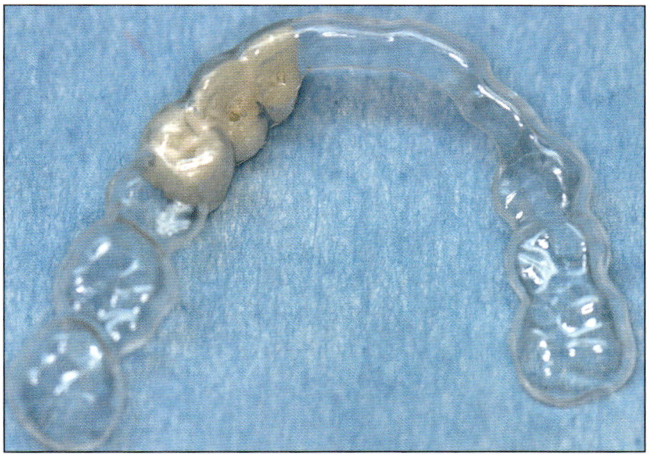

Fig 4-9i ScannoGuide, occlusal view.

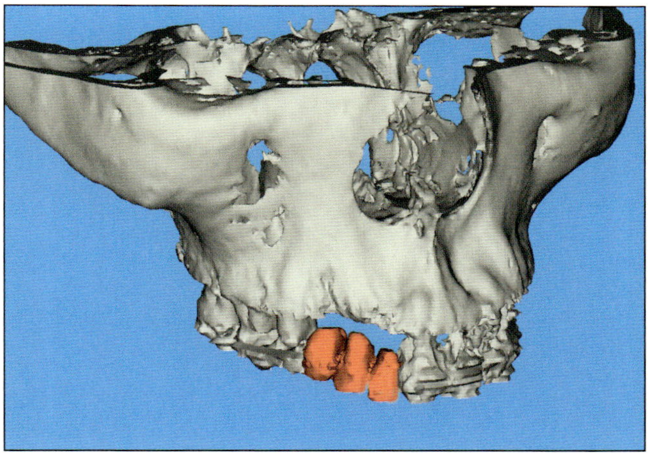

Fig 4-9j 3D representation of the ScannoGuide and bone.

Appearance of the appliance in the CT images

The scanning appliance is viewed as for edentulous cases. Because of the radiopacity of the appliance, the teeth can be clearly visualized in the 3D reconstruction (Fig 4-9j).

Virtual Teeth

The Virtual Tooth feature allows 2D and 3D imaging of the planned definitive restoration without the use of a scanning appliance (Fig 4-10a).

Virtual teeth are placed on the patient's jaw by *(1)* opening the Virtual Tooth tool; *(2)* selecting the teeth to be replaced; and *(3)* adjusting the height, length, and curve of the teeth (Figs 4-10b to 4-10f).

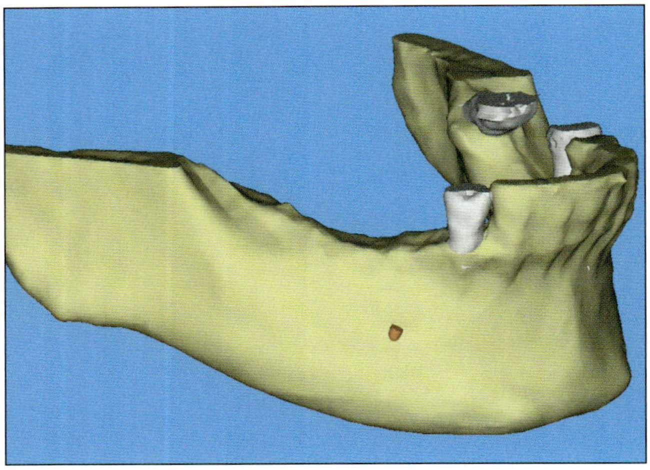

Fig 4-10a Initial appearance of the jaw showing the mandibular right edentulous ridge. Four teeth from the first premolar to the second molar need to be replaced.

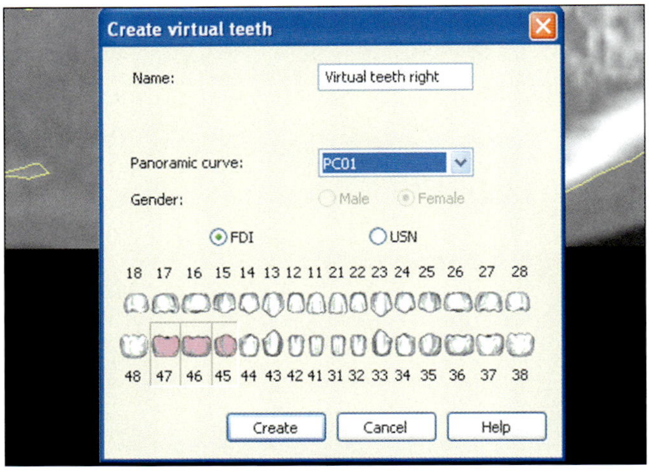

Fig 4-10b Virtual Tooth wizard.

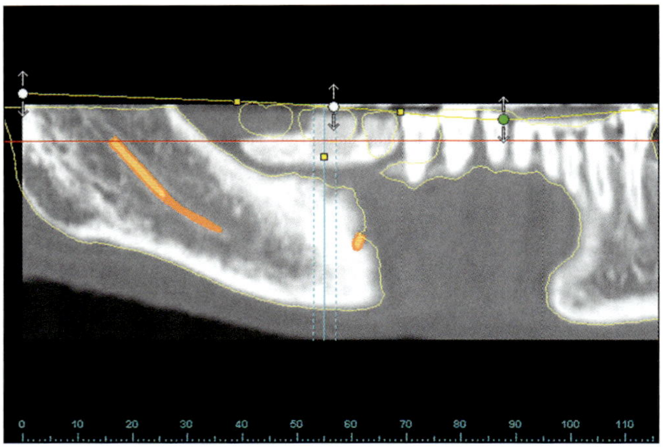

Fig 4-10c Adjustment of the virtual teeth in the panoramic view.

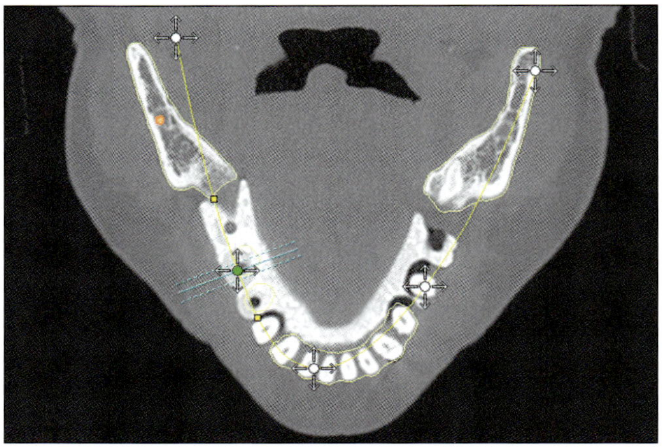

Fig 4-10d Evaluating the panoramic curve in the axial view.

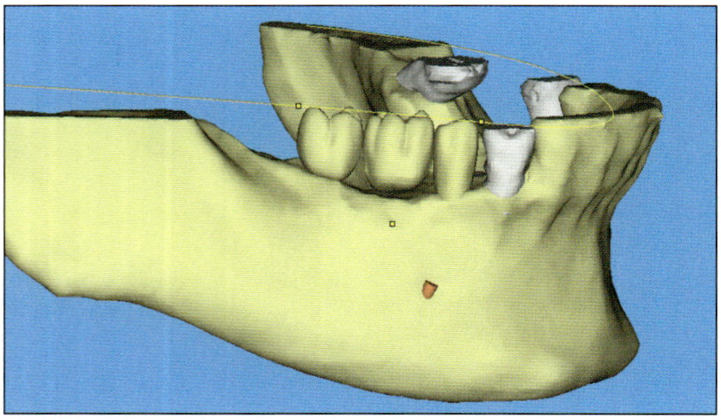

Fig 4-10e Manipulating the virtual teeth in the 3D reconstruction.

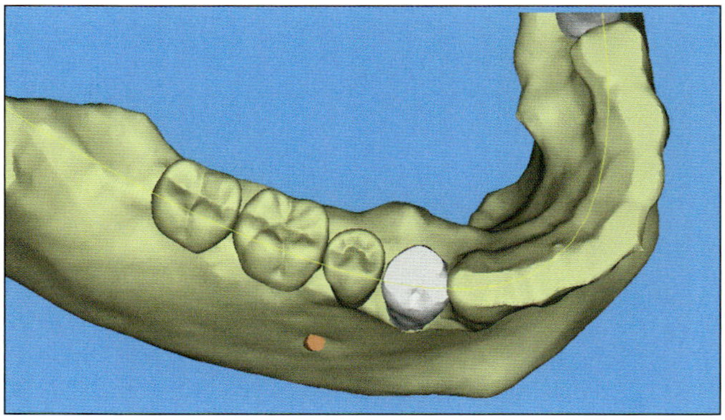

Fig 4-10f Alignment of the virtual teeth with existing teeth.

A benefit of this tool is that it minimizes the number of appointments needed and eliminates the fabrication time. Virtual teeth can be used for cases in which the image and the position of the opposite arch are not essential, for example, when dealing with localized and limited tooth and bone loss. While the Virtual Tooth tool does not replace an appliance, a clinical assessment can identify those situations in which it is applicable. In some instances, virtual teeth can help determine tooth position when radiographic artifacts would otherwise have interfered.

The limitations of the Virtual Tooth include the inability to determine the maxillomandibular relationship; the inability to capture soft tissue position, which could affect the vertical position of the implants; and the inability to preoperatively verify implant positioning.

5

AXIAL IMAGE CONVERSION AND SEGMENTATION

Ellen Dhoore, MSc

This chapter reviews the process of converting the native computed tomography (CT) images and the preparation of the three-dimensional (3D) planning environment. It is necessary to convert the stack of axial images into a format that is compatible with SimPlant (Materialise). Coronal and sagittal reconstructions are created from the axial images. The data are also processed into 3D representations of chosen regions of interest (ROI). The software allows for segmentation of information, such as bone, implants, metal structures, tooth roots, and the scanning appliance. A 3D object can be generated for each segmented part, and the objects can be viewed individually or in combination. Structures of no interest—for example, the spine, mandibular rami, and skull base—can be separated from the ROI and eliminated from the 3D objects.

Conversion of CT Images to a SimPlant-Compatible Format

Axial images in native CT format must be imported into SimPlant and converted to a new proprietary format. The import feature supports a wide range of scanner and image formats. The native CT data can be transferred via a variety of methods (hard disk, CD-ROM, optical disk, or tape) or sent via a DICOM network.

The number of axial slices per scan varies depending on the patient's anatomy, the referring clinician's ROI, and the thickness of each slice. As a basic rule, the scope of the scan should cover all bony anatomy in the jaw of interest, all tooth information, and the entire scanning appliance (if available). For the maxilla, the height of the scan into the sinus and orbit region should be within the range outlined in the scanning protocol and verified with the referring clinician. For patients where long zygoma or pterygoid implants are planned, the scope of the scan range needs to be modified.

The image selector tool allows identification of the exact images wanted for the CT study. If images for both the maxilla and mandible are included, the data should be separated into two studies. When all of the necessary orientation information about the images is known, the project is displayed in three panes, showing axial, coronal, and sagittal images. Each image is cross-referenced in the other images with color-coded reference lines (Fig 5-1).

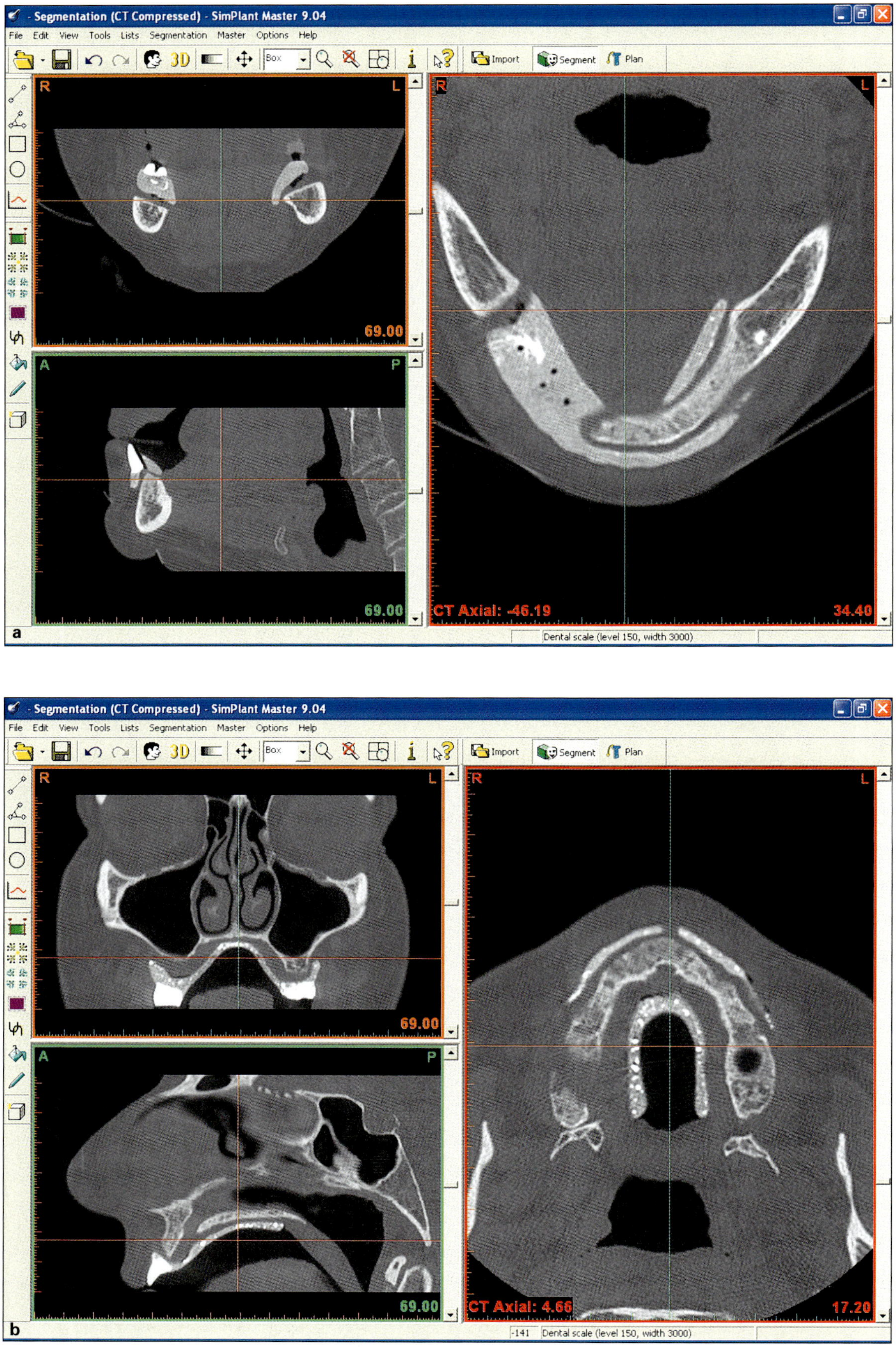

Fig 5-1 *(a)* Edentulous mandible and scanning appliance with axial image bordered in red, coronal image bordered in green, and sagittal images bordered in orange. *(b)* Edentulous maxilla and scanning appliance.

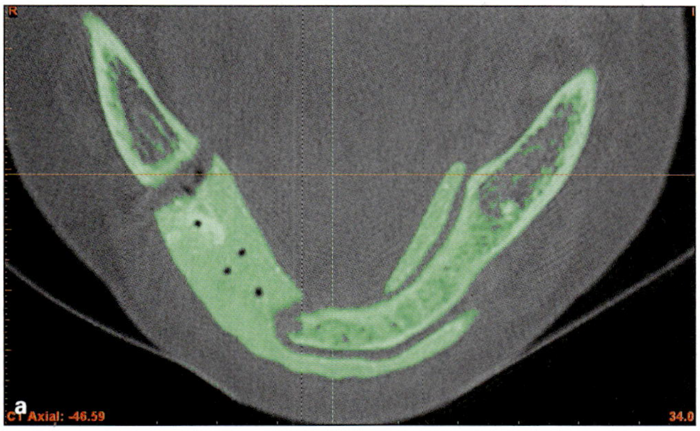

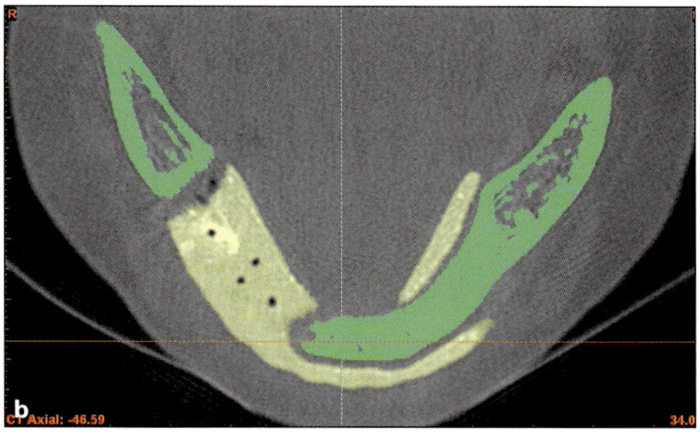

Fig 5-2 *(a)* Before region growing: mandible bone and scanning appliance in one mask. *(b)* After region growing: mandible bone in green mask and scanning appliance in yellow mask.

Segmentation of 2D Images for Representation as 3D Objects

Segmentation is the process of separating objects within the patient's 2D images to create 3D objects. The steps involved are: *(1)* thresholding, *(2)* region growing, *(3)* manual editing, and *(4)* 3D calculation.

Thresholding

When setting a threshold for segmentation, the user identifies a range of pixels to be included in the segmented object. The segmented object, represented by a colored mask, will contain only those pixels within the range. The software incorporates default settings for the maxilla and mandible that offer a good starting position; however, the final threshold should be evaluated case by case. A good threshold should reduce the noise (extraneous pixels) around bone while preserving the sharp bone edges.

Region growing

The original mask can be split into new, separate masks through region growing, which creates a new mask from pixels in the connecting region. Individual structures can thus be separated into their own masks. Both region growing and manual editing are required to separate connected objects (Fig 5-2).

Manual editing

Tools for erasing, drawing, and applying a local threshold can be used on the active mask. The manual editing function is used to separate connected objects before region growing, and the eraser tool is used to eliminate metal scatter or artifacts. The editing tools affect only the mask that will later be calculated into a 3D object. The original CT information does not change.

3D calculation

3D objects can be calculated with different quality levels—low, medium, or high—and all 3D parameters can be customized. With each separated 3D object, the referring clinician can better determine a treatment plan, because additional data can be evaluated.

The value of 3D objects is in their representation of the patient's bony anatomy as well as tooth anatomy, the radiologic scanning appliance, and more. With each separated 3D object, the referring clinician can better treatment plan for dental implants.

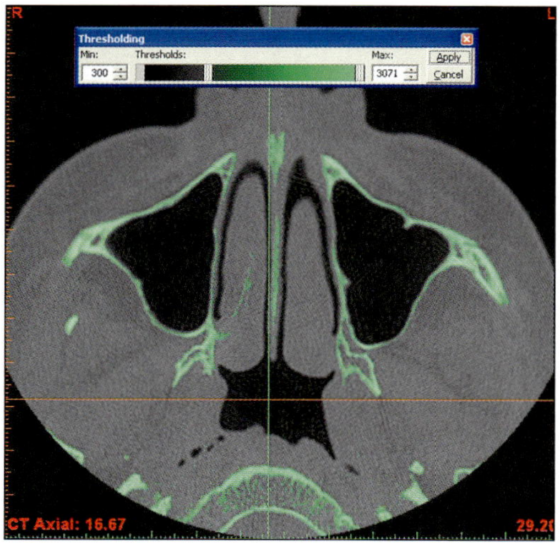

Fig 5-3 Thresholding set at 300 HU for maxillary bone. The result is displayed in the green mask.

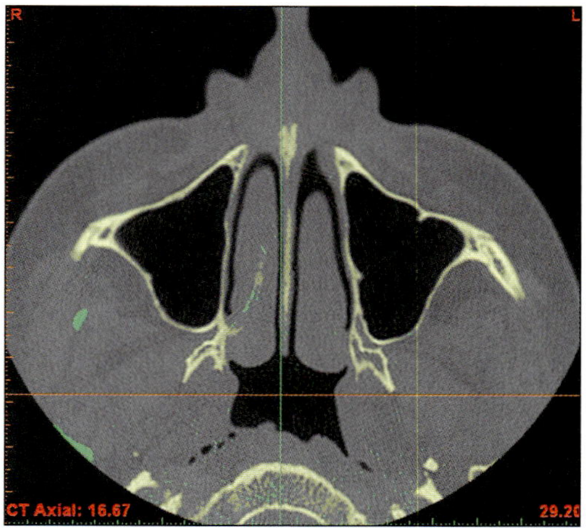

Fig 5-4 Region growing in the green mask in the ROI. The result is displayed in the yellow mask.

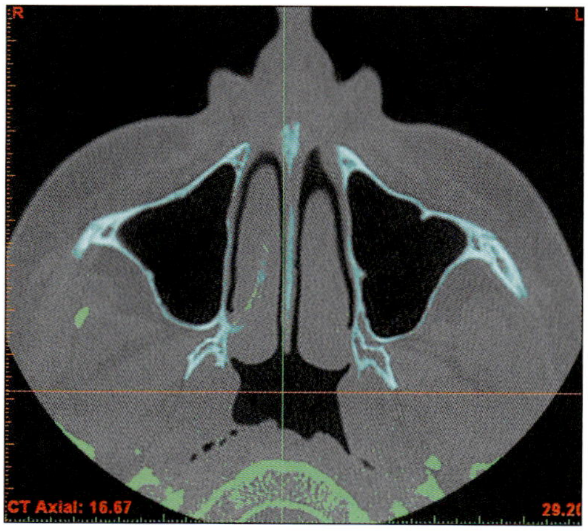

Fig 5-5 The result of region growing: mask with maxilla and scanning appliance.

Segmenting an Edentulous Maxilla with a Radiologic Scanning Appliance

- To reduce the noise but preserve sharp bone edges, a threshold of 300 Hounsfield units (HU) is used for the maxillary bone (Fig 5-3).
- Region growing in the ROI of the green mask is shown in Fig 5-4. The resulting yellow mask contains not only maxillary bone but also the scanning appliance, spine, and mandibular rami information. To limit the size of the maxillary model behind the pterygoid wings, all of the information in the coronal images has to be removed, and region growing is repeated.
- The skull, spine, and mandible have been removed from the mask, leaving only the maxilla and scanning appliance after region growing is performed (Fig 5-5). This mask is retained for later use, and a duplicate is made for manual editing.
- Using manual editing, the maxilla is separated from the scanning appliance by removing all contact points between the scanning appliance and maxilla (Fig 5-6) while region growing several times in between. After the alterations, the maxilla will be separated from the scanning appliance.
- The resulting mask (Fig 5-7) contains only the maxillary bone and can be used to calculate a 3D image of the maxilla.
- The scanning appliance is then isolated and divided into two parts: teeth and denture plate (Figs 5-8 and 5-9).

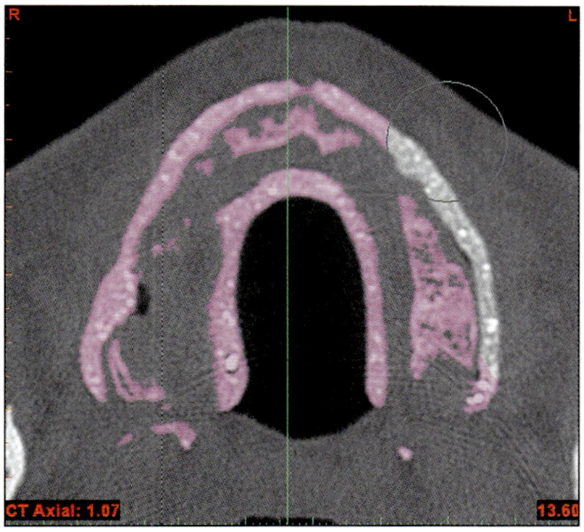

Fig 5-6 Manual editing is used to separate the maxilla and scanning appliance.

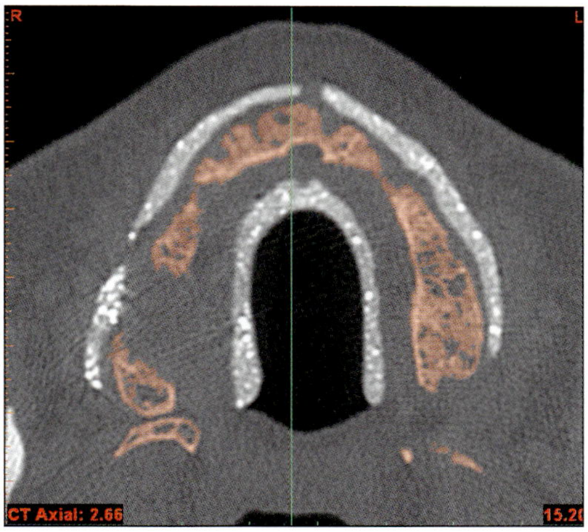

Fig 5-7 The maxillary bone remains.

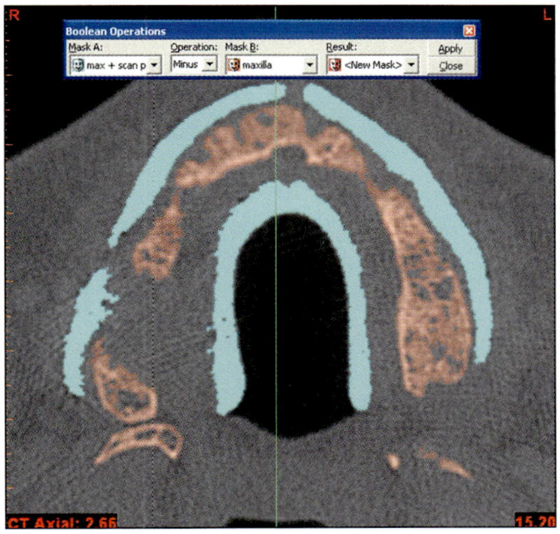

Fig 5-8 The scanning appliance is separated into teeth and denture plate.

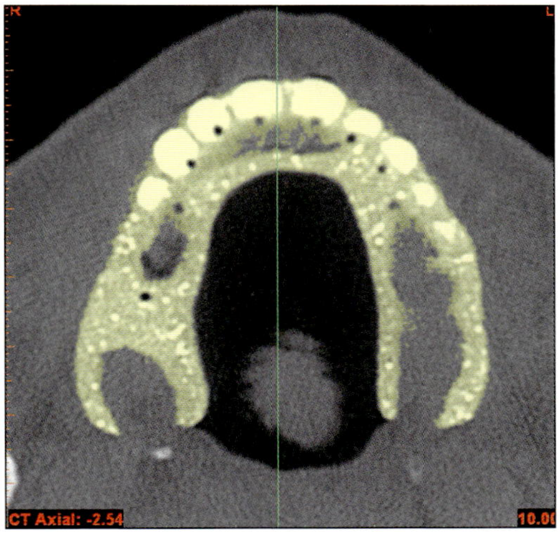

Fig 5-9 Scanning appliance, denture plate, and teeth.

To separate the scan prosthesis, the Boolean operation *mask of* scanning appliance + *maxilla – mask of maxilla* is used.

- The result of the Boolean operation is the scan prosthesis, denture plate, and teeth, with some artifacts present (see Fig 5-9). This mask is retained for future use.
- A new mask and threshold are created for the teeth in the scanning appliance. Because of the high concentration of barium sulfate in the appliance, the threshold can be much higher than for bone (Fig 5-10). In this case, the threshold is around 1,300 HU.
- Region growing results in a mask of the teeth in the scanning appliance, including negligible artifacts and excess information, which can be removed with manual editing (Fig 5-11).
- To separate the denture plate of the scanning appliance, a final Boolean operation is performed: subtraction of teeth mask from the mask with the complete scanning appliance, denture plate, and teeth (Fig 5-12).
- Final editing is then done on the mask of the denture plate, and all excess information is removed (Fig 5-13).
- A 3D representation of all 3D models: Maxilla and scanning appliance, denture base, and teeth are separated in different 3D objects to enhance visualization during implant planning (Fig 5-14).

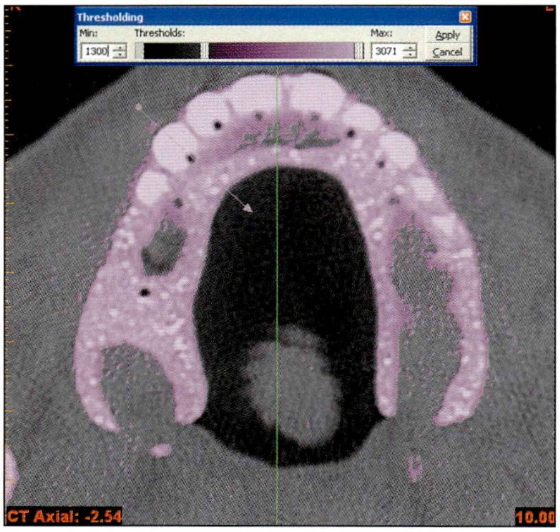

Fig 5-10 Mask for prosthetic teeth (threshold, 1,300 HU).

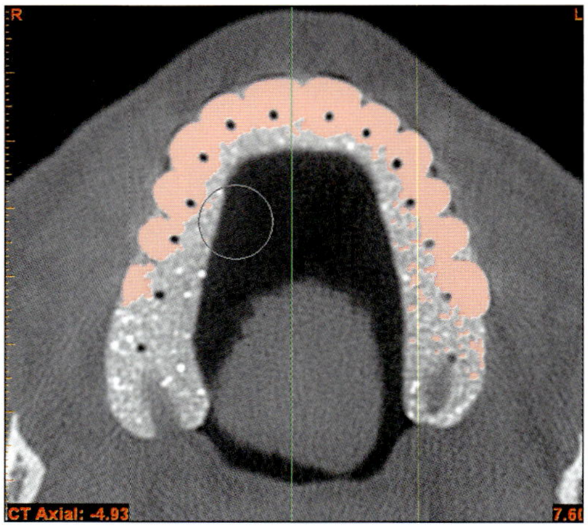

Fig 5-11 Mask of teeth in the scanning appliance.

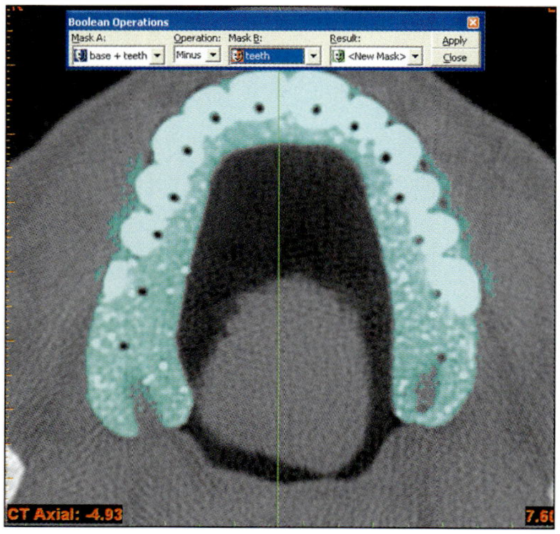

Fig 5-12 Separating denture plate from scanning appliance.

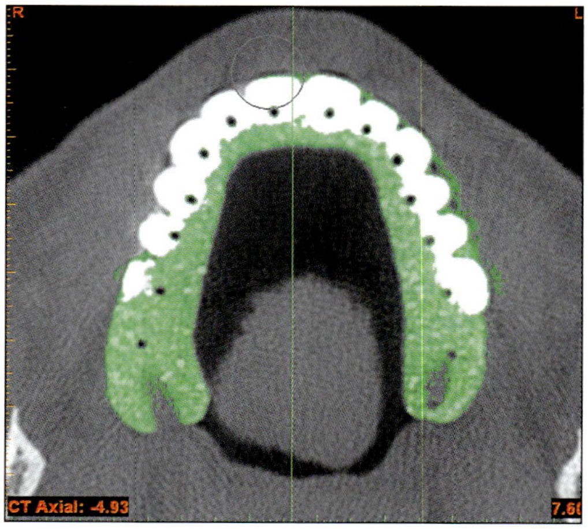

Fig 5-13 Final editing.

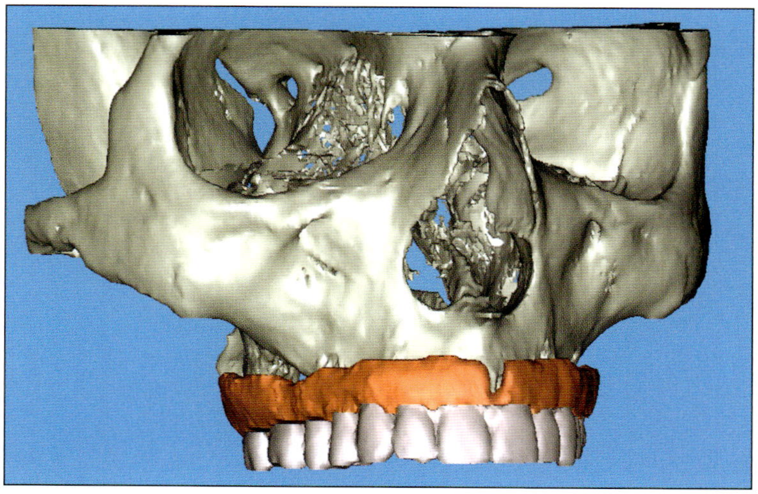

Fig 5-14 3D representation of all models.

Limiting the influence of artifacts

Since most artifacts are located on the level of teeth or implants, the CT data are generally of sufficient quality for implant planning. The patient's plaster cast can be used in combination with the CT data for template design. An optical scanner can digitize the information from the plaster cast. Then the digital information is united with the corresponding segmented data, and a surgical guide can be produced.

6

SURGIGUIDE OPTIONS

George A. Mandelaris, DDS, MS
Alan L. Rosenfeld, DDS, FACD

For most clinicians, implant placement has been and continues to be intuitively guided, and this can lead to less-than-optimal implant positioning. While suboptimal implant placement may seem insignificant at the time of surgery, the impact of the discrepancy and the magnitude of prosthetic compensation required can lead to an unsatisfactory prosthetic outcome, complicating patient care.[1]

Recent technologic advances allow for osteotomy site preparation and implant positioning to be computer guided rather than intuitively driven.[2] This process is prosthetically driven and requires the use of scanning appliances designed to transfer the prosthetic outcome information to the computed tomography (CT) study.[2,3]

Management of diagnostic and clinical information using computer software enables the restorative dentist to set the surgical performance standard. The use of stereolithographic medical modeling coupled with three-dimensional (3D), patient-specific CT information makes it possible to fabricate bone-, tooth-, tooth and mucosa–, and exclusively mucosa-supported surgical guides (ie, SurgiGuides). SurgiGuides allow osteotomy site preparation to be performed in a more precise and efficient manner and, in certain instances, with less patient discomfort than conventional implant surgery.[3]

With the advent of sophisticated scanning appliances, rapid prototype medical modeling, and the construction of computer-generated surgical guides that accurately reflect the prosthetic outcome to submillimeter accuracy, the restorative dentist has the opportunity to assume a collaborative leadership role in implant dentistry.[4–6]

Rapid Prototyping and Medical Modeling

The techniques and applications of rapid prototype medical modeling and the process of stereolithography are covered in detail in chapter 9. Briefly, rapid prototyping is a method of producing solid physical copies of human anatomy from 3D computer data.[7] All rapid prototyping techniques are based on the same principle of constructing a 3D structure in layers. The direct benefits to the dental implant patient include *(1)* a better understanding of the treatment requirements and commitment needed for successful therapy; *(2)* a significant reduction in surgical time and a proportional decrease in postoperative pain, discomfort, and swelling; and *(3)* a better understanding of anticipated outcomes and alternative types of treatment.

Medical modeling has several important applications.[8–10] First, it enables visualization of anatomic features such as tumor size and location, bone morphology, and orientation of vital structures. Second, it facilitates communication between surgical team members, restorative dentists, and the patient. Third, it enables the rehearsal of surgical procedures, such as osteotomy preparation, implant positioning, abutment selection, and implant provisionalization. Complex surgical intervention can be performed on a medical model and a dress rehearsal performed prior to patient intervention. Fourth, future component prototypes can be designed easily and used on medical models.

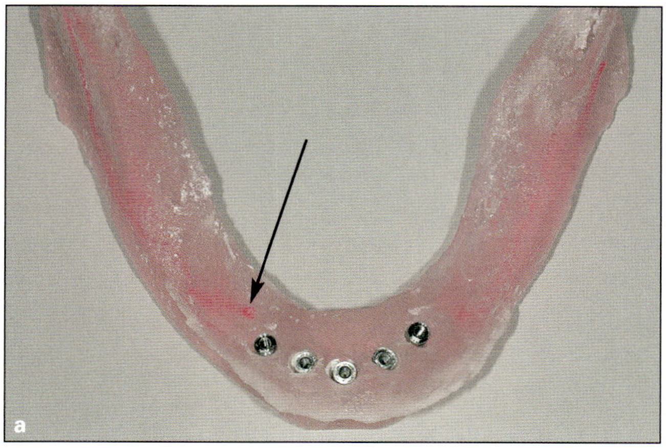

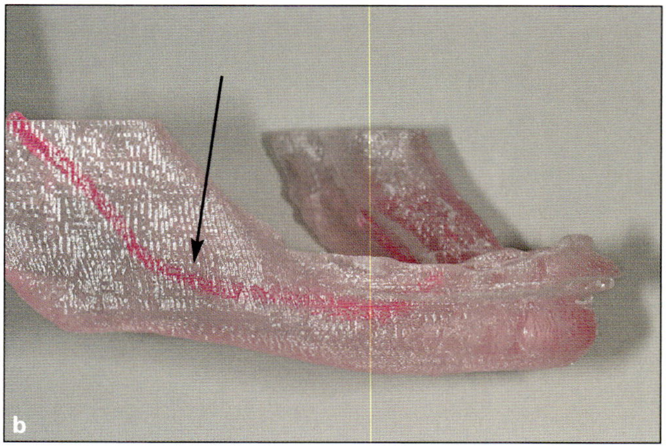

Figs 6-1a and 6-1b Stereolithographic mucosa medical model constructed with five osteotomy site preparations at planned implant positions. Laboratory analogues have been placed. Abutments are selected preoperatively for a "dress rehearsal" of proposed implant treatment. Note colorization of the inferior alveolar nerve and mental foramen *(arrows)*.

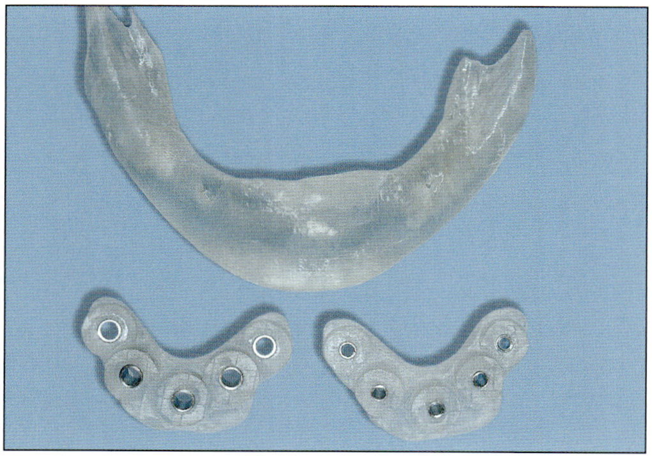

Fig 6-2 Stereolithographic bone model of the mandible with computerized extractions. Bone-supported SurgiGuides are based on the 3D implant plan. *Left*, 3.2 mm SurgiGuide; *right*, 2.2 mm SurgiGuide.

Stereolithography

Stereolithography is the most widely known and used rapid prototyping technique[7,11] and the one most often used to generate medical models and computer-generated surgical guides for osteotomy site preparation in dental implant surgery.[9,11] Accuracy and reliability are two of the distinguishing characteristics of the stereolithographic process.[12] Stereolithography can be used to generate medical models that are transparent, selectively colored according to region of visual interest, constructed in a timely manner, and cost effective[13] (Figs 6-1a and 6-1b). Anatomic skull replicas derived from 3D CT imaging using the rapid prototyping technique of stereolithography have been shown to have submillimeter dimensional accuracy.[3,14–16]

SurgiGuides

SurgiGuides (Materialise) are the computer-designed and stereolithography-generated surgical guides used during osteotomy site preparation (Fig 6-2). Stereolithography interfaces a patient's 3D CT study with the SimPlant plan. Made of acrylic resin, SurgiGuides contain one or more steel drilling sleeves, each of a defined diameter and with minimal tolerance, to control and ensure the accuracy of each osteotomy site preparation in two planes—buccolingually and mesiodistally.

SurgiGuide design is based on the presurgical 3D positioning of implant icons using SimPlant (Materialise) interactive software, which transfers the prosthetically driven

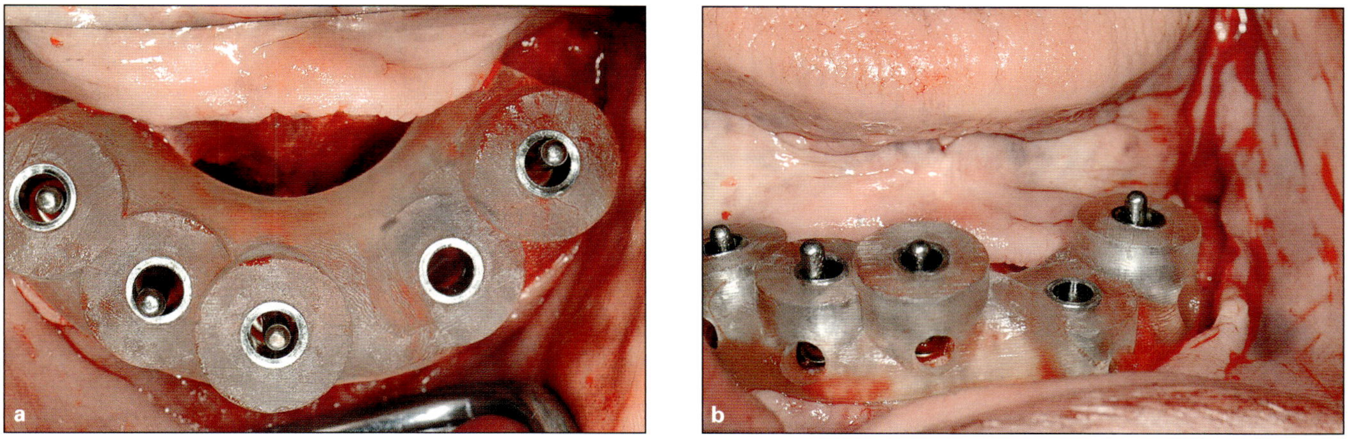

Figs 6-3a and 6-3b Bone-supported SurgiGuide on the patient's mandible with four guide pins in planned osteotomy sites.

surgical treatment plan onto the CT. SurgiGuides can be supported by bone, teeth, teeth and mucosa, mucosa, or supragingival pre-existing dental implant components and mucosa.

Each SurgiGuide features a defined number of steel tubes corresponding to the number of desired osteotomy preparations and the specific drill diameters. The 3D axial position of each drilling tube is based on the implant position determined during the software treatment planning process. The diameter of each steel tube depends on the diameter of the twist drill used for osteotomy site preparation. Typically, the diameter of the drilling tube is 0.2 mm greater than that of the twist drill. The drilling tubes are selected based on the manufacturer's twist drill specifications (which is indicated at the time of SurgiGuide ordering). Each drill diameter requires fabrication of a separate SurgiGuide, which is checked for accuracy on the stereolithographic model and through surgical dress rehearsals, if necessary. The stability of the guide is directly proportional to the surface area upon which it is seated.

Implant Site Preparations Requiring Bone Exposure

Bone-supported SurgiGuides

Bone-supported SurgiGuides are designed to conform precisely to the patient's full or partially edentulous jawbone to facilitate planned osteotomy site preparation (Figs 6-3a and 6-3b). Advantages of using bone-supported SurgiGuides include preoperative delivery of a 3D medical model of the patient's jawbone, the ability to visualize the surgical field, a stable fit, and improved space availability for drill use (compared to mucosa-supported SurgiGuides). A disadvantage is the need for bone exposure, and therefore this surgical guide option is most advantageous when an open flap technique is required to accomplish the planned surgical outcome (eg, bone recontouring to establish proper ridge morphology for implant placement, the need for bone harvesting and/or bone grafting in conjunction with implant surgery, etc). An open flap technique might also be necessary when accessing adjacent teeth to treat periodontal defects by guided tissue regeneration, providing functional crown lengthening, assisting in surgical management of the biologic width around the natural dentition, or managing peri-implant mucogingival tissues that cannot be adequately managed by a closed approach.

The use of bone-supported SurgiGuides requires at least 30 mm of supporting mesiodistal bone surface. Since each SurgiGuide obtains stability by surface area contact with bone, the surgical field must be sufficiently broad to allow access for guide insertion as well as stability. In general, the more surface area contact with bone, the less potential for guide dislocation during osteotomy preparation.

Bone fixation pins can be used to help stabilize each SurgiGuide when surface area is limited. Since multiple guides are used during osteotomy site preparation, the diameter and position of the pins should be varied with successive SurgiGuides to avoid instability caused by bone elasticity. Incorporating fixation pins is most ideal when the SAFE System guide is used (Figs 6-4a and 6-4b). Since the SAFE System requires only one SurgiGuide to be used during osteotomy site preparation, the added stability pro-

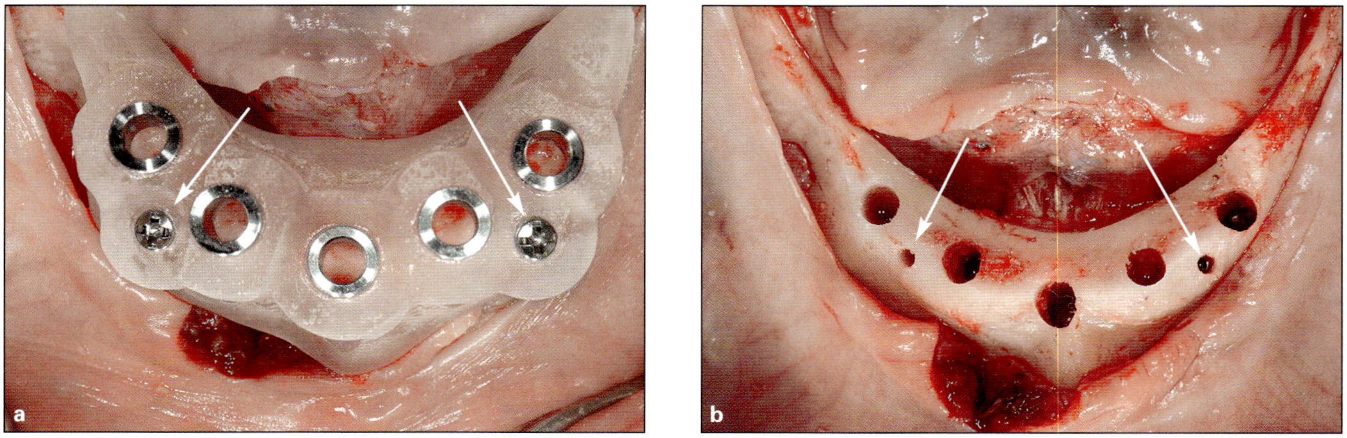

Figs 6-4a and 6-4b *(a)* Bone-supported SAFE SurgiGuides with two fixation pins to further stabilize the guide on the patient's mandible. *(b)* Following osteotomy site preparation, the guide and fixation pins are removed to examine the prepared sites and pin positions *(arrows)*.

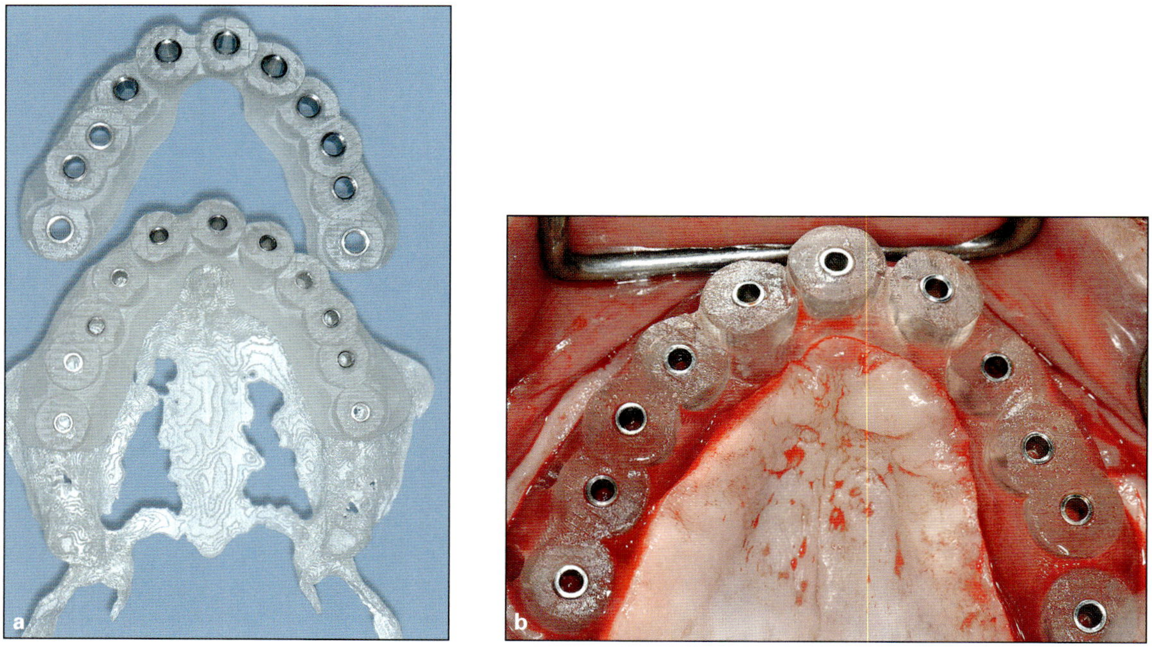

Figs 6-5a and 6-5b Bone-supported SurgiGuides based on the 3D implant plan. *(a)* 3.2-mm SurgiGuide *(top)* and 2.2-mm SurgiGuide upon the stereolithographic bone model *(bottom)*. *(b)* Bone-supported SurgiGuide (2.2 mm) on the patient's maxilla for the preparation of 11 osteotomy sites.

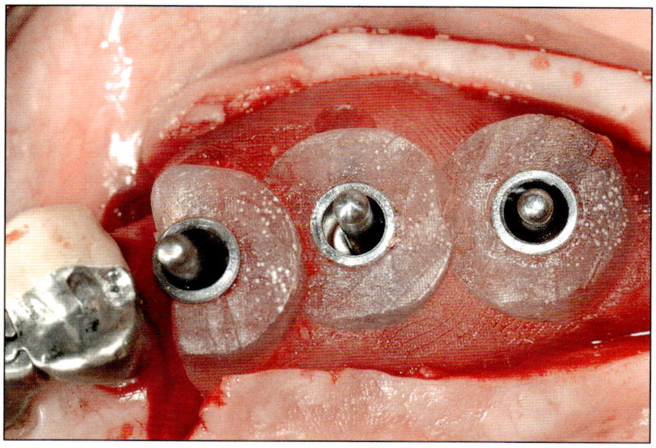

Fig 6-6 Bone-supported SurgiGuide (3.2 mm) on the patient's partially edentulous maxillary posterior bone for the preparation of three osteotomy sites. Guide pins demonstrate osteotomy site orientation and angulation.

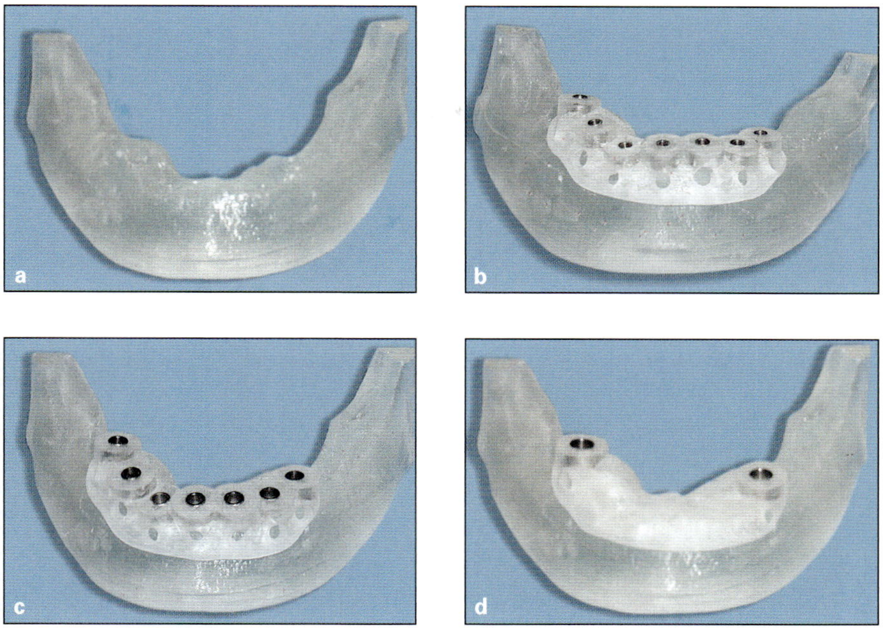

Figs 6-7a to 6-7d *(a)* Stereolithographic bone model of the mandible. *(b–d)* Successive bone-supported SurgiGuides based on the 3D implant plan.

vided by fixation pins is maximized. Bone-supported SurgiGuides are ideal for use in fully edentulous case types (Figs 6-5a and 6-5b). They can also be used in the partially edentulous patient (Fig 6-6), often with design modifications to compensate for the insufficient amount of surface area available for guide support.

Once the surgical field is defined and exposed, the guide is placed on the patient's jawbone to assess its stability. It is imperative to ensure adequate flap reflection for guide insertion and to completely eliminate all residual tissue tags that may adhere to the underlying bony cortex and extraction deformities. Because SurgiGuides consist of several successive drill diameter osteotomy site preparation guides (Figs 6-7a to 6-7d), it is important to make sure that all guides demonstrate proper fit. A tactile assessment for proper positioning of each guide will help ensure correct guide alignment for successive osteotomy preparations when increasing the diameter at each osteotomy position.

For situations in which the bone crest must be reduced prior to osteotomy site preparation, a computer-generated bone reduction guide can be fabricated to direct the surgeon in reducing a specific amount of undesirable bone. Bone reduction is generally needed to create a bone crest that is wide enough to initiate osteotomy site preparation and position implant platforms of a relative uniform vertical dimension. Bone reduction guides allow a precise amount of osteoplasty to be performed that would otherwise preclude the full depth of the planned osteotomy sites from being created with a SurgiGuide. Thin crestal bone and tooth extraction cases are two examples of situations where a bone reduction guide may be useful (Figs 6-8a to 6-8d).

Within each SurgiGuide is a drilling cylinder with a diameter slightly larger than that of the twist drill to be used for preparation of that particular osteotomy site. A typical osteotomy site preparation for a standard-sized implant (4.0-mm diameter), for example, would require a 2.0 mm twist drill using a SurgiGuide with a 2.2 mm drilling tube diameter followed by a 3.0 mm twist drill using a SurgiGuide with a 3.2 mm drilling tube diameter. The use of pilot drills is unnecessary with SurgiGuide-assisted osteotomy site preparation. Countersinking, if performed, is accomplished after the final diameter of the osteotomy site has been prepared and without the use of a guide.

If the bone-supported SurgiGuide closely approximates an adjacent tooth, the closest drilling tube may need to be elongated to bypass the vertical height of the tooth (Figs 6-9a and 6-9b). The extent to which the tube is elongated may prevent the surgeon from being able to create the full depth of the desired osteotomy site if the required drilling length surpasses the available drill lengths. In this case, the final depth of the osteotomy site would need to be determined with mental navigation. If the patient is partially edentulous, a tooth-supported SurgiGuide is another option to partially overcome this problem.

It is important to remember that time spent in preoperative treatment planning correlates with a reduction in surgical treatment time. Prosthetically directed surgical planning is completed on the computer. Also, because

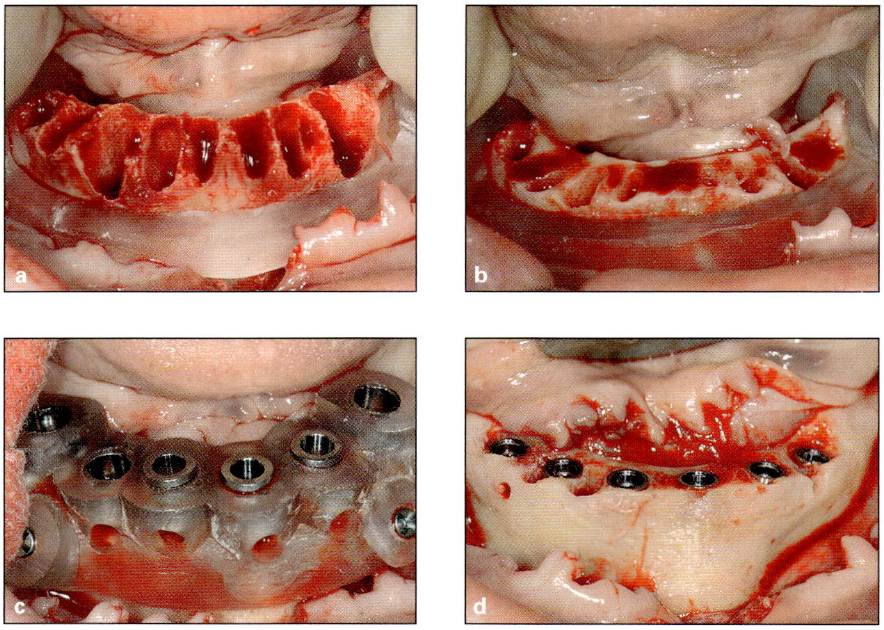

Figs 6-8a to 6-8d *(a)* Bone reduction guide in place following extraction of remaining mandibular teeth. *(b)* Osteoplasty completed using bone reduction guide. *(c)* SAFE SurgiGuide in place for osteotomy site preparation. *(d)* Final implant positioning at planned vertical positions.

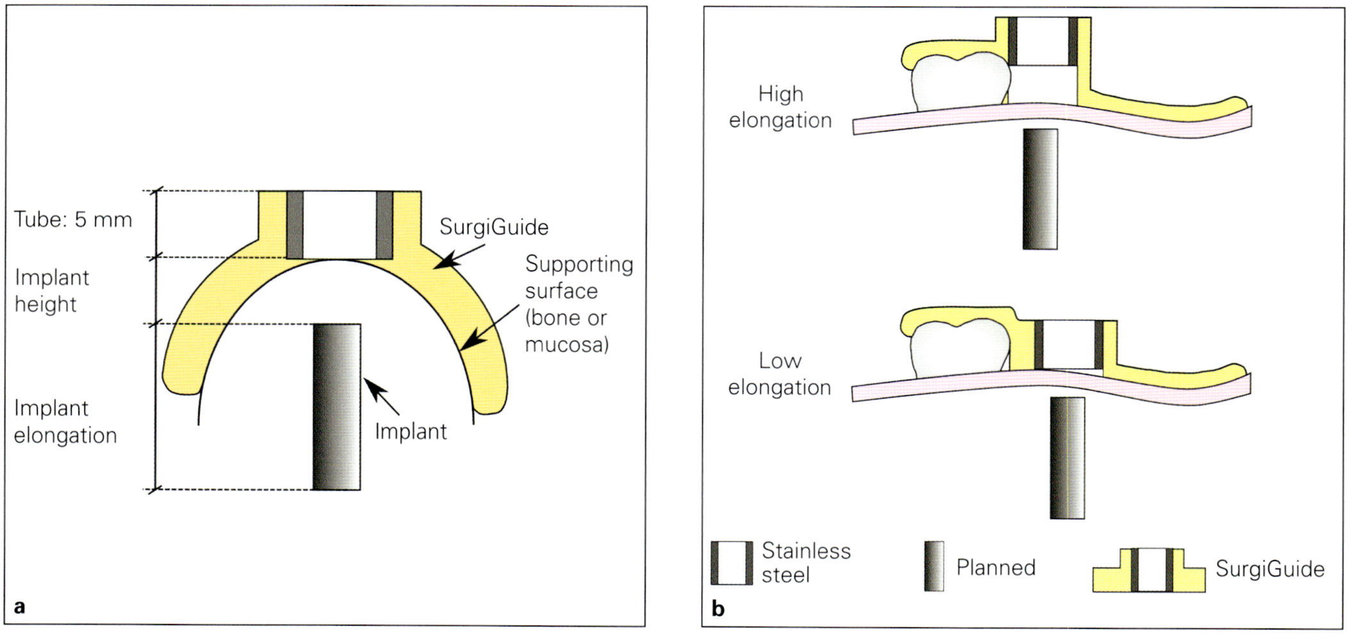

Figs 6-9a and 6-9b Drilling tube elongation. *(a)* The drilling tube is positioned above the planned implant position at the highest point of the bone crest. The drilling tube elongation represents the distance from the planned implant platform determined by the largest-diameter SurgiGuide and then used for each SurgiGuide in the case. *(b)* When an implant is positioned close to an adjacent tooth, it may not be possible to place the tube next to the tooth and instead must be positioned above the tooth. This is known as a *high tube elongation*.

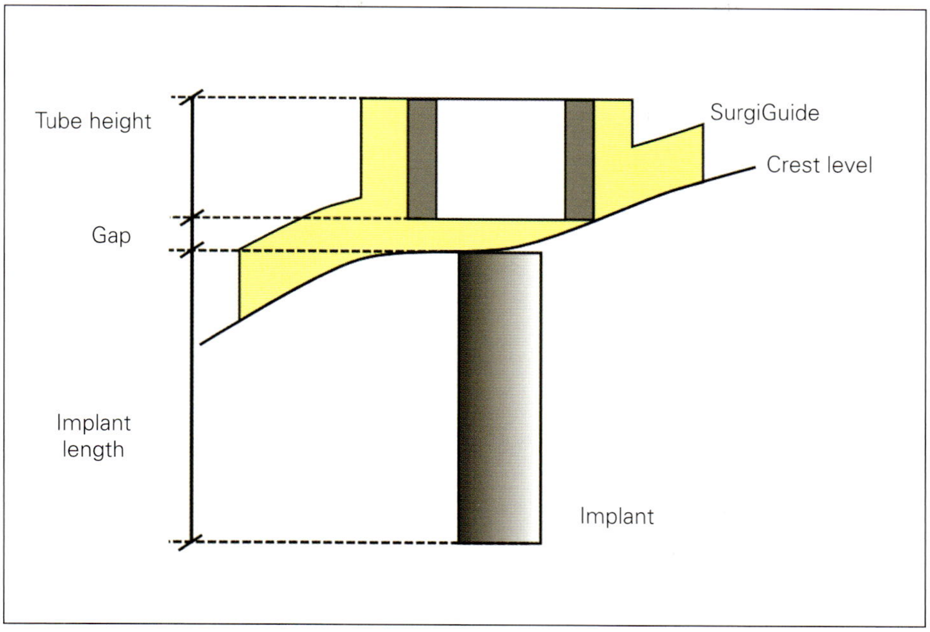

Fig 6-10 Drilling depth for SurgiGuide-assisted osteotomy site preparation. Drilling length = implant length + gap + tube height.

there is no representation of final tooth position in space with the SurgiGuides, the ability to verify precise positioning by the surgeon at the time of surgery demands a transfer of trust and confidence in the technology. This underscores the importance of accurate diagnostics and prosthetically directed implant planning by the interdisciplinary team and, in part, reinforces the concept of collaborative accountability.[5]

SurgiGuides and Depth Control

Vertical positioning is not controlled with conventional SurgiGuides. Local and regional anatomy influence the operator's vertical positioning of osteotomy sites when using conventional SurgiGuides. True vertical depth control directly by the SurgiGuide system is possible only when the SAFE system and associated drills are used. Therefore, careful intraoperative vertical measurements of the guide in conjunction with the patient's native bone availability, regional anatomy, and the planned implant length need to be made.

With regard to vertical depth, the basic rule in designing SurgiGuides is to position the drilling tube as close as possible to the supporting crest identified on the SimPlant study. The supporting crest might be the bone or mucosa, depending on the type of SurgiGuide used.

Three important points should be considered when determining tube height. First, the tube should be positioned at the most coronal position of the bone or mucosal crest that is coronal to the implant. To account for the vertical stacking height, the following formula can be used: implant length + gap + tube height = total drilling length (Fig 6-10).

Second, all drilling tubes should be vertically positioned at the height of the largest-diameter drilling tube required for the desired osteotomy site. That is, smaller-diameter SurgiGuide tubes are set at the same vertical position established for the largest-diameter SurgiGuide to avoid interference when seating the guide at the crest.

Third, proximity to natural teeth can result in excessive tube elongation. A minimum of 4 mm of space is needed from the lateral border of a natural tooth to the planned center of a conventional 4.0-mm-diameter implant. The "restorative space" feature in SimPlant can help avoid positioning errors.

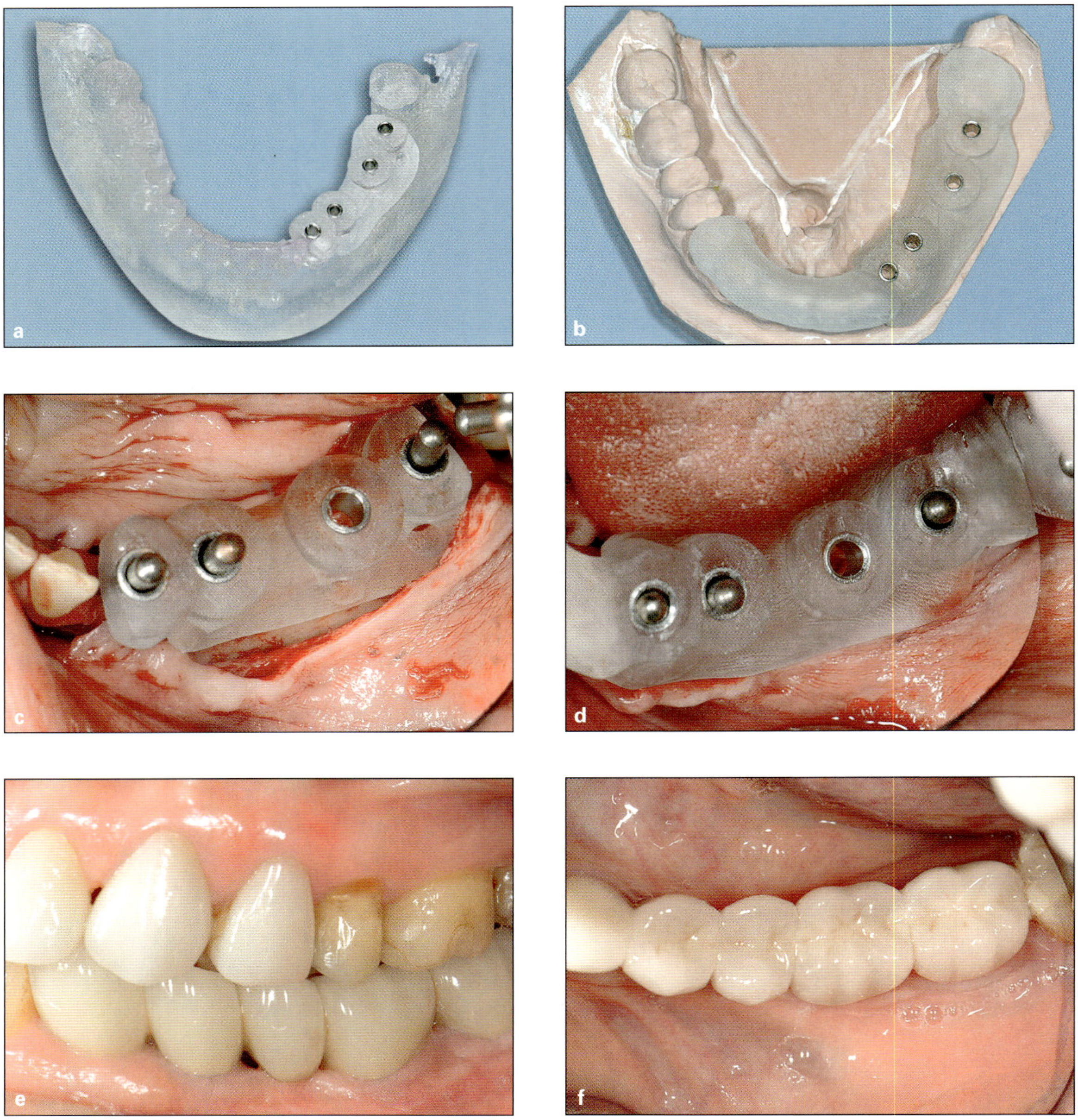

Figs 6-11a to 6-11f *(a)* Bone-supported SurgiGuide created using a stereolithographic acrylic resin bone model. *(b)* Tooth-supported SurgiGuide on optically scanned hard stone mandibular cast. *(c)* Bone-supported pins in place to identify the prepared osteotomy sites. *(d)* Tooth-supported SurgiGuide seated on the patient's mandible with the same guide pins used in the bone-supported SurgiGuide. *(e,f)* Final prosthetic outcome. (Courtesy of Dr Robert Gordon, Glenview, IL.)

Implant Site Preparation Without Bone Exposure

Tooth- or tooth and mucosa–supported surgical guides

For implant site preparation without bone exposure in partially edentulous patients, the stereolithographic surgical guide is designed to fit precisely on the dental structures. To test the clinical efficacy of implant placement without bone exposure, both bone-supported and tooth-supported surgical guides were fabricated for use in the same patient based on a SimPlant software treatment plan. A stereolithographic bone-supported model was fabricated and surgical guides were constructed according to the treatment plan. In addition, an optically scanned cast of the teeth and jaw enabled fabrication of a tooth-

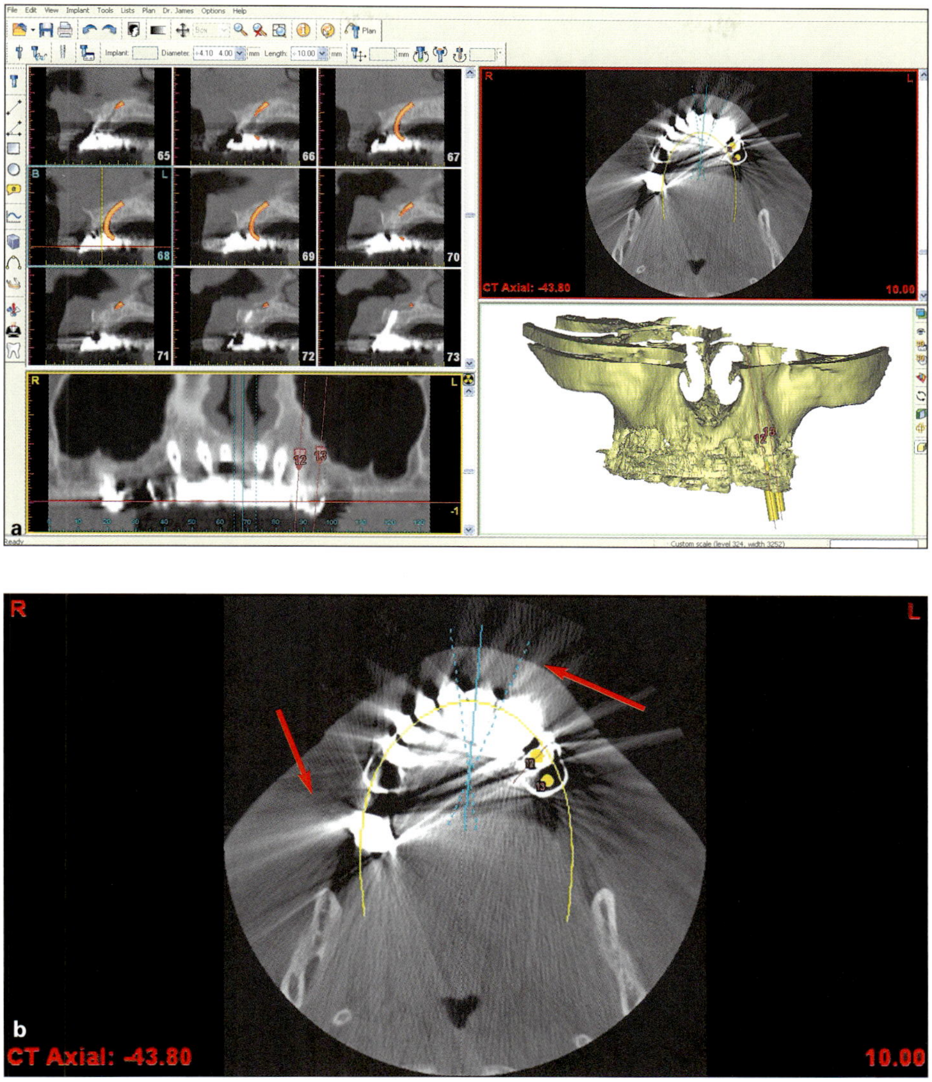

Figs 6-12a and 6-12b *(a)* SimPlant study of patient who previously had five maxillary implants placed. Additional implants are planned for the left first and second premolar sites. The panoramic view *(bottom left)* identifies the vertical positioning *(red line)* and correlates with the axial view *(top right)*. *(b)* Axial view enlarged. Note the intense amount of imaging artifact *(red arrows)* created by the patient's metal-ceramic prostheses and interfering with attempts to triangulate a reproducible image plane.

supported surgical guide. The osteotomy preparations were completed using the bone exposure approach. With guide pins in position, the tooth-supported guide was effortlessly inserted (Figs 6-11a to 6-11f).

Although the treatment-planning process closely follows that of the bone-supported guide, several important points must be made. First, imaging artifact caused by any metal prostheses worn by the patient may interfere in the triangulation of a reproducible image plane. Without the ability to reproduce a consistent image plane, it would be impossible to build a stable tooth-supported SurgiGuide (Figs 6-12a and 6-12b). Should this occur, a bone-supported guide remains an option. Second, a quality impression and hard stone cast of the scanned arch is needed. An optical scan of the hard stone cast is registered to the CT image to create alignment between the computer-generated treatment plan and the tooth-supported guide (Figs 6-13a to 6-13c)

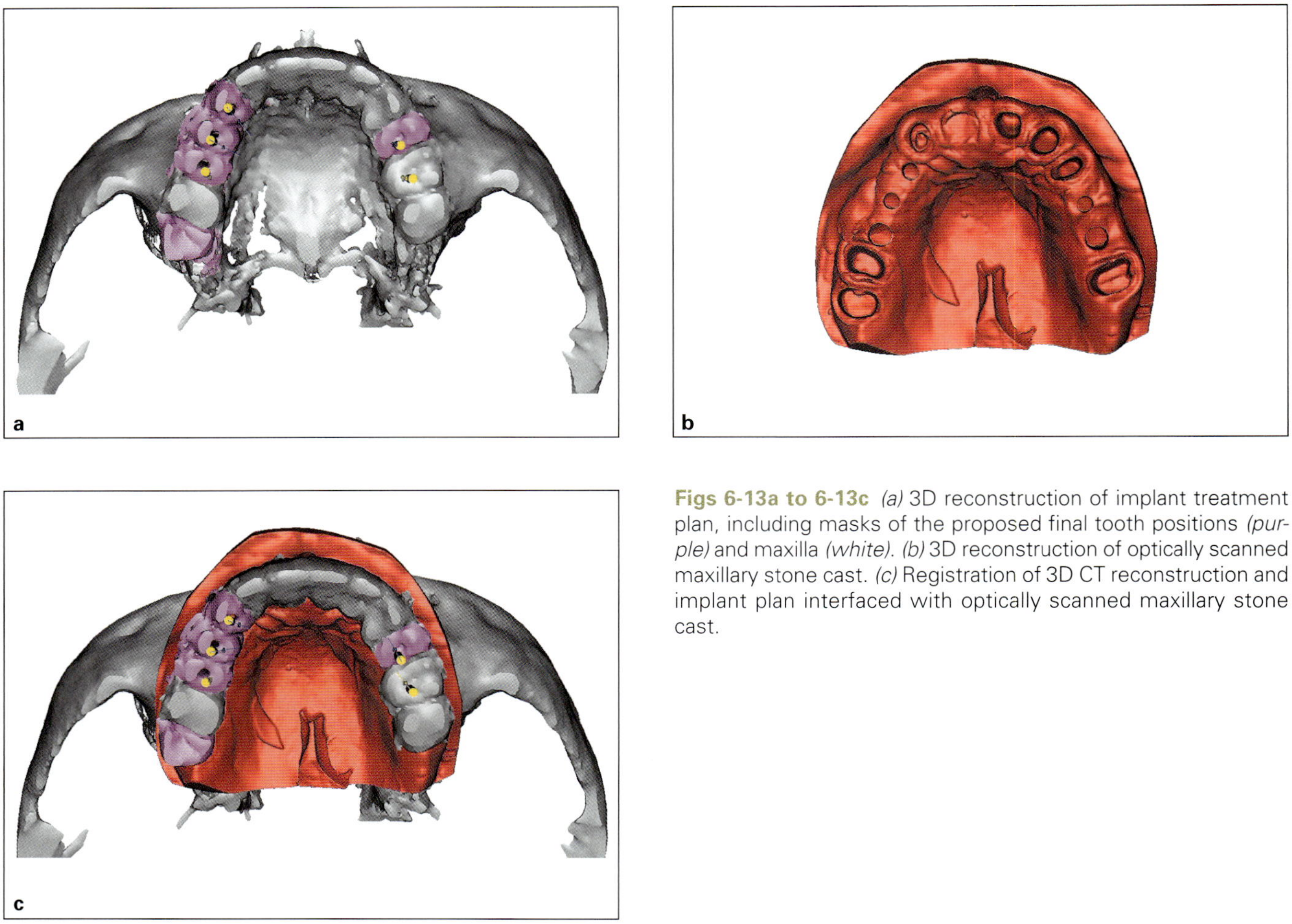

Figs 6-13a to 6-13c *(a)* 3D reconstruction of implant treatment plan, including masks of the proposed final tooth positions *(purple)* and maxilla *(white)*. *(b)* 3D reconstruction of optically scanned maxillary stone cast. *(c)* Registration of 3D CT reconstruction and implant plan interfaced with optically scanned maxillary stone cast.

For patients in orthodontic therapy, tooth movement must cease from the time the CT scan is taken until SurgiGuide-assisted implant surgery is completed to ensure a stable fit of the guide and the precision of the planned osteotomy preparation. To eliminate the effect of any artifact caused by the orthodontic hardware, brackets and archwires should be removed for the CT study and SurgiGuide use during implant surgery. However, many adult patients are provisionalized during orthodontic therapy or have minimal artifact-producing metal-ceramic prostheses (crowns/bridges); therefore, the risk vs benefit of removing the orthodontic appliances must be judged independently in each case. In the authors' experience, artifact created by orthodontic hardware has not been a limitation. Because the vertical height of any artifact-producing orthodontic hardware is relatively small compared to the total number of axial images that comprise a CT study in either jaw, the quality of the images is not significantly degraded (Figs 6-14a to 6-14c). In general, orthodontic appliances do not degrade the interpretive quality of the CT.

It is often more difficult to capture a quality impression and fabricate a useful diagnostic model during orthodontic therapy, but these steps are critical if a stable guide is to be fabricated. If orthodontic appliances are maintained during the CT study and diagnostic model acquisition, the brackets and archwire can be masked in the CT study (Fig 6-15). A tooth-supported SurgiGuide is created using combination palatal mucosal tissues and the incisive third of the maxillary dentition as well as any other positive retention–bearing surfaces available (Figs 6-16a and 6-16b). In such cases, using the SAFE SurgiGuide system may hold certain advantages resulting from the use of only one guide, which can be fixated to enhance stability. However, as with any tooth-supported SAFE case, required tube elongation may exceed the available drill length.

Use of the tooth-supported guide is similar to that of the bone-supported guide. This design is often chosen to reduce the size of the surgical field, which minimizes or eliminates the need for bone exposure (Figs 6-17a to 6-17g), and allows for enhanced guide stability if the edentulous space is small. Obviously, the more surface area

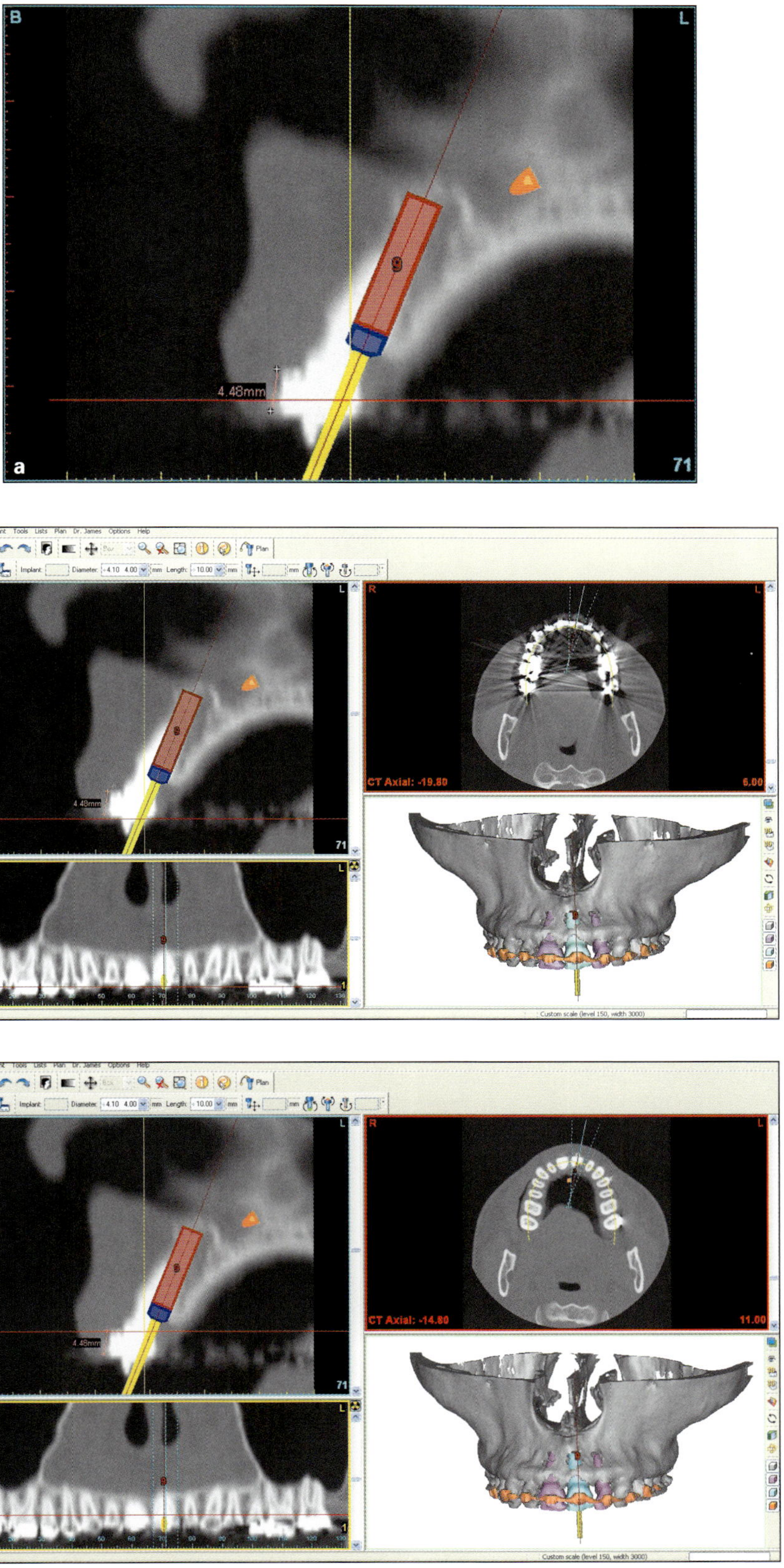

Figs 6-14a to 6-14c *(a)* Cross-sectional view of the planned implant position. Note the vertical measurement (4.48 mm) of the orthodontic bracket *(red circle)*. *(b)* SimPlant plan at incisal edge of bracket. Note corresponding axial view demonstrating imaging artifact. *(c)* Same SimPlant plan at the apical extent of the orthodontic bracket. Note the reduction of imaging artifact produced in the axial view.

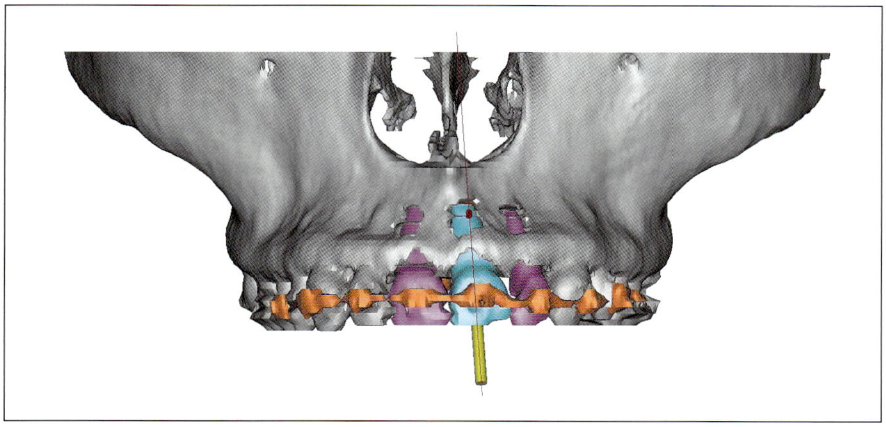

Fig 6-15 3D reconstruction of the maxilla in an orthodontic patient. The left central incisor is planned for an immediate implant. Masks of the maxilla, the natural central incisors and left lateral incisor, and the orthodontic hardware are visible.

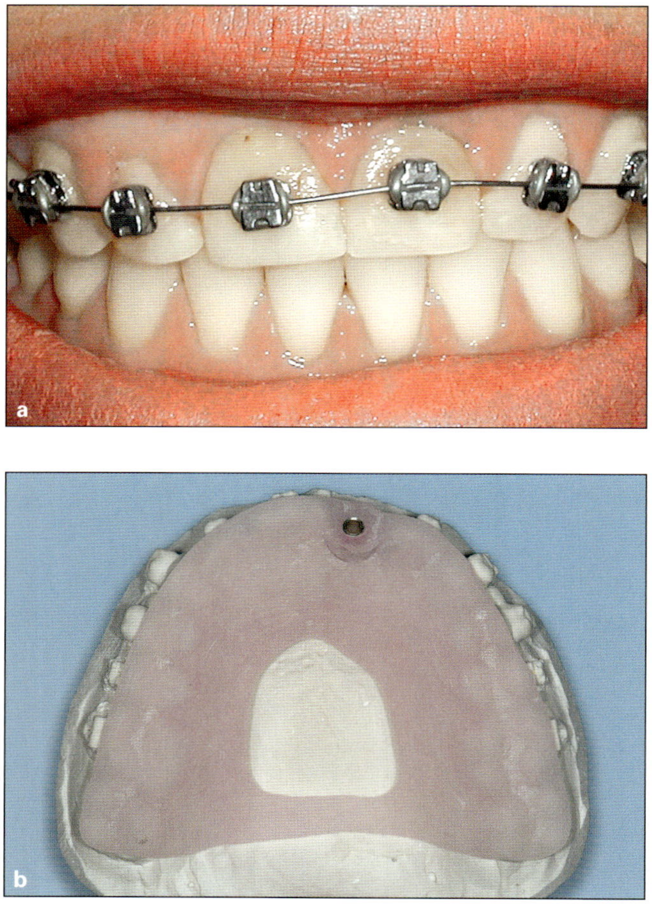

Figs 6-16a and 6-16b *(a)* Clinical view of an orthodontic patient with an ankylosed left central incisor. An immediate implant is planned. *(b)* Tooth-supported SurgiGuide seated on optically scanned hard stone cast of the maxilla to facilitate osteotomy site preparation.

that is used for the tooth-/tooth and mucosa–supported SurgiGuide, the more enhanced the stability. As with any SurgiGuide design that is not fixated, it is beneficial that the surgeon stabilize the guide by hand during utilization to resist any lateral moments on the guide, which could destabilize it during osteotomy preparation. If a non–bone exposure approach is taken in the partially edentulous patient, peri-implant mucogingival considerations and associated management can be addressed preoperatively.

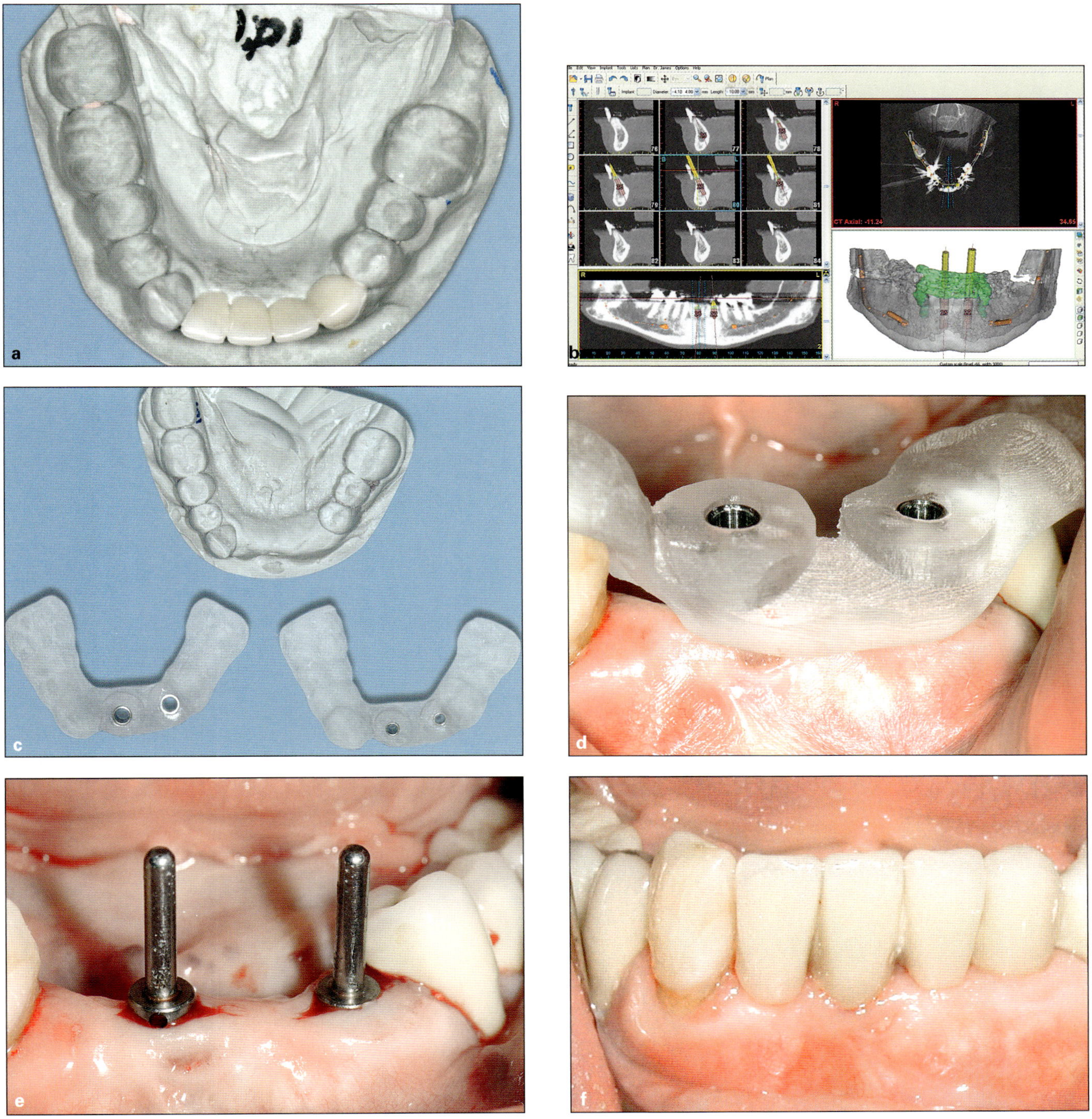

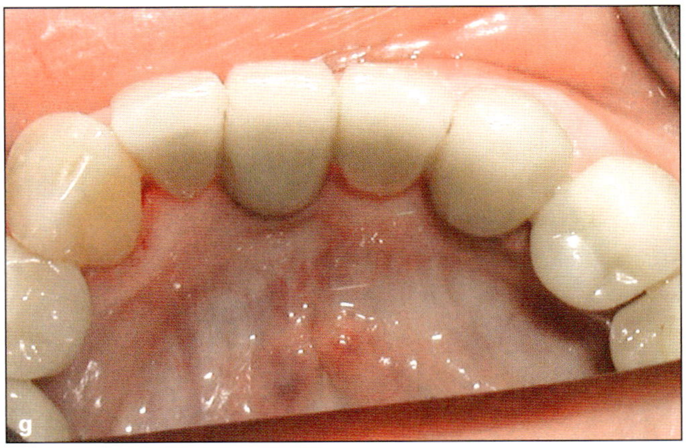

Figs 6-17a to 6-17g Implant treatment planning for medically compromised patient. *(a)* Diagnostic waxup. *(b)* SimPlant plan. *(c)* Tooth-supported SurgiGuides (*left*, 3.2 mm; *right*, 2.2 mm) fabricated from optically scanned hard stone cast of the mandible. *(d)* 2.2-mm SurgiGuide seated on the mandible for minimally invasive osteotomy site preparation. *(e)* 3-mm level osteotomy site preparation with guide pins in position. *(f,g)* Final prosthetic outcome. (Courtesy Dr Kevin Krug, Lombard, IL.)

Mucosa-supported SurgiGuides

Mucosa-supported surgical guides are designed to intimately fit over the soft tissue surface of the completely edentulous patient. Similar to bone-supported SurgiGuides, these surgical guides are of successive diameter for the preparation of osteotomy sites. In completely edentulous cases, the patient's soft tissue surface can be identified by the use of a third-generation scanning appliance known as the ScannoGuide (Figs 6-18a to 6-18c).

ScannoGuide and masks

The ScannoGuide is a unique scanning appliance composed of varying concentrations of barium in the denture base and teeth—typically, 10% and 30% by weight, respectively. The optimal final tooth position represented in the ScannoGuide is determined by the prosthetic outcome requirements. The ScannoGuide, thus representing the final prosthetic outcome relative to tooth position and oromuscular support, becomes the basis for prosthetically directed surgical treatment planning.

The ScannoGuide appliance allows for segmentation of the different structural densities that can be distinguished on the CT study, and segmentation of differing radiodensities is the basis for developing visual masks. Examples of masks would be natural tooth crowns, roots of natural teeth, existing dental implants, denture teeth, and the denture base of the scanning appliance. These masks can be toggled on and off in the effort to evaluate the impact of various structures in 3D using the SimPlant interactive software. Masks are created using SimPlant Master or Pro software and are based on the defining of objects by their varying densities. This means that each segment or structure of interest can be visualized independently and interactively.

The majority of mucosa-supported SurgiGuides are used in the fully edentulous case type. For treatment planning in these cases especially, masks allow for the appreciation of a patient's underlying bony skeletal relationship and the impact of postextraction resorption patterns against the final tooth or final prosthesis position in space. Skeletal jaw relationships can be understood more clearly with this technology and their associated impact on prosthesis design identified before intervention (Figs 6-19a to 6-19h).

A mucosa medical model of the patient's jaw can be created by the stereolithographic rapid prototyping process, and a mucosa-supported surgical guide can be fabricated (Fig 6-20). To ensure accuracy, it is imperative that the ScannoGuide is fully seated with minimal compression during the CT scanning process. Bilateral placement of cotton rolls is the simplest method to secure the guide and open the vertical dimension necessary to avoid interarch jaw superimposition. Another option is to use a radiolucent occlusal registration material. Failure to ensure complete seating of the ScannoGuide will result in the formation of air pockets between the soft tissue and the denture base. This disruption in turn interferes with the accuracy of the stereolithographic mucosa medical model and mucosa-supported surgical guide. Conversely, if the ScannoGuide is seated too firmly during CT imaging, excessive tissue compression can occur, reflecting an inaccurate resting dimensional status of the mucosa and negatively affecting the fit of the SurgiGuide.

For locating the precise center of each tooth, a 1- to 2-mm-diameter hole is placed in the cingulum and central fossa of each tooth. This hole appears as a negative (black) image on the CT scan and enables axial alignment of implants for each tooth. The negative image targets should ideally define the desired emergence position of the implant(s) in relation to the final prosthesis design. In the case of a fixed restoration, this may be the central fossa of the prosthetic tooth. In the design of a removable prosthesis, the desired emergence may be more lingual. It is critically important for all members of the team (surgeon, restorative dentist, and laboratory technician) to perform a balanced and objective review of the diagnostic workup, scanning appliance, and CT study/plan prior to medical model and SurgiGuide construction. The 3D implant plan and its associated spatial positioning of implants defines the surgical performance standards required for the plan's success.

During surgery, it is helpful to manually immobilize the mucosa-supported guide to resist any lateral moments that could destabilize it during osteotomy site preparation. Attaching fixation screws to the underlying bone is another method of stabilizing the guide. However, because mucosa-supported SurgiGuides consist of successive surgical guides, the same fixation screw–stability issues described in the section on bone-supported SurgGuides also apply here.

The major advantage of the mucosa-supported SurgiGuide is the flapless nature of the surgical procedure. As noted earlier, the mucosa-supported SurgiGuide option is used most often in the completely edentulous patient. Eliminating flap reflection allows for the periosteum to be maintained, improving the available blood supply during initial wound healing. Other advantages of a flapless approach to implant surgery are less pain, swelling, and postoperative discomfort; shorter and less invasive surgery; a simpler operative procedure; elimination of the

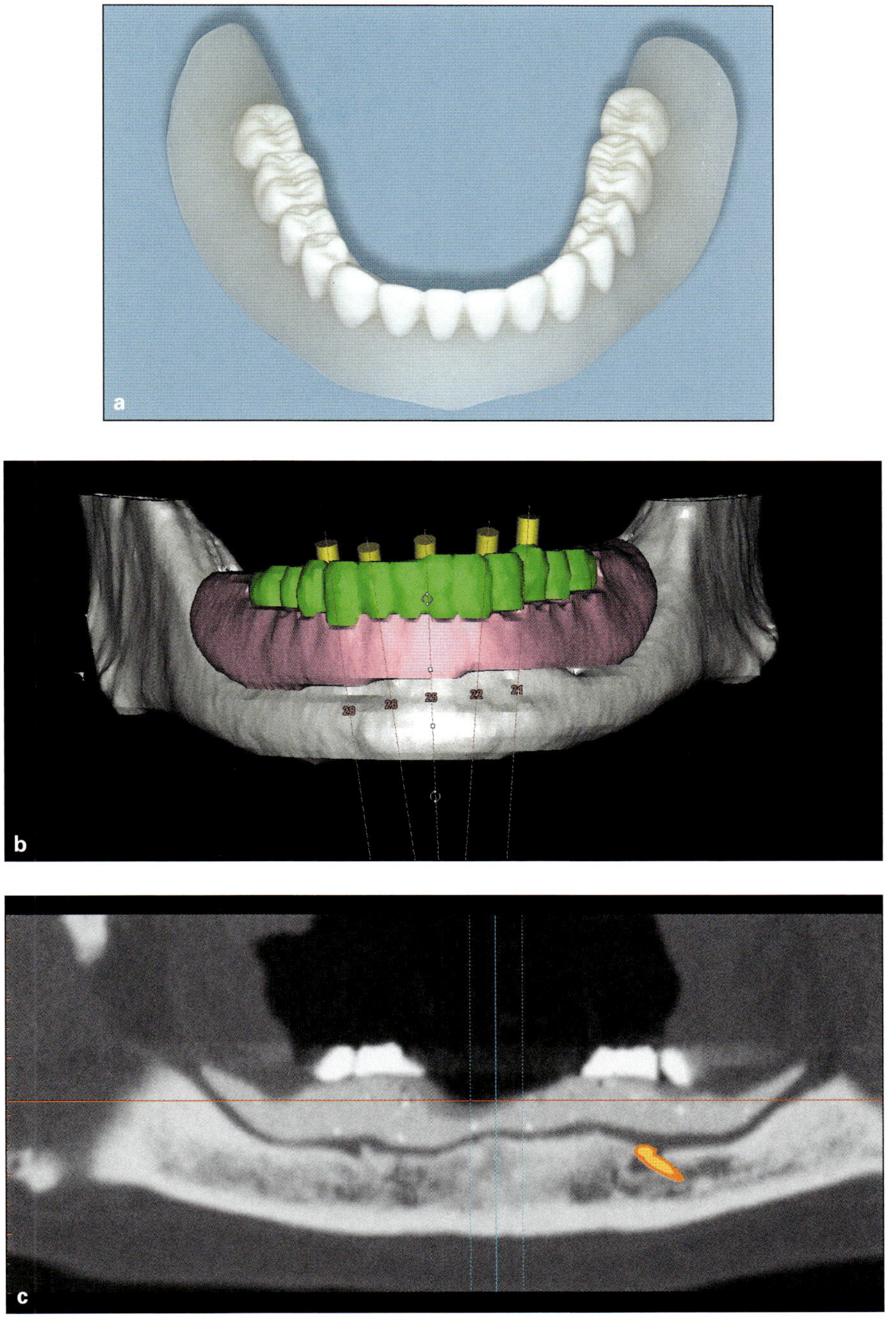

Figs 6-18a to 6-18c *(a)* Barium differential gradient ScannoGuide. *(b)* 3D CT reconstruction of patient with complete edentulism of the mandible, imaged with a ScannoGuide. Masks of the mandible, inferior alveolar nerves, denture base, denture teeth, and proposed implants are visible. *(c)* Panoramic view of SimPlant analysis of patient's mandibular CT scan. The ScannoGuide is in place, demonstrating the differential barium concentration gradient in the denture base and mandible, suggesting accurate adaptation of the ScannoGuide to the mucosa.

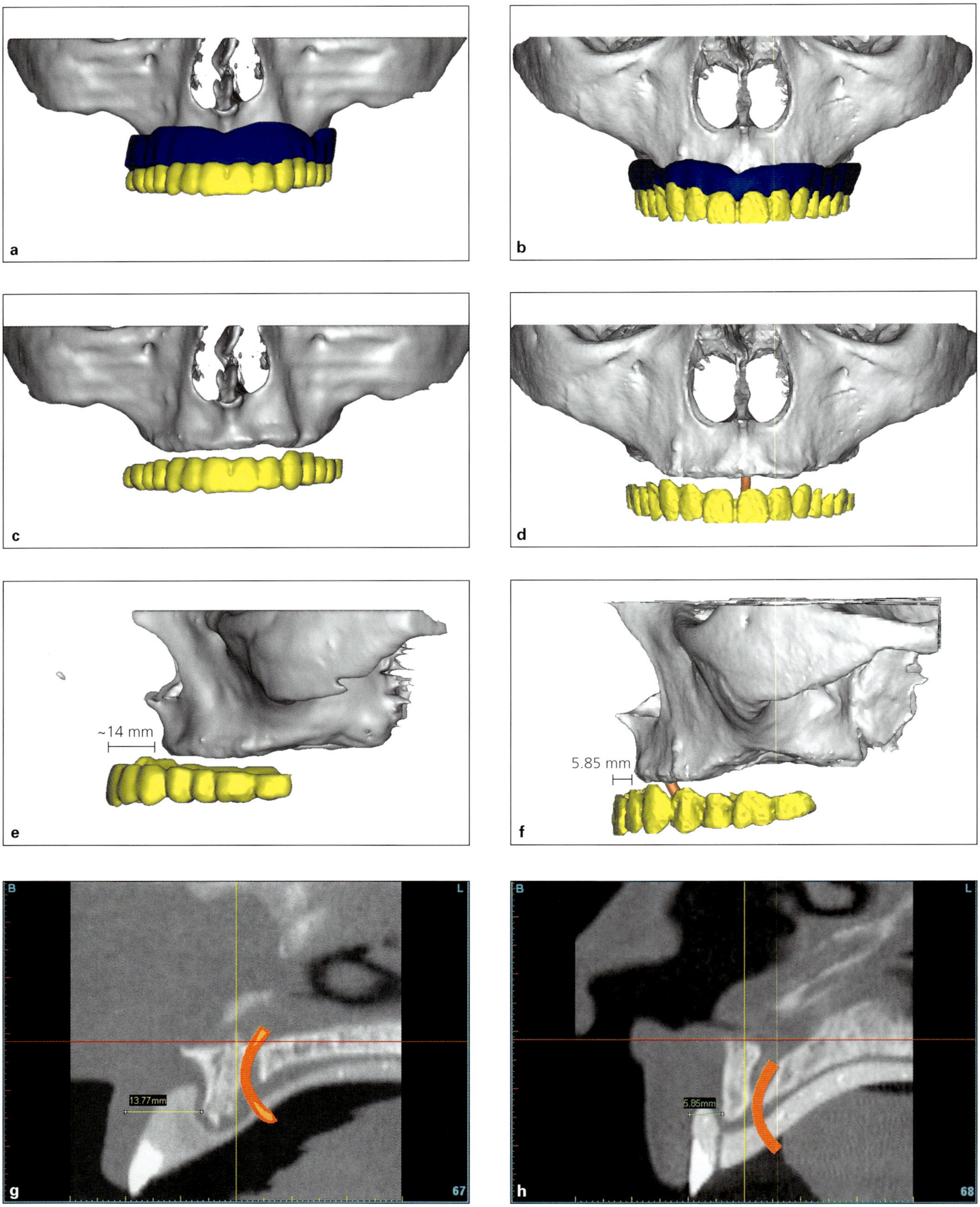

Figs 6-19a to 6-19h *(a,b)* Images of two patients with maxillary complete edentulism taken with a ScannoGuide. For each patient, masks of the maxilla, denture base, and teeth are visible. *(c–f)* Skeletal relationship of the patients compared to optimal tooth position for an implant prosthesis. *(g,h)* Cross-sectional images at the maxillary midline demonstrating significantly different cantilever effect of desired prosthesis between the two patients as a result of skeletal differences (approximately 14 mm versus 5.85 mm).

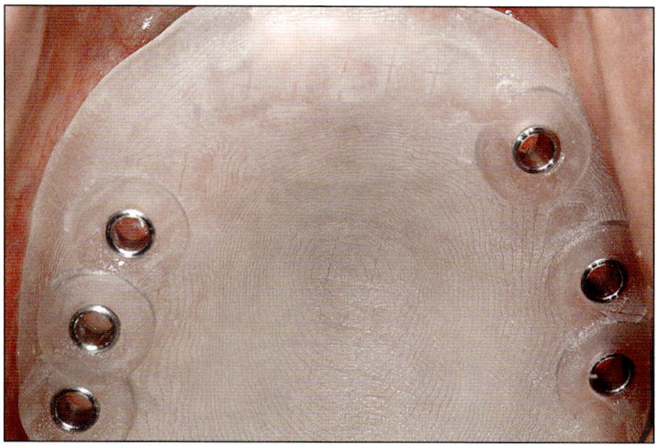

Fig 6-20 Patient with maxillary complete edentulism. Entirely mucosa-supported SurgiGuide seated on patient's edentulous maxilla.

need for sutures; faster healing times; and the possibility of a more esthetic outcome. In cases where a flapless and staged approach to implant placement have been planned, the same SurgiGuide can often be used at stage 2 surgery (uncovering procedure) to identify the positioning of the submerged implants and uncover them via a minimally invasive technique.

Disadvantages of the mucosa-supported SurgiGuide approach to surgery are the inability to view crestal and lateral bone positions during implant placement and the inability to manage mucogingival considerations at the time of implant surgery.

Specialized SurgiGuide Design Options

In certain clinical situations, specialized guides can be used. For example, a SurgiGuide can be designed to fit on existing natural tooth/teeth and supragingival implant components (such as a healing abutment) for a patient who has previously undergone implant therapy. Another option for a patient who has previously had implant therapy but has no natural dentition remaining would be a SurgiGuide designed to be supported by the existing supragingival implant components and the patient's mucosa. If stability is a concern, the use of fixation screws should be given consideration. To allow such a SurgiGuide to be constructed, an accurate cast would be optically scanned, and the process of guide construction would be similar to that of tooth-supported SurgiGuides. Because significant radiographic artifact may result around an existing implant body, accurate bone-supported SurgiGuides may not be possible.

Creation of a true tooth and bone–supported SurgiGuide is not an option because of residual error inherent in matching teeth from a diagnostic cast with bone from a CT scan. Despite the extremely low level of residual error in the interfacing process between these two surfaces, guide instability and inaccuracy are unavoidable. However, in the construction of a bone-supported SurgiGuide, if the adjacent teeth are artifact free, an "attachment" to the tooth can be made. This may be of benefit when surface area contact of bone is compromised.

Tube elongation at planned osteotomy sites that proximate adjacent teeth is sometimes problematic. Careful planning to ensure the lateral positioning of implants to natural teeth is paramount to maintain proper interproximal bone and blood supply. The "restorative space" feature in SimPlant can assist the surgeon in avoiding this problem. As noted earlier, the more elongated the drilling tube, the greater the probability that the final osteotomy depth will need to be created by mental navigation. In the case of the SAFE System SurgiGuides, associated drills may not be long enough and could lose vertical depth control in osteotomy site preparation. In such cases, two guide designs may be needed to complete the case. For example, a SAFE SurgiGuide could be constructed for posterior implant positions where tube elongation is not an issue, and a separate conventional SurgiGuide could be created for the anterior osteotomy site position where the tube elongation is more problematic. In this scenario, the twist

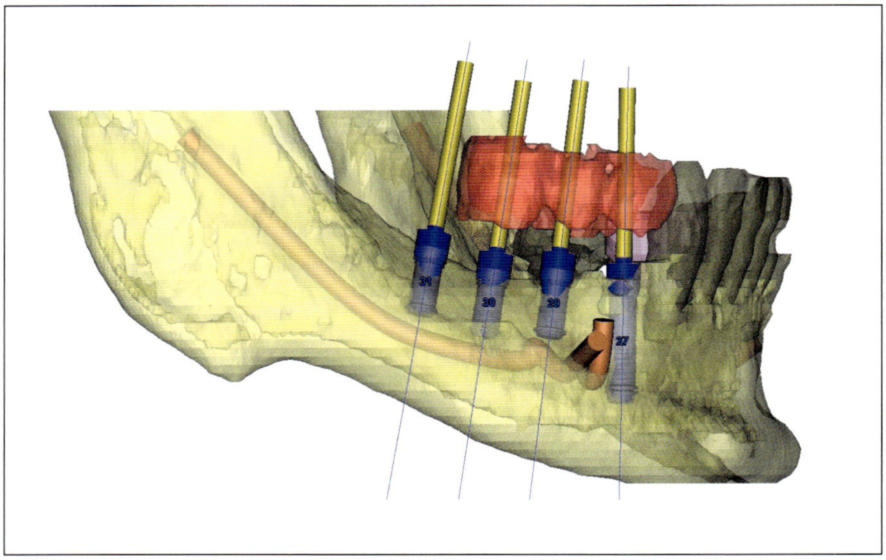

Fig 6-21 3D reconstruction and SimPlant plan for implant therapy in the posterior right mandible. Tube elongation will occur at the first premolar site due to its proximity to the canine site.

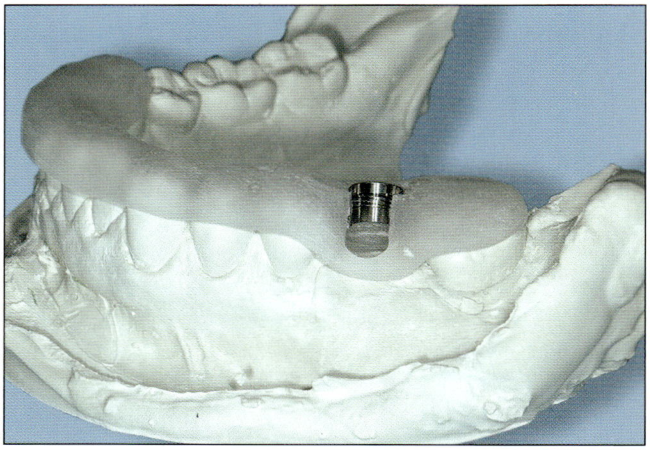

Fig 6-22 Tooth-supported SurgiGuide on optically accurate stone mandibular cast to facilitate osteotomy site preparation. A lateral entrance sleeve, to which the drilling tube and twist drill will be introduced, is created to help accommodate guided osteotomy site preparation in anatomically challenging areas.

drill length required to complete the osteotomy site will also determine guide choice (Fig 6-21).

Finally, lateral entrance sleeves (Fig 6-22) can be incorporated into guiding cylinders to allow the drilling cylinder and twist drill to be introduced more easily. This design is advantageous in areas such as the posterior mandible, where access is more challenging.

Figures 6-23a and 6-23b demonstrate pathways to facilitate SurgiGuide selection opportunities based on the clinical situation of the dental implant patient.

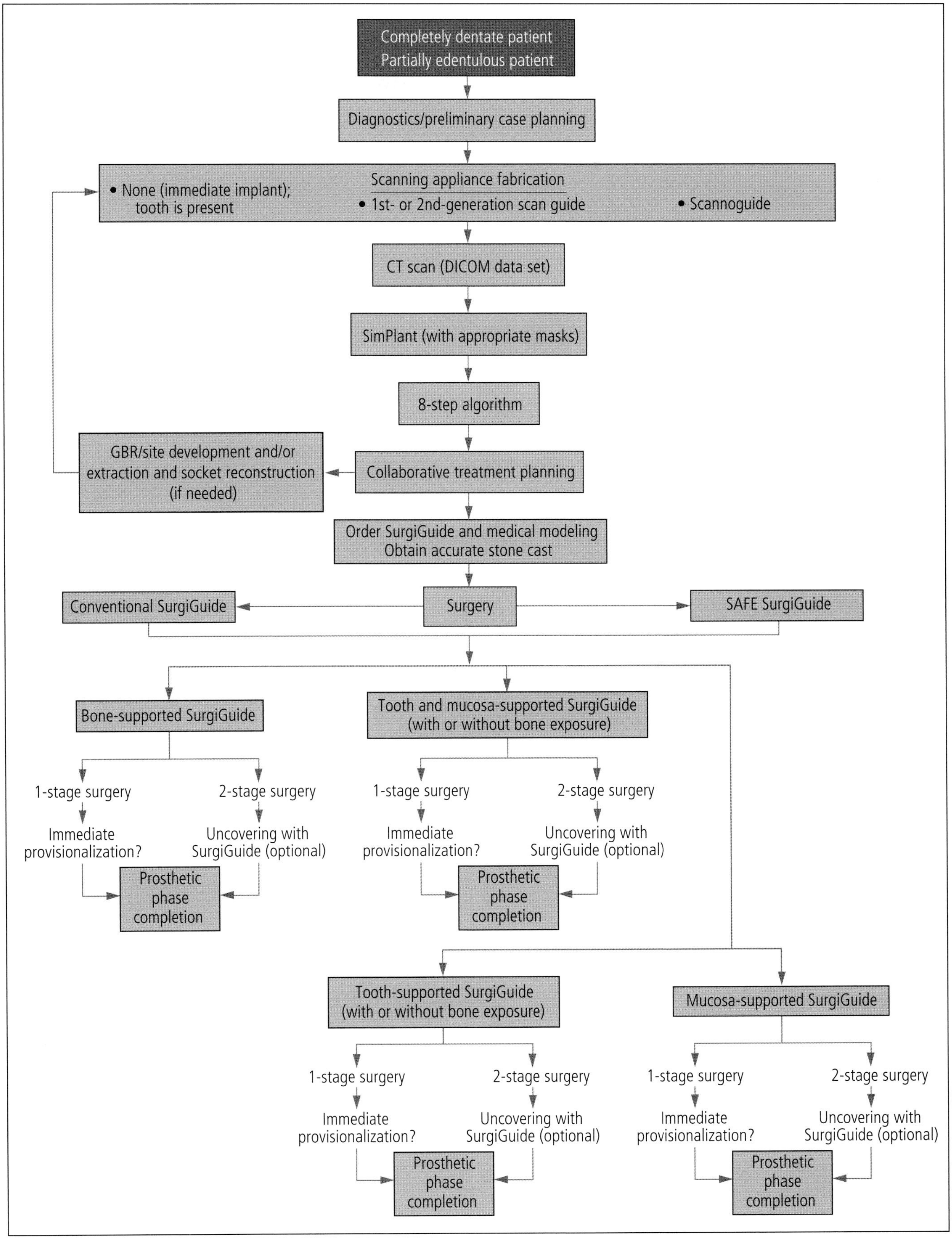

Fig 6-23a SurgiGuide application in the partially edentulous or completely dentate patient. GBR = guided bone regeneration.

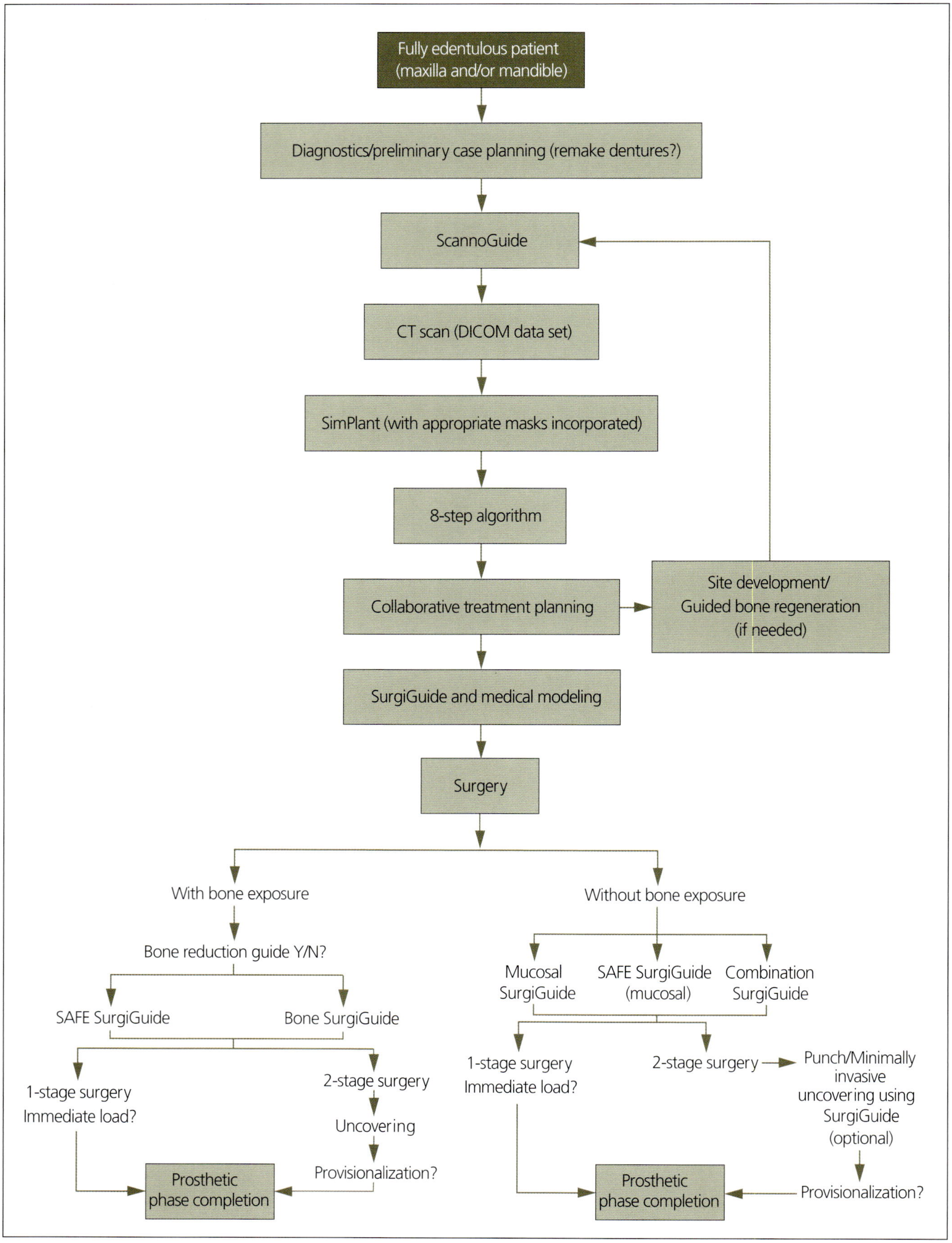

Fig 6-23b SurgiGuide application in the completely edentulous patient.

Benefits of SurgiGuide Use in Dental Implant Surgery

The most important aspect of patient care is an accurate diagnosis and treatment strategy that addresses the needs and concerns of both the patient and the implant team. The ability to incorporate the prosthetic outcome into a CT dataset represents a collaborative breakthrough between the implant surgeon and restorative dentist, allowing roles and responsibilities to be clearly defined. This is the fundamental basis for a paradigm shift in implant dentistry. The concept of collaborative accountability will become the standard of care.

For any therapeutic intervention, the possibility of an adverse outcome generally poses a greater or lesser risk according to the time of discovery. For implant therapy, this discovery can be made preoperatively, intraoperatively, or postoperatively. The time of discovery can often have far-reaching implications that may involve treatment cost, professional integrity, and loss of patient confidence. Certainly, an unanticipated treatment outcome affects doctor-patient, doctor-doctor, and doctor-technician relationships, and it ultimately impacts the dental profession as a whole. Anticipated treatment outcomes will only strengthen these relationships and enhance the confidence of the treatment population (patients) who benefits from oral implantology.

The use of surgical guides reduces the amount of time required for surgery. Patient comfort is greatly improved by a reduction in time of bone exposure. Another major advantage is a reduction in interoperator variability, the so-called talent gap. By standardizing the method of prosthetically directed osteotomy preparations, patients benefit by treatment consistency.

Perhaps the most underappreciated benefit is the ability to conduct the process of informed consent in an atmosphere of complete disclosure. Once patients begin to appreciate the time and effort spent in the preparation of their care, treatment acceptance often improves.

Use of CT scanning technology is not limited to complex cases. Every implant surgery has unique nuances that affect treatment outcome, involving factors such as bone density, regional anatomy, bone resorptive patterns, root angulation, localized pathology, guided bone regeneration requirements, and the selection of site-specific implant designs. The ability to interpret CT radiographs is proportional to familiarity and its clinical application is related to experience.

Reports have shown a reduction in laboratory cost overruns resulting from poor implant placement via traditional "mental navigation" by up to 30% when compared to computer-guided implant placement.[1]

Conclusions

1. Interactive CT technology is the only diagnostic method that allows for the incorporation of prosthetic information established by the restorative dentist to be superimposed directly onto a CT study and analyzed three-dimensionally against the patient's existing regional anatomy before surgical intervention.
2. Collaborative accountability represents a leadership breakthrough for the restorative dentist.
3. Preoperative performance standards can be established prior to treatment intervention.
4. Rapid prototype medical modeling and the science of stereolithography has application in implant dentistry. Through this process, the era of minimally invasive surgical treatment has now extended beyond medicine and into dentistry.
5. Stereolithographic medical modeling is accurate and applicable to prosthetically directed implant surgery.
6. SurgiGuides enable more precise osteotomy preparation with a reduction in surgical equipment and standardization of treatment outcomes.
7. SurgiGuides allow for the execution of a collaboratively based treatment plan.
8. The opportunity to offer patients the option of minimally invasive or flapless surgery is a desirable benefit. The ability to deliver an immediate-load prosthesis is greatly simplified with this technology.
9. The ability to conduct the process of informed consent in an atmosphere of complete disclosure is perhaps the most underappreciated benefit of this technology.

References

1. Beckers L. Positive effect of SurgiGuides on total cost. Materialise Headlines 2003;1:3.
2. Sarment D, Al-Shammari K, Kazor C. Stereolithographic surgical templates for placement of dental implants in complex cases. Int J Periodontics Restorative Dent 2003;23:287–295.
3. Sarment D, Sukovic P, Clinthorne N. Accuracy of implant placement with a stereolithographic surgical guide. Int J Oral Maxillofac Implants 2003;18:571–577.

4. Rosenfeld A, Mandelaris G, Tardieu P. Prosthetically directed implant placement using computer software to insure precise placement and predictable prosthetic outcomes. Part I. Diagnostics, imaging, and collaborative accountability. Int J Periodontics Restorative Dent 2006;26:215–221.
5. Rosenfeld A, Mandelaris G, Tardieu P. Prosthetically directed implant placement using computer software to insure precise placement and predictable prosthetic outcomes. Part II. Rapid prototype medical modeling and stereolithographic drilling guides requiring bone exposure. Int J Periodontics Restorative Dent 2006;26:347–353.
6. Rosenfeld A, Mandelaris G, Tardieu P. Prosthetically directed implant placement using computer software to insure precise placement and predictable prosthetic outcomes. Part III. Stereolithographic drilling guides that do not require bone exposure and the immediate delivery of teeth. Int J Periodontics Restorative Dent 2006;26:493–499.
7. Popat A. Rapid prototyping and medical modeling. Phidas Newsletter 1998;1:10–12.
8. Erickson D, Chance D, Schmitt S, Mathis J. An opinion survey of reported benefits from the use of stereolithographic models. J Oral Maxillofac Surg 1999;57:1040–1043.
9. Swaelens B. Drilling templates for dental implantology. Phidas Newsletter 1999;3:10–12.
10. Webb P. A review of rapid prototyping (RP) techniques in the medical and biomedical sector. J Med End Technol 2000;24:149–153.
11. Poukens J, Haex J, Verdonck H, Riediger D. Study on the accuracy of stereolithographic surgical guides in dental implantology. Phidas Newsletter 2002;8:8–14.
12. Barker T, Earwaker W, Lisle D. Accuracy of stereolithographic models of human anatomy. Australian Radiol 1994:38:106–111.
13. Wouters K. Colour Rapid Prototyping. An extra dimension for visualizing human anatomy. Phidas Newsletter 2001;6:4–7.
14. Wulf J, Vitt K, Gehl H-B, Busch L. Anatomical accuracy in medical 3D modeling. Phidas Newsletter 2001;7:1–2.
15. Vrielinck L, Politis C, Schepers S, Pauwels M, Naert I. Image based planning and clinical validation of zygoma and pterygoid implant placement in patients with severe bone atrophy using customized drill guides. Preliminary results from a prospective follow-up study. Int J Oral Maxillofac Surg 2003;32:7–14.
16. Tardieu P, Vrielinck L. Implantologie assistée par ordinateur: Le programme SimPlantSurgiCase et le SAFE System. Cas clinique: Mise en charge immédiate d'un bridge mandibulaire avec des implants transmuqueux. Implant 2003;19:15–28.

7

COMPUTER-GUIDED IMPLANT TREATMENT PATHWAY

Richard Mecall, DDS, MS

The purpose of this chapter is to provide an integrative approach to computer-guided implant planning by merging prosthetic and surgical information into a universal pathway (Fig 7-1). This conceptual framework allows the dental implant team the opportunity to achieve consistent diagnoses and treatment. While each patient may have a unique problem, an algorithmic approach allows the clinician to anticipate a sequence of treatment and to improve communication with the team members as well as the patient.

To develop an algorithmic approach to implant treatment, there must be a standardized method for evaluating diagnostic information and developing a treatment plan.

The basic treatment pathway consists of the following phases:

I. Initial diagnostics
II. Scanning appliance fabrication
III. CT scan and SimPlant conversion
IV. Eight-step treatment-planning process and patient consultation
V. Medical modeling
VI. Surgery
VII. Definitive restoration and supportive maintenance

PHASE I

Initial Diagnostics

- Clinical exam (face and mouth)
- Radiographic exam
- Determination of case type
- Patient consultation
- Resolution of any clinical and radiographic diagnostic inquiries
- Diagnostic waxup

↓

PHASE II

Scanning Appliance Fabrication

- Selection of scanning appliance
- Fabrication in laboratory
- Delivery to patient

↓

PHASE III

CT Scan and SimPlant Conversion

- CT scans with scanning appliance in place
- Conversion of digital files to SimPlant format
- Segmentation and creation of masks for relevant anatomic structures

↓

PHASE IV

Eight-Step Treatment-Planning Process

- Treatment planning using CT scans and 3D models in SimPlant
- Resolution of any physical and radiographic diagnostic inquiries
- Preoperative patient consultation
- Order placement for surgical guide

↓

PHASE V

Medical Modeling

- Surgical guide fabrication
- Construction of implant master model and provisional restoration if immediate loading is planned

↓

PHASE VI

Surgery

- Flap creation or tissue punch, as indicated
- Surgery using surgical guide
- Placement of implants and abutments
- If using immediate loading, placement of provisional restoration

↓

PHASE VII

Definitive Restoration and Supportive Maintenance

- Placement of definitive prosthesis following appropriate healing period
- Patient follow-up and maintenance of restoration

Fig 7-1 Computer-guided implant treatment pathway.

PHASE I

Initial Diagnostics

Box 7-1 Considerations in emergency and nonemergency initial assessment

Emergency
- Tooth removal/infection control
- Debridement
- Socket preservation
- Ovate pontic
- Provisional fixed or removable prosthesis

Nonemergency

Patient problems
- Periodontal disease
- Periapical pathology
- Dental caries
- Acute trauma
- Developmental abnormality
- Missing teeth

Patient concerns
- Financial
- Esthetics
- Function
- Time
- Fear

Box 7-2 Areas of clinical assessment

Face
- Facial symmetry
- Lip symmetry
- Lip movement
- Dentofacial midline
- Proclination or retroclination of teeth

Mouth
- Maxillary incisal edge position
- Mandibular incisal edge position
- Posterior occlusal plane
- Tooth proportions
- Soft tissue quantity and quality
- Biologic width
- Bone height, width, and angle

Entry into the pathway begins with an assessment of the need for emergency or nonemergency care (Box 7-1). While nonemergency treatment allows for collaborative decision making, emergency treatment requires immediate decisive action. For this reason, infection control takes precedence, but its clinical management may vary. Preservation of tissue form and volume in addition to insertion of an interim provisional restoration are essential. In nonemergency care, identification of the patient's needs and concerns is mandatory. The restorative approach is determined through the process of examination and consultation. Knowing the type of definitive restoration that will be used guides the diagnostic and treatment processes.

A standardized method for evaluating diagnostic information and developing a treatment plan requires a hierarchy of diagnostic investigation and decision making. This begins with a determination of the patient's needs, concerns, and desired restorative approach, which is achieved during initial clinical and two-dimensional (2D) radiographic exams. These exams uncover any existing problems that must be resolved before moving forward in the pathway.

Clinical and radiographic diagnostic exams

Investigating diagnostic inquiries as they arise during a patient's treatment and resolving them using appropriate methods (called *critical actions*) is part of the evaluate-and-manage approach of the pathway. For the purposes of this text, a *diagnostic inquiry* is an investigation of a patient's pathologic condition that requires reconciliation during treatment. Such investigations must be made on an ongoing basis throughout treatment. There are three basic types of diagnostic inquiries: clinical, radiographic, and physical. Physical diagnostic inquiries, as well as further radiographic inquiries, are discussed later in the text.

Clinical diagnostic inquiries

Clinical diagnostic inquiries are made to discover restorative information essential to constructing a scanning appliance and are identified using a thorough clinical examination of the face and mouth (Box 7-2). The

PHASE I

Table 7-1 Most common clinical diagnostic inquiries and associated critical actions	
Clinical diagnostic inquiries	**Critical actions**
Gingival margin asymmetry	Orthodontic eruption, root coverage, crown lengthening, soft tissue ridge augmentation, soft tissue grafting, prosthetic molding
Interdental papilla deformity	Orthodontic eruption, restoration of coronal form
Interradicular space limitations	Orthodontics, space enlargement or closure
Facial plate integrity (fistula, dehiscence, fenestration)	Bone graft (autograft, allograft, xenograft)
Skeletal malocclusion	Orthodontics, restorative dentistry
Abnormal intermaxillary relationships	Orthodontics, restorative dentistry
Occlusal plane irregularities, vertical dimension occlusal instability	Orthodontics, restorative dentistry
Crown length deficiency neighboring an implant	Osseous surgery
Physiologic or pathologic limitation upon opening	Physical therapy, short implants, lateral access surgical guides
Unstable occlusion	Occlusal analysis and treatment

most common clinical diagnostic inquiries and associated critical actions are listed in Table 7-1. Correction and resolution of all clinical inquiries should be completed before fabrication of a scanning appliance.

The face

An investigation of clinical diagnostic inquiries begins with an assessment of the patient's dental anatomy, which includes the dentofacial musculature in regard to facial symmetry, lip length, lip mobility, closest speaking space, and proclination or retroclination of teeth.[1] Facial symmetry, dentofacial midline, lip symmetry, lip movement, and *s* clearance sounds are directly influenced by anterior tooth position and the amount of tooth and soft tissue visible during function.[2] Proclination or retroclination of teeth influences lip support and may contribute to the presence of a thin facial plate that is unable to repair following tooth removal (Figs 7-2 and 7-3). Proclination or retroclination of teeth may also contribute to cantilevering of the tooth in the alveolar process. This tooth–alveolar housing abnormality creates a discrepancy between the long axis of the tooth and the alveolar process, which complicates prosthetically optimal implant placement.[3]

The mouth

Examination of the mouth can be subdivided into defining the optimal tooth position, establishing tooth proportions, and determining quantity and quality of the soft tissue and length of gingival attachment.[4] Crestal bone height is examined as it relates to the cementoenamel junction in the partially edentulous patient and residual ridge in the completely edentulous patient. This is especially crucial in patients with a high lip line (Fig 7-4). Lastly, vertical dimension, cuspal form, occlusal landmark relationships, and anterior guidance all influence implant position and must be incorporated into the scanning appliance design.[4–5]

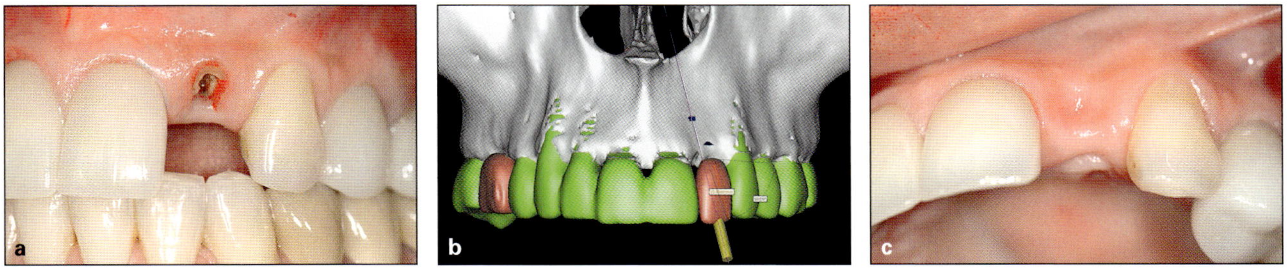

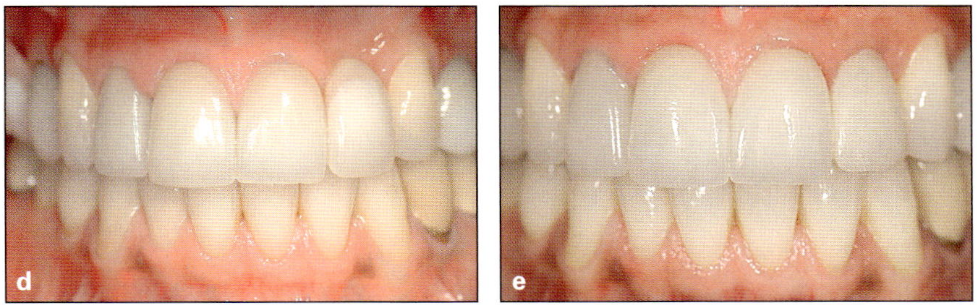

Fig 7-2 *(a)* Proclination of teeth and thin facial plate evidenced on clinical presentation. *(b)* Note anatomic fenestrations in anterior maxillary region on 3D model. *(c, d)* Anatomic fenestrations have led to aggressive postextraction resorptive patterns in spite of socket preservation and insertion of an ovate pontic interim restoration. *(e)* The clinical diagnostic inquiry was resolved using connective tissue grafting during implant placement.

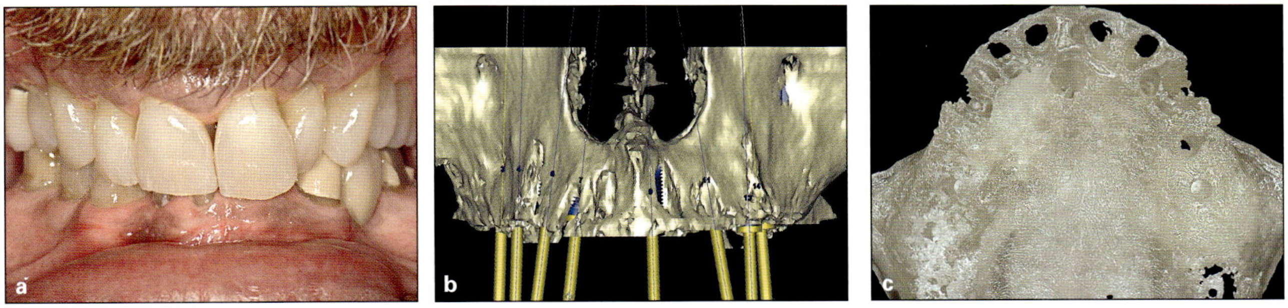

Fig 7-3 *(a)* Note retroclination of anterior teeth. *(b)* 3D model reveals anatomic fenestrations and thin facial plate. *(c)* Facial fenestrations are also evident on the anatomic model. Socket preservation procedures were completed at the time of extraction, but additional corticocancellous bone grafting was necessary to address the clinical diagnostic inquiry.

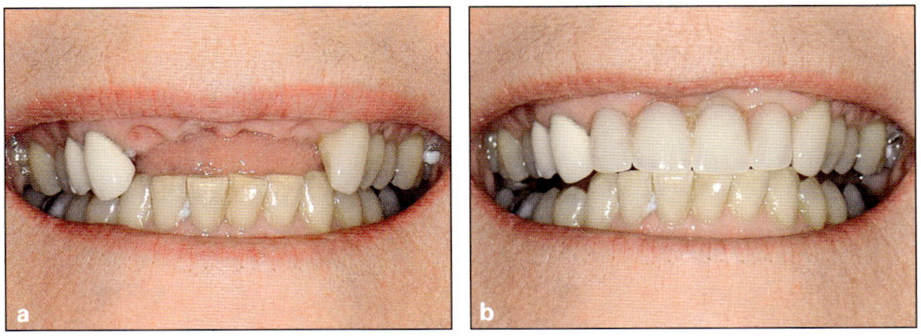

Fig 7-4 *(a)* Note the visibility of soft tissue below the high lip line in full smile. *(b)* Note the relationship between the cervical area of the teeth, ridge mucosa, and lip. Evaluating this relationship is important in determining the ability to develop an optimal emergence profile and the need to lengthen interproximal contacts or replace lost tissue with restorative material. The lip–ridge mucosa relationship can often dictate the design of the definitive restoration (eg, multiple-unit implant-supported, bar-supported overdenture, or fixed hybrid restoration) and should be incorporated in the design of the scanning appliance.

PHASE I

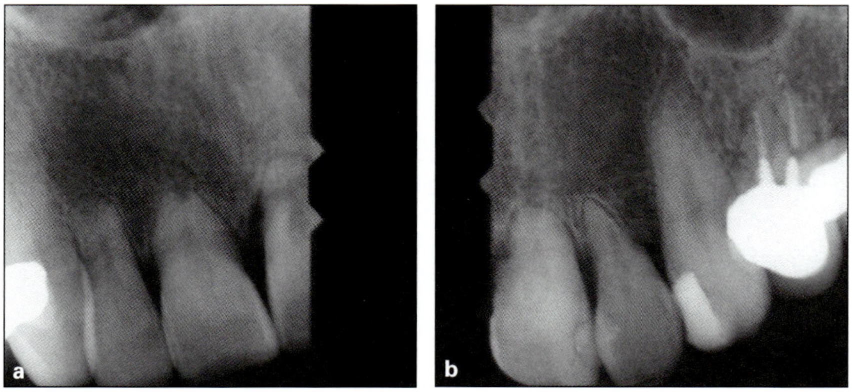

Fig 7-5 *(a, b)* Periapical radiographs revealing external root resorption and resultant disuse atrophy of the ridge in the region no longer occupied by a natural tooth root. The composite Hounsfield density is 294 HU, which is consistent with type 4 bone. Management of this inquiry would require an implant suited for poor-quality bone and modification of osteotomy site preparation to achieve primary implant stability.

Table 7-2 Most common radiographic inquiries and associated critical actions

Radiographic diagnostic inquiry	Critical action
Tooth alveolar housing relationships	Orthodontics, bone graft*
Ridge resorption (height and width)	Bone graft, zygomal or pterygoid plate implant, vertical ridge reduction when appropriate
Sinus pneumatization	Bone graft*
Nerve proximity	Short implant, nerve repositioning, bone graft
Bone quality	Bone graft*
Root resorption	Bone graft, osteotomy site modification

*Autograft, allograft, xenograft, or composite.

Radiographic diagnostic inquiries

Radiographic diagnostic inquiries require the use of the most appropriate 2D radiographs, ie, periapical, panoramic, or tomographic, to assess the bony anatomy (Fig 7-5). Examples of the most common radiographic inquiries and the associated critical actions are listed in Table 7-2. Since 2D radiography often does not reveal enough information, it is strongly recommended that further radiographic inquiries be made in phase IV using computed tomography (CT). Frequently, information critical to decision making that could not have been visualized using 2D radiographic methods is revealed using 3D radiography.[6]

Case type patterns and treatment

The initial clinical and radiographic exams allow the clinician to detect certain diagnostic patterns and then assign a patient to a basic case type, which helps guide the choice of treatment modalities and restorative approaches. Understanding similarities between patient case patterns can provide the clinician with a preview of the treatment objectives and procedures that will be necessary to manage the patient's problem. Case type patterns are an important part of the pathway since they provide a language with which the clinician can accurately communicate with the dental laboratory, specialists, and office personnel. In addition, it allows the clinician the opportunity to provide the patient with a realistic estimate of the total treatment cost early in the process. Since resolution of diagnostic inquiries often carries a significant cost, it is essential that financial aspects be addressed with the patient before any treatment begins. It is helpful to develop a fee worksheet that lists all possible treatment measures and their associated fees, which the clinician can use to quickly calculate a total cost. In this manner, case pattern analysis provides a cost-effective method for delivering elective dental implant treatment and allows the patient to make an informed decision. Case type patterns and treatment procedures common to each are identified in Table 7-3 and illustrated in Figs 7-6 to 7-10.

Table 7-3 Case types and corresponding treatment

Case type	Description	Treatment
1	• Acceptable tooth position • Favorable gingival symmetry, volume, and color • Normal bone height and width • Occlusal stability	Immediate dental implant and restoration
2	• Gingival asymmetry or color alteration • Evidence of early facial bone loss • Possible mucogingival abnormalities or thin biotype • Possible occlusal instability	Orthodontic forced eruption, soft tissue grafting, connective tissue grafting, dental implant
3	• Predominantly horizontal and some vertical bone loss • Altered occlusal vertical dimension • Reduced mesiodistal space • Possible occlusal instability	Bone graft, sinus augmentation, soft tissue ridge augmentation, provisionalization/crown lengthening, conventional fixed or buccal lingual cantilevered implant restoration
4	• Predominantly vertical and some horizontal bone loss • Altered occlusal vertical dimension • Reduced mesiodistal space • Possible occlusal instability	Bone graft, sinus augmentation, soft tissue ridge augmentation, implant-supported overdenture or hybrid prosthesis, Immediate Smile or staged treatment
5	• Significant vertical and horizontal bone loss • Loss of perioral musculature support • Possible occlusal instability	Bone graft, sinus augmentation, implant-supported overdenture or hybrid prosthesis, Immediate Smile or staged treatment

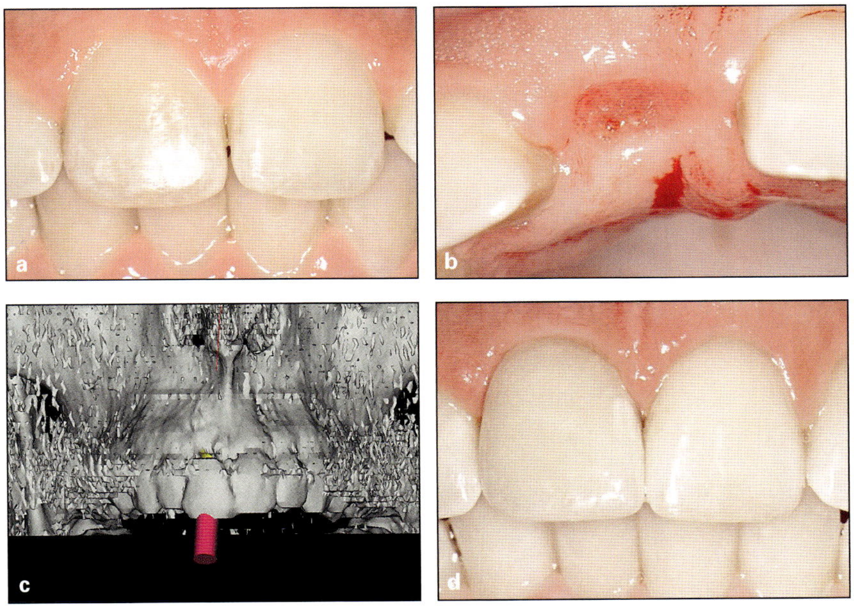

Fig 7-6 Case type 1. *(a)* A maxillary right central incisor requires extraction as a result of acute trauma. *(b)* Note the tissue volume and papilla form in the extraction site. *(c)* 3D model with proposed implant placement. *(d)* Clinical result following tooth whitening and placement of an implant and a single-tooth restoration.

PHASE I

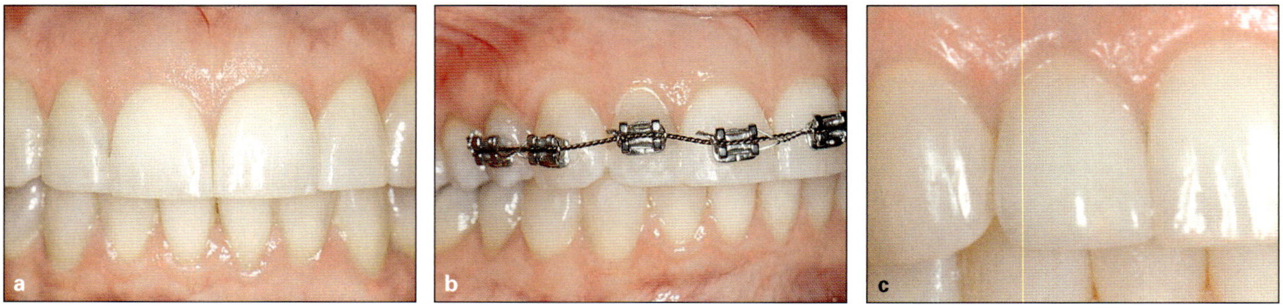

Fig 7-7 Case type 2. *(a)* Note the gingival margin position of the maxillary right lateral incisor, which is apical to that of the adjacent central incisor. The required extraction of the lateral incisor will exacerbate this relationship. *(b)* Gingival asymmetry is managed using orthodontic forced eruption prior to extraction and implant placement. *(c)* Following placement of an implant and the definitive restoration, a normal gingival relationship is present.

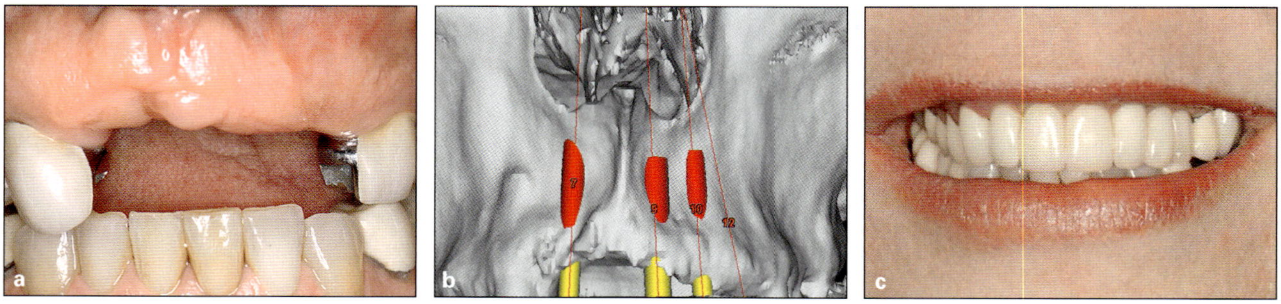

Fig 7-8 Case type 3. *(a)* Early vertical and advanced horizontal bone loss. Note how the presence of horizontal bone loss can affect the circumference or linear length of the edentulous area and reduce space available for implant placement. *(b)* 3D model showing more palatal implant placement, which decreases the arch length and affects the interimplant distances. *(c)* Clinical results following corticocancellous bone graft, soft tissue ridge augmentation, and placement of implants and a conventional fixed prosthesis from the maxillary right lateral incisor to the left second premolar.

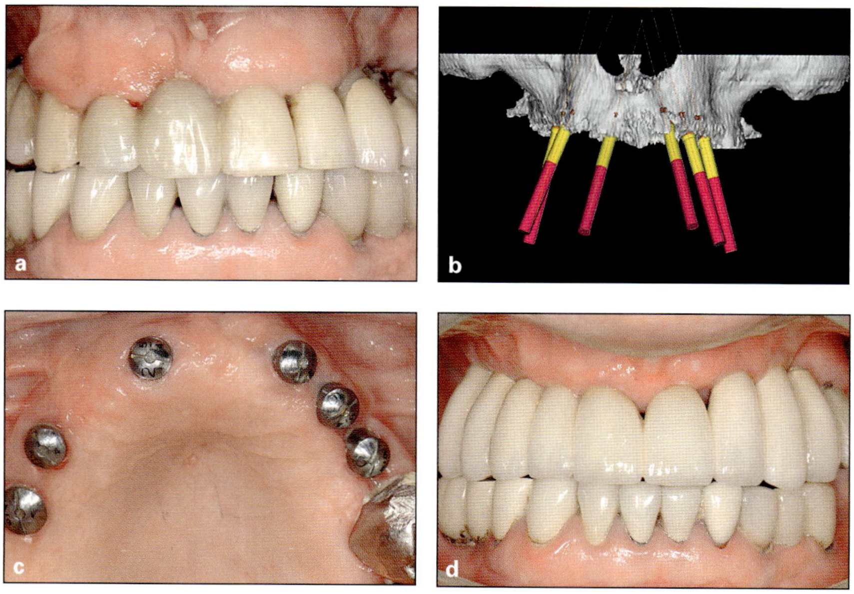

Fig 7-9 Case type 4. *(a)* Predominantly vertical, and some horizontal, bone loss. Note the impact of vertical bone loss on clinical crown length. This vertical bone loss can influence esthetics, speech patterns, and ultimately the type of definitive restoration. *(b)* 3D model with proposed implant placement. *(c)* Occlusal view of maxilla following implant placement. *(d)* Definitive restoration.

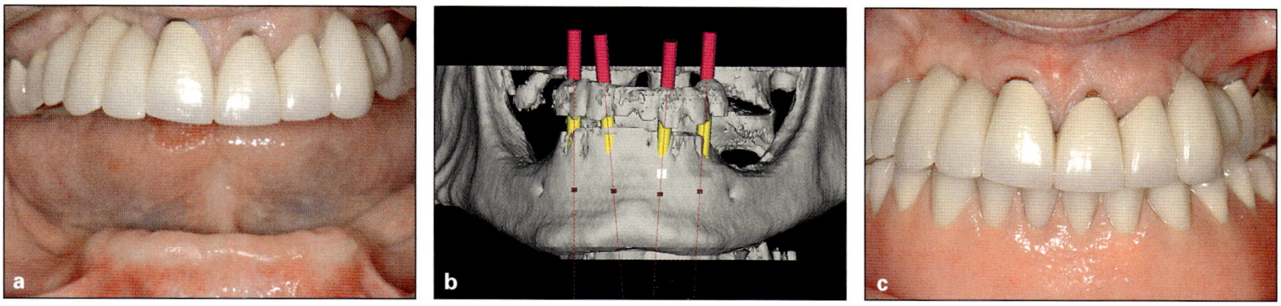

Fig 7-10 Case type 5. *(a)* Advanced vertical and horizontal bone loss. Edentulism has led to disparity in bone height anterior to and posterior to the mental foramina. Availability of bone for implant placement is limited to the anatomic region between the mental foramina. Number, length, and distribution of implants impact the extent of posterior cantilevering that can be used to provide posterior function. *(b)* 3D model with proposed implant placement. *(c)* Clinical view following placement of implants and implant-supported overdenture, which provides perioral musculature support.

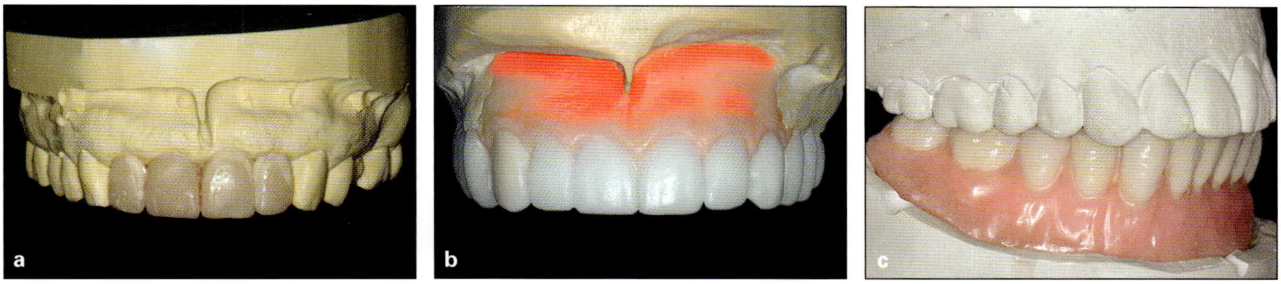

Fig 7-11 Types of waxups: tooth-form *(a)*, full-contour *(b)*, and trial tooth setup *(c)*.

Table 7-4 Types of diagnostic waxups and their indications

Type of waxup	Indications
Tooth-form	Dental and surgical anatomy within normal limits. Tooth landmark relationships, proportions, or vertical dimension require modification.
Full-contour	Dental anatomy within normal limits; determination of the volume of hard and soft tissue augmentation for optimal final tooth position required.
Trial tooth setup	Complete edentulism; dental and possibly also surgical anatomy require modification.

Selecting and performing the diagnostic waxup

The types of diagnostic waxups (Fig 7-11) and their indications are listed in Table 7-4. A diagnostic waxup must be created in order to fabricate the scanning appliance as well as a provisional restoration (if necessary).

PHASE II

Scanning Appliance Fabrication

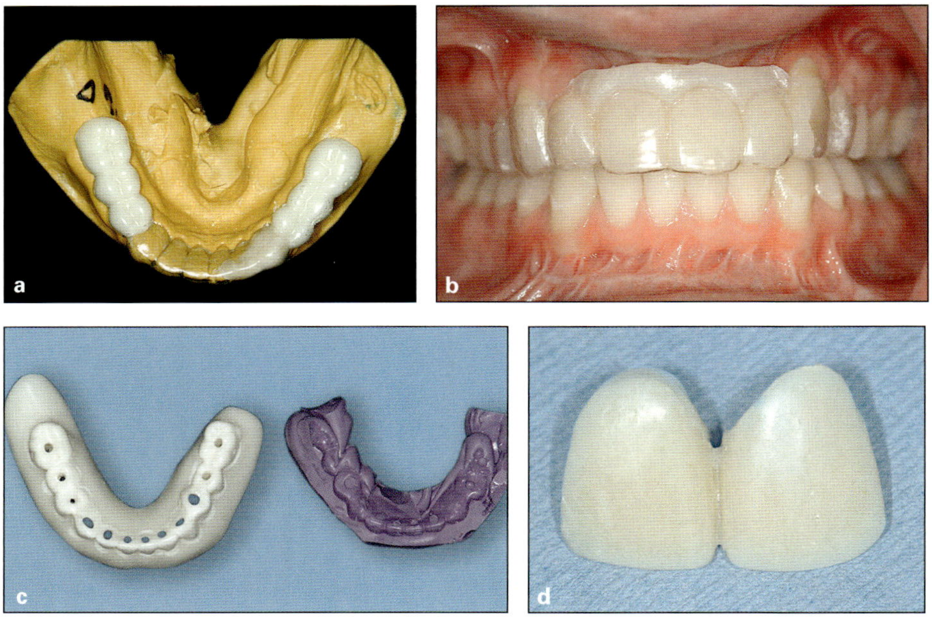

Fig 7-12 Types of scanning appliances: tooth-form *(a)*, full-contour *(b)*, complete denture *(c)*, and provisional restoration *(d)*.

Table 7-5 Types of scanning appliances with associated waxup and indications

Type of scanning appliance	Type of waxup	Indications
Tooth-form	Tooth-form	Dental and surgical anatomy appear within normal limits
Full-contour	Full-contour	Dental anatomy within normal limits but surgical anatomy requires augmentation and volume of tissue needs to be determined
Complete denture	Trial tooth setup	Surgical and dental anatomy require modification
Provisional restoration	Tooth-form	Dental anatomy only requires modification

Box 7-3 Scanning appliance fabrication considerations

1. **Type of scanning appliance** (see Table 7-5).
2. **Contrast medium for soft tissue representation:** In all scanning appliances, 30% barium is used to represent the teeth; for full-contour and complete denture templates, 10% barium is used to enable identification of the soft tissue portion as well.
3. **Inspection windows:** All templates for partially edentulous cases (tooth-form, full-contour, and provisional restoration) require an inspection window for seating verification.
4. **Radiolucent interocclusal record:** When immediate provisional restorations are planned or complete edentulism or a Kennedy Class II situation exists, interocclusal record using a radiolucent material must be performed to ensure repeatability of the positioning of the template.
5. **Surgical guide fixation:** A decision should be made regarding whether the surgical guide will be fixated using screws or 0.010 ligature wire. The scanning appliance must include sufficient regional anatomy to allow for the possibility of screw fixation.

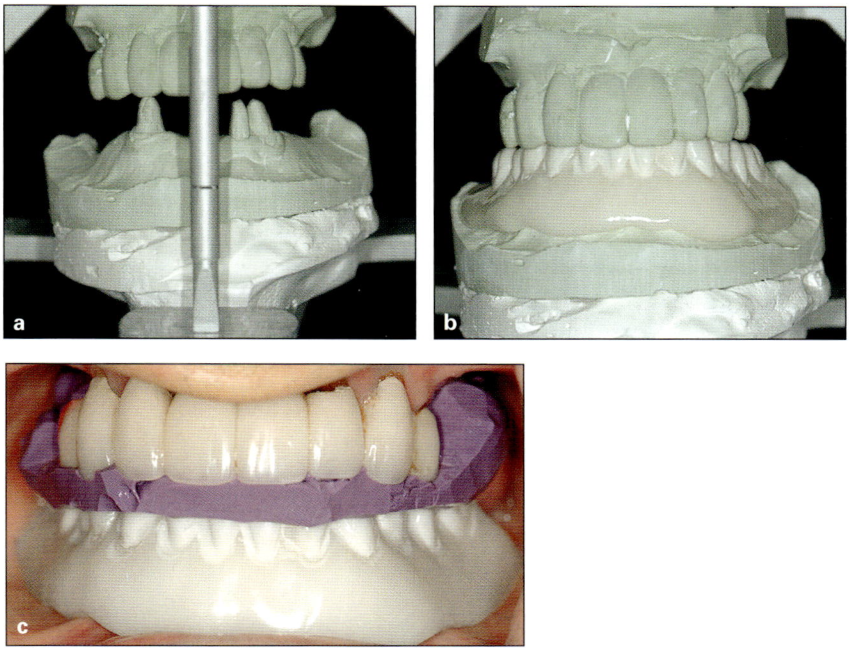

Fig 7-13 Laboratory procedures for fabrication of a full-contour scanning appliance. *(a)* Casts mounted in the articulator. *(b)* Fabrication of the full-contour scanning appliance supported by teeth and mucosa, containing 30% barium in the tooth portion and 10% barium in the soft tissue portion. *(c)* Delivery of scanning appliance with radiolucent interocclusal record, which was created in the laboratory, to ensure proper positioning of the scanning appliance. The patient is ready for imaging.

The type of scanning appliance must be selected (Fig 7-12) based on the type of waxup created in the previous phase (Table 7-5). Other considerations for the fabrication of scanning appliances are listed in Box 7-3. Laboratory procedures for fabrication of a full-contour scanning appliance are shown in Fig 7-13.

PHASE III CT Scan and SimPlant Conversion

Once the CT scans have been taken, the resulting DICOM files are processed into the SimPlant format. At this point, masks of specific anatomic structures are created in a process called *segmentation*. This is done to facilitate manipulation of anatomic structures on the 3D image viewed in the software. The most common masks are listed in Box 7-4.

Box 7-4 Common masks created in SimPlant

- Maxilla
- Mandible
- Scanning appliance
- Gingival surface of denture
- Denture base
- Existing dental implants
- Natural dentition
- Groups of axial and frontal views of the maxillary sinus*
- Groups of axial and frontal views of the mandibular canal*

*Less frequently used. These masks require a significant amount of time to create but are available when needed.

PHASE IV

Eight-Step Treatment-Planning Process

An eight-step method is used to plan treatment. Radiographic inquiries not visible with standard dental radiographs are investigated at this time (see Table 7-2).

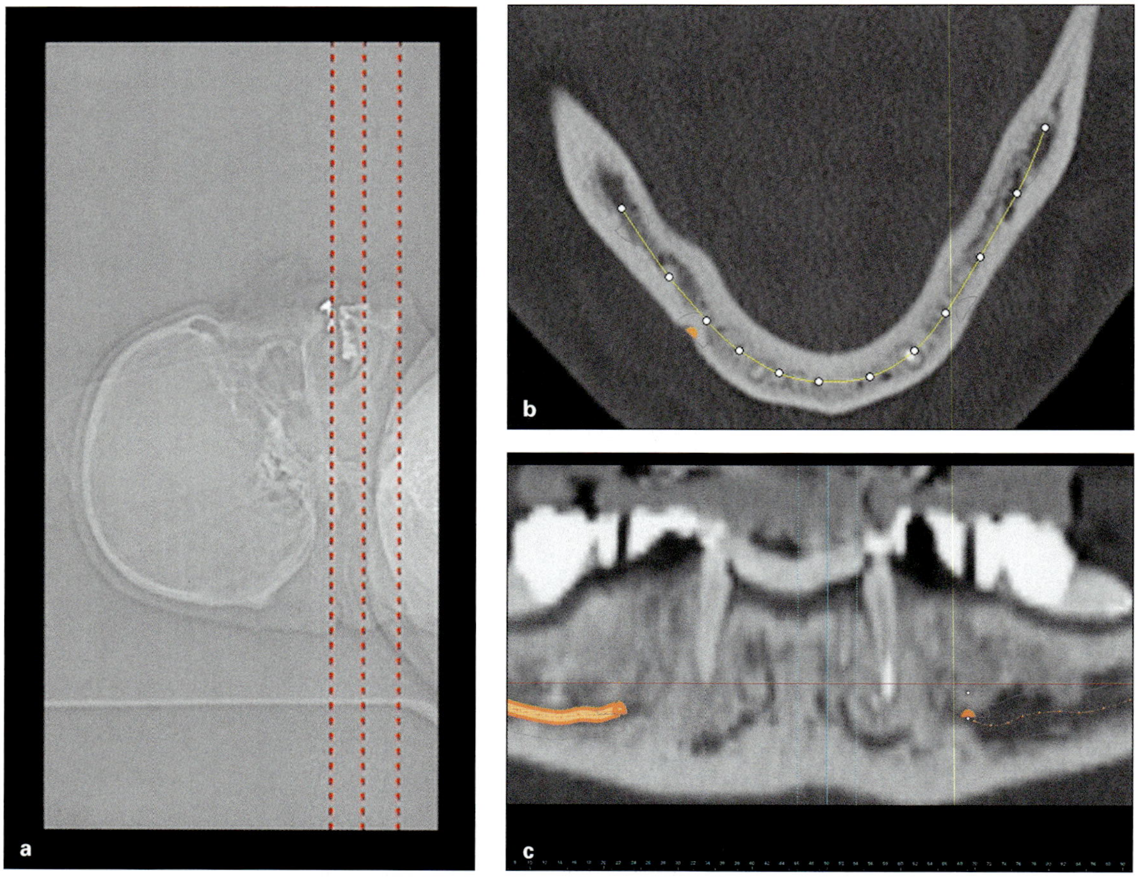

Fig 7-14 Step 1. *(a)* Axial image should be parallel to occlusal plane. *(b)* Panoramic curve drawn on axial image. *(c)* The nerve drawn on the image.

1. Determine the accuracy of the CT study

The first step is to review the setup film to *(1)* confirm that the axial image is parallel to the occlusal plane (Fig 7-14a); *(2)* draw the panoramic curve on the axial image at the sinus floor (in the maxilla) or the roof of the mandibular canal (in the mandible) (Fig 7-14b); and *(3)* draw the nerve (Fig 7-14c).

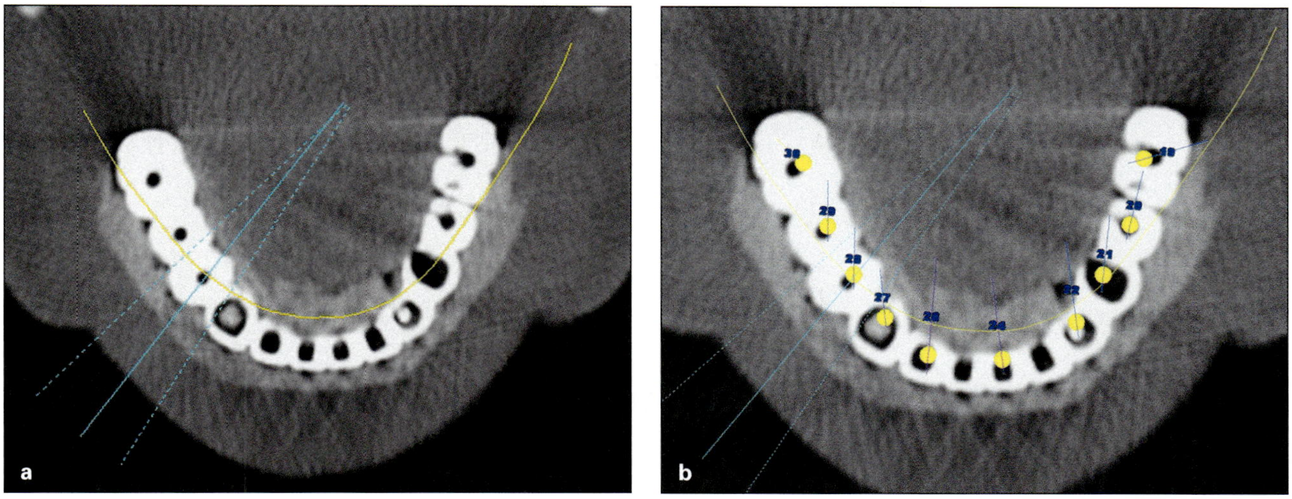

Fig 7-15 Step 2. *(a)* Emergence axis located on axial image. *(b)* Implants have been placed into negative space markers for each proposed implant site.

Fig 7-16 Step 3. Implant viewed in cross section. The implant has been manipulated into its optimal position with the implant-planning software. Completion of step 3 gives the clinician the opportunity to evaluate whether the optimal surgical position is compatible with the image of the proposed definitive restoration. Clinical crown length, emergence angle, buccal lingual cantilever, and tissue depth are all evaluated.

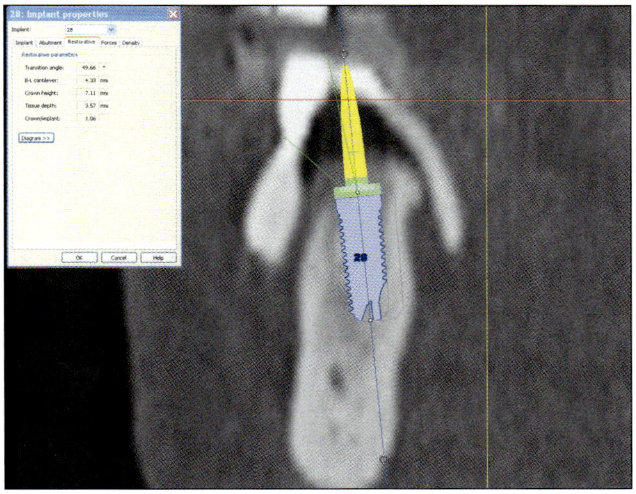

2. Locate emergence axis and place implant

The next step is to locate the emergence axis on the axial plane at the level of the occlusal table or incisive edge of the tooth (Fig 7-15a), and place the implant into the negative space markers (Fig 7-15b).

3. View implants in cross section

The implant should be placed on cross-sectional view to verify platform position, restorative assessment, cantilever, and emergence profile (Fig 7-16). This procedure should be repeated for each implant site.

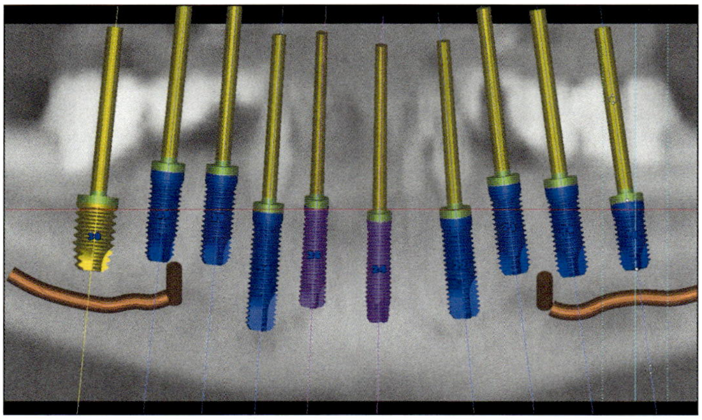

Fig 7-17 Step 4. Parallelism of implants and adjacent teeth is verified on the panoramic view. Parallelism in 2D and later in 3D is important as it relates to the path of insertion for the provisional and definitive restorations. Information gathered in steps 4 and 5 provide insight for abutment selection and the need to control hex timing during the medical modeling and implant placement phases of the treatment pathway. These decisions may influence the choice of implant system.

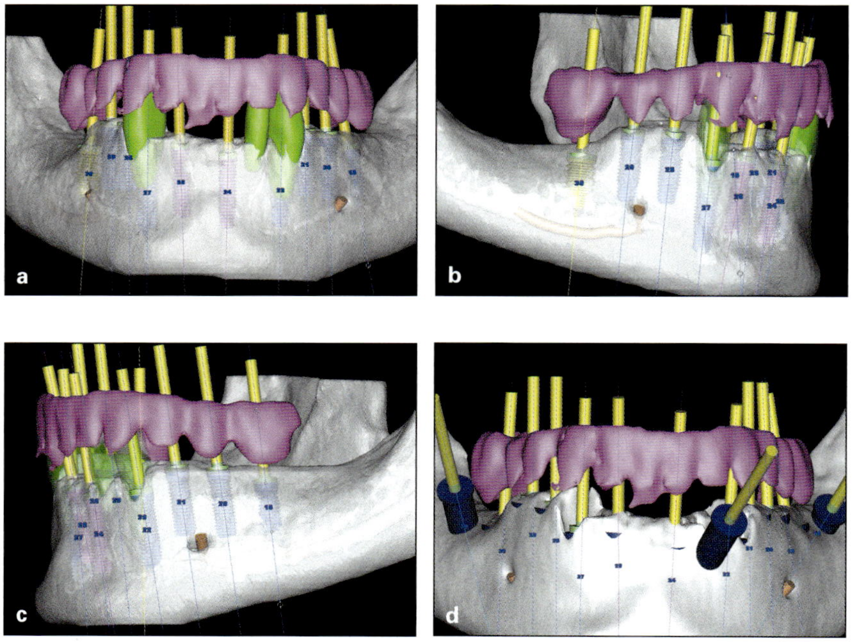

Fig 7-18 Step 5. *(a–c)* The mandible has been made transparent to allow assessment of the parallelism of the implants. The natural teeth *(green)* assisted in the support of the scanning appliance. *(d)* The mask of the natural teeth has been turned off since they will be extracted. The screw fixation sites are determined, ensuring they do not interfere with implant placement.

4. Verify parallelism of implants and adjacent teeth

The parallelism of implants and adjacent teeth can be verified using the panoramic view (Fig 7-17).

5. View implants and scanning appliance in 3D

Using the 3D view, the parallelism of the implants is confirmed, vital structures are evaluated for potential injury, and surgical guide fixation screws are inserted if necessary (Fig 7-18). Path of withdrawal for the definitive restoration can be verified since the scanning appliance is its replica.

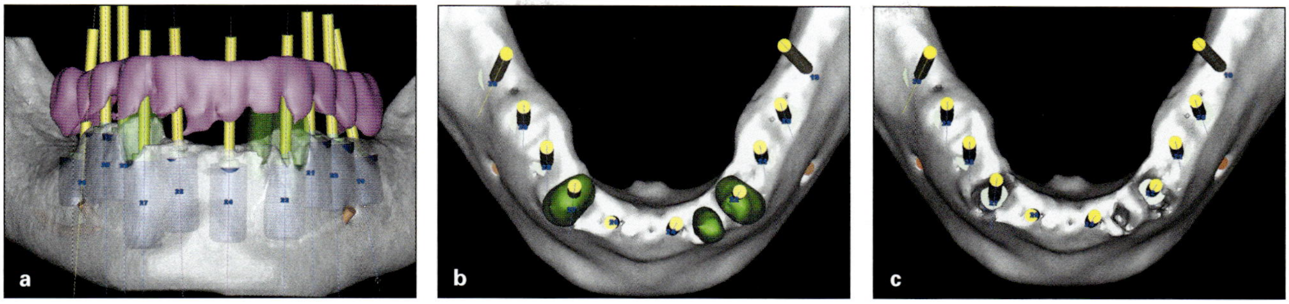

Fig 7-19 Step 6. *(a)* In transparency mode, the fenestration tool is used to create an enlarged diameter of predetermined size around the planned implants *(dark blue)* to assess the potential for fenestration or dehiscence of the bone. *(b)* Teeth *(green)* in place. *(c)* When the mandibular left lateral incisor and canine were removed from the model, a large gap was revealed, indicating the need for bone augmentation.

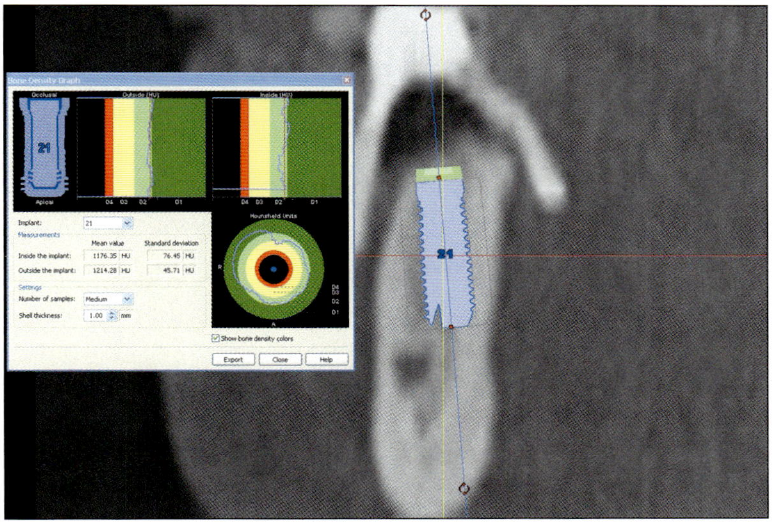

Fig 7-20 Step 7. In this case, a bone density of 1,250 HU was found, which indicates that bone augmentation and modification of the osteotomy site preparation will be required.

6. Evaluate for possible fenestrations of the cortical plates

The cortical plates are evaluated for possible fenestrations (Fig 7-19a). In addition, discrepancy between the morphology of the bone in an extraction site and the diameter of the implant can be assessed (Figs 7-19b and 7-19c).

7. Determine bone density

The density of the bone is determined (Fig 7-20). Step 7 provides presurgical information related to the method of osteotomy site preparation. The ability to determine an average HU value can also influence whether implant treatment is staged or an immediate load provisional restoration can be selected.

PHASE IV

Table 7-6 Most common physical diagnostic inquiries and associated critical actions

Physical diagnostic inquiry	Critical action
Metallic artifact	Model-based guide construction for tooth- or bone-supported guide
Surgical access limitations	Short implants, lateral access surgical guides
Excessive elongation	Bone or mucosal guide
Collision of cylinder with retained tooth or another cylinder	Modify treatment plan, increase elongation within limits of surgical system and access

8. Preview and order surgical guide

The clinician should preview the surgical guide, address any physical diagnostic inquiries, and consult with the patient before ordering the surgical guide.

Physical diagnostic inquiries

Physical inquiries are addressed following completion of a treatment plan prior to selection of the most appropriate surgical guide (Table 7-6). The most common inquiry is the presence of metal restorations or endodontic metal posts, which can create artifacts on the CT image, affecting interpretation. Limited surgical access is another common problem. In some cases the overall vertical height of the guided implant placement system, as required by the specific anatomic situation, will exceed the maximum drill length of the guidance system (Figs 7-21a to 7-21d). In addition, limited space between implant sites or between retained teeth and an implant site may not provide enough clearance for the guiding cylinders (Fig 7-21e). These issues must be resolved before the surgical guide is ordered (Figs 7-21f and 7-21g).

Patient consultation

The preoperative patient consultation occurs when all of the surgical and prosthetic planning has been completed. At this time, the patient is fully informed of the treatment plan, any additional needs and concerns of the patient are addressed, and the patient's consent for treatment is obtained. Full and complete disclosure and management of patient expectations is crucial at this stage.

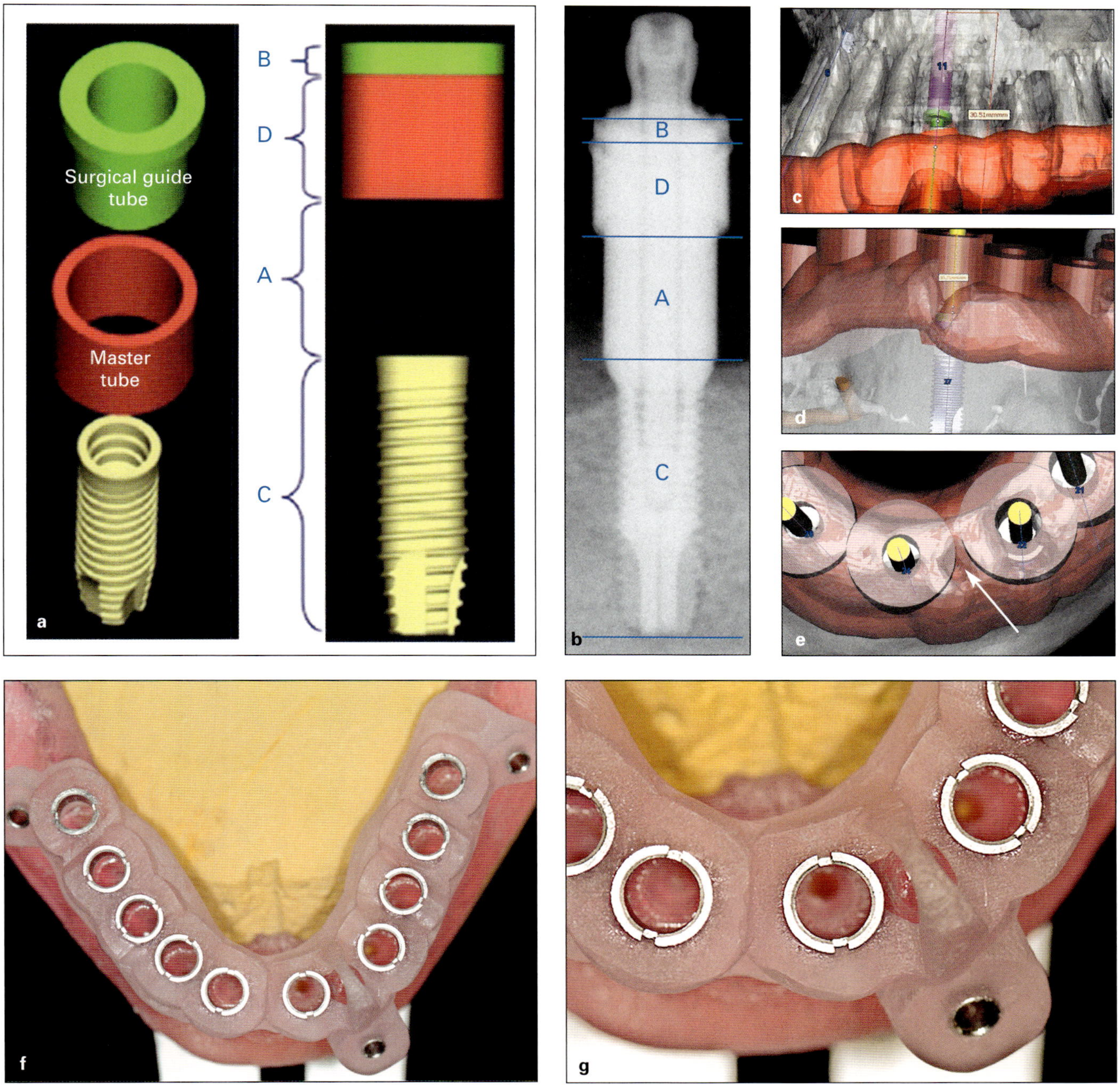

Fig 7-21 Step 8. Addressing physical inquiries before ordering the surgical guide. *(a, b)* Components of guide system that contribute to total height. A = distance from the implant seating surface to the bottom of the guiding cylinder; B = thickness of the flange on the drilling cylinder; C = implant length; D = height of the guiding cylinder. *(c)* Vertical stacking height of guide measured in the 3D model. *(d)* Potential excessive elongation. *(e)* The guiding cylinder for the implant at the mandibular left canine position is in close proximity to the left lateral incisor *(arrow)*, which will be retained to assist in the support of the surgical guide. *(f)* A bone-supported guide can be used to reduce elongation of the guide system. *(g)* The lateral incisor will be reduced prior to surgery; however, resin still had to be trimmed from the adjacent cylinders to allow space for the tooth. To increase stability, resin is placed to overlap the retained tooth.

PHASE V

Medical Modeling

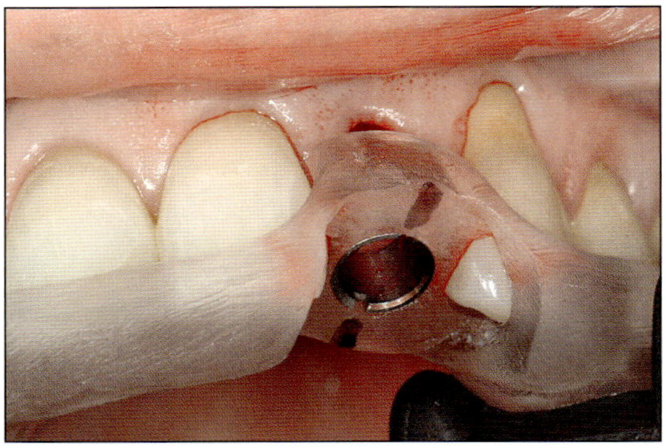

Fig 7-22 Tooth-supported surgical guide.

If immediate loading is not planned, only the production of the surgical guide ordered in the previous phase occurs in this phase. However, if immediate loading is planned, a master model and provisional restoration must be fabricated at this stage. The steps required vary depending on the type of surgical guide to be used, as described below.

Construction of implant master model and immediate load provisional restoration

Tooth-supported guides

A plaster cast of the patient's dentition can be used unless there are teeth to be extracted at the time of surgery. In this situation, a digital model with extracted teeth and prepared implant analogue sites incorporated should be used.

The required components are:

- Tooth-supported surgical guide (Fig 7-22)
- Stone cast or digital model with extracted teeth
- Interocclusal record in repeatable treatment position

The remount procedure is completed as follows:

1. Remount digital model or stone cast into the articulator with scanning appliance interocclusal record.
2. Insert implant analogues using the surgical guide with laboratory analogue mounts or guide sleeves and fabricate implant master model.
3. Establish hex timing with insertion of analogues into model.
4. Attach temporary cylinders and fabricate abutment seating index to maintain hex timing.
5. Fabricate provisional restoration.

Bone-supported guides

When bone-supported guides are to be used, the required components are:

- Digital copy of scanning appliance with receptor sites for vertical remount studs (Fig 7-23a)
- Original scanning appliance interocclusal record in repeatable treatment position
- Anatomic bone model with vertical remount studs (Fig 7-23b)
- Bone-supported surgical guide

The remount procedure is completed as follows:

1. Place digital copy of scanning appliance with vertical remount stud sites on anatomic bone model (Fig 7-23c).
2. Remount in articulator with scanning appliance interocclusal record (Fig 7-23d).
3. Remove remount studs from anatomic bone model (Fig 7-23e) and seat surgical guide (Fig 7-23f).
4. Insert implant analogues into surgical guide with laboratory analogue mounts or guide sleeves and fabricate implant master model (Fig 7-23g).
5. Establish hex timing with insert of analogues into model (see Fig 7-23g).
6. Attach temporary cylinders and fabricate abutment seating index to maintain hex timing (Figs 7-23h to 7-23k).
7. Fabricate provisional restoration (Figs 7-23l and 7-23m).

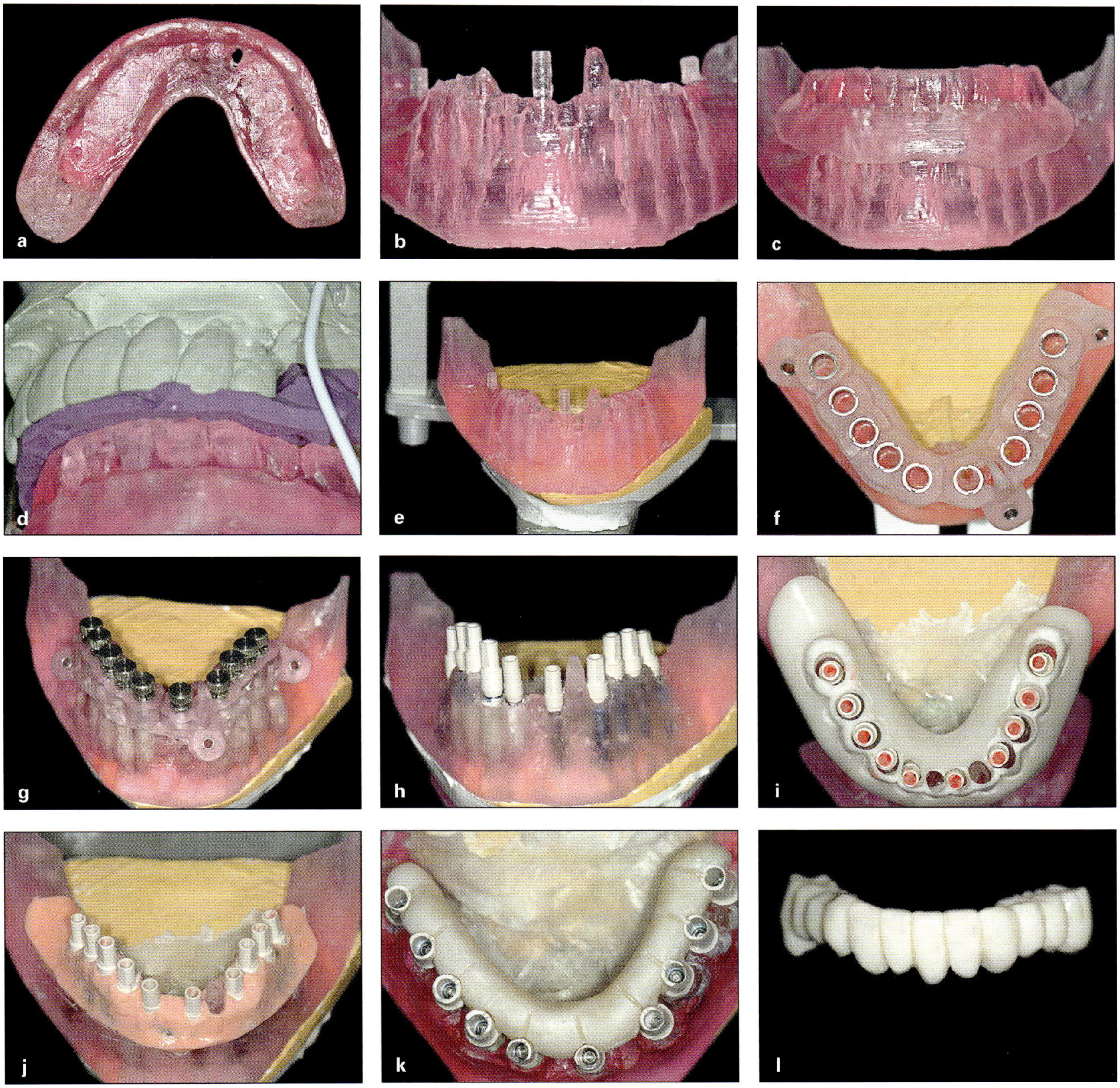

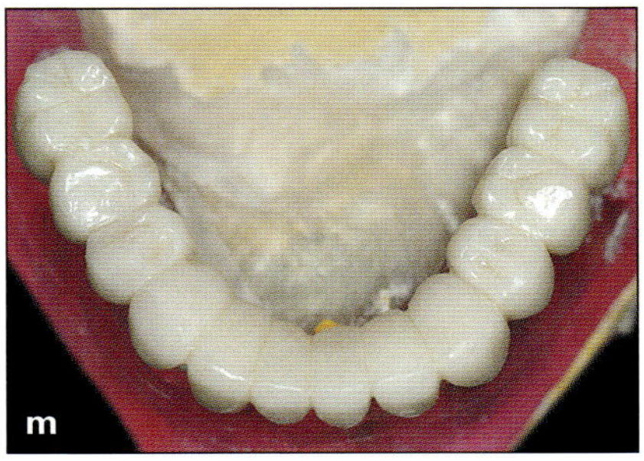

Fig 7-23 Construction of immediate-load provisional restoration when bone-supported guides are used. *(a)* Mucosal surface of digital copy of scanning appliance with receptor sites for vertical remount studs. *(b)* Anatomic bone model with vertical remount studs used to support the digital copy of the scanning appliance. *(c)* Digital copy of scanning appliance seated on remount studs of anatomic bone model. *(d)* Digital copy of scanning appliance and anatomic bone model mounted to opposing cast with original interocclusal record. *(e)* Remount studs removed from bone model. *(f)* Bone-supported surgical guide seated on anatomic bone model. *(g)* Using the surgical guide, implant analogues are inserted into the bone model, and hex timing is established. *(h)* Temporary abutments inserted into implant analogues of bone model. *(i)* Using the scanning appliance, a soft tissue model has been created on the articulator. *(j)* A master model with soft tissue has been created, allowing the abutments to be prepared. *(k)* A hex timing index has been fabricated in the articulator for orientation of abutments at the time of surgery. *(l, m)* Prefabricated provisional restoration, which will be placed and adjusted as necessary at the time of surgery.

PHASE V

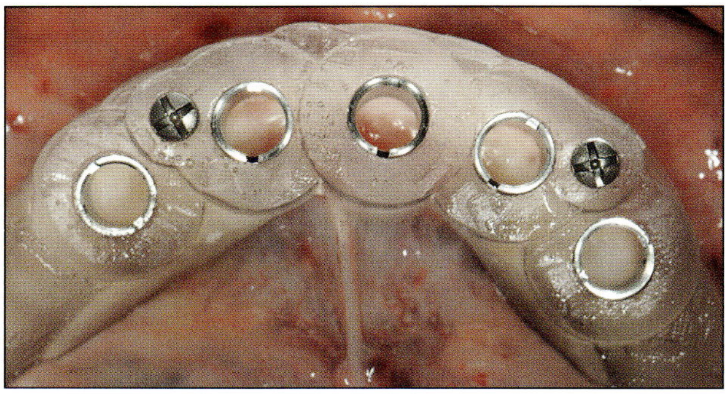

Fig 7-24 Mucosa-supported surgical guide with screw fixation.

Mucosa-supported guides

The required components for constructing an implant master model when using a mucosa-supported guide are:

- Digital copy of scanning appliance
- Original scanning appliance interocclusal record in repeatable treatment position
- Anatomic mucosal model
- Mucosa-supported surgical guide (Fig 7-24)

The remount procedure is completed as follows:

1. Remount mucosal model with digital copy of scanning appliance and scanning appliance interocclusal record into the articulator in repeatable treatment position.
2. Insert implant analogues into surgical guide with laboratory analogue mounts or guide sleeves and fabricate implant master model.
3. Establish hex timing with insert of analogues into model.
4. Attach temporary cylinders and fabricate abutment seating index to maintain hex timing.
5. Fabricate provisional restoration.

PHASE VI Surgery

The first decision that must be made is whether it is possible to use a flapless approach. Indications for preparing a mucosal flap versus using a flapless approach are presented in Box 7-5. If a flap is prepared, it is important to use broad flap reflection (Fig 7-25a). Also, when possible, it is helpful to retain the teeth neighboring the surgical site in order to orient the guide upon insertion (Fig 7-25b). If a flapless approach is used, it is best to create the opening using a tissue punch.

The guide is inserted, with the seating confirmed using inspection windows or interocclusal record, and then fixed using either 0.010 wire or bone fixation screws (Fig 7-25c). The hex timing is set using the surgical guide. Tissue punch (if using a flapless approach) and drilling are performed through the surgical guides. The implants are placed (Figs 7-25d to 7-25g) and the abutments seated using the hex timing verification index (Figs 7-25h and 7-25i). If an immediately loaded provisional restoration is planned, it is placed and either cement- or screw-retained (Figs 7-25j to 7-25m).

Box 7-5 Indications for mucosal flap preparation versus a flapless approach

Mucosal flap preparation

- Clinical and radiographic inquiries suggest hard or soft tissue augmentation needed
- Metallic artifact present at crown axial level on scan
- Edentulous space is 30 mm or greater
- Excessive elongation can be diminished by seating surgical guide on bony ridge

Flapless approach

- Adequate zone of keratinized tissue
- Acceptable elongation distance
- Tooth- or mucosa-supported guide

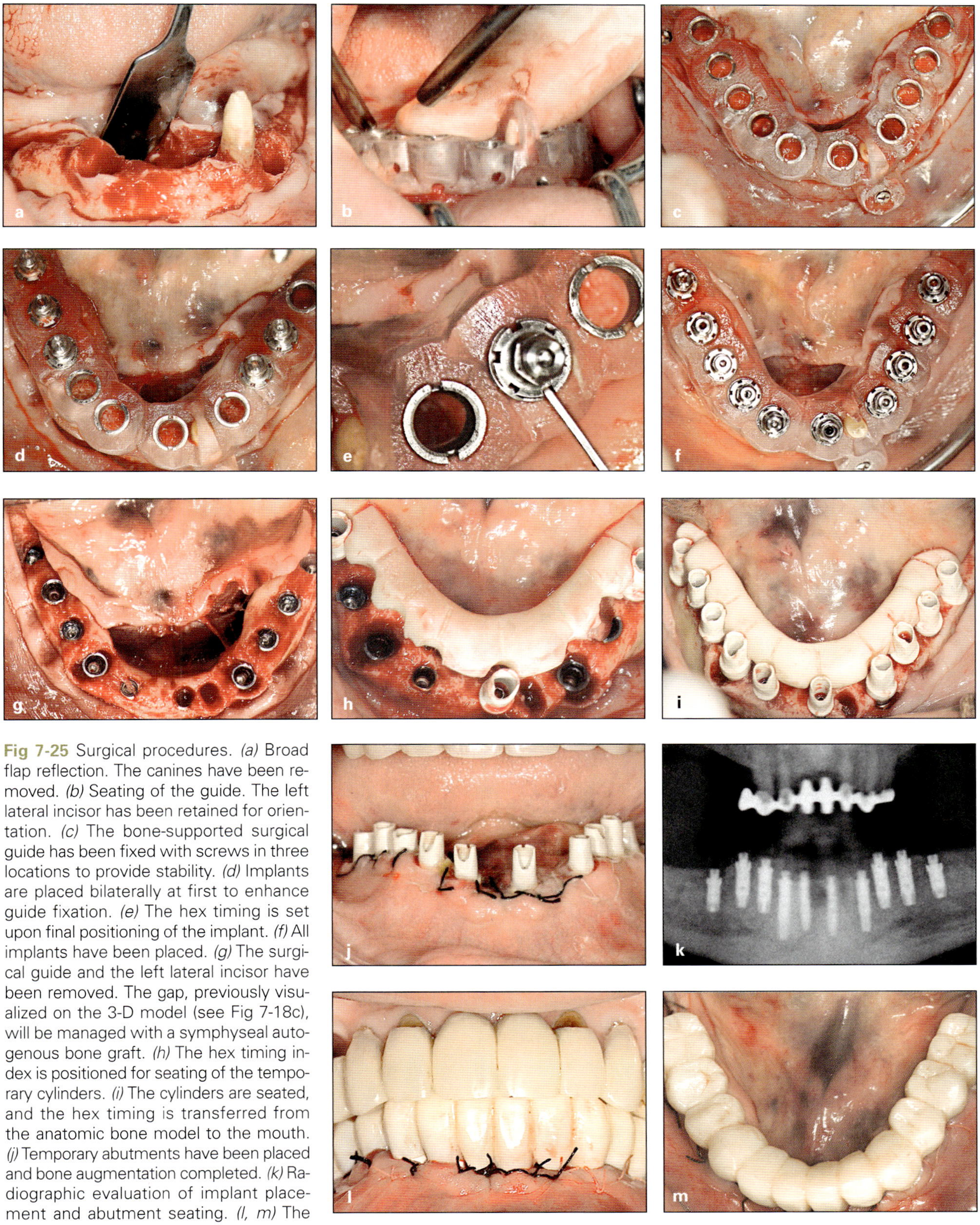

Fig 7-25 Surgical procedures. *(a)* Broad flap reflection. The canines have been removed. *(b)* Seating of the guide. The left lateral incisor has been retained for orientation. *(c)* The bone-supported surgical guide has been fixed with screws in three locations to provide stability. *(d)* Implants are placed bilaterally at first to enhance guide fixation. *(e)* The hex timing is set upon final positioning of the implant. *(f)* All implants have been placed. *(g)* The surgical guide and the left lateral incisor have been removed. The gap, previously visualized on the 3-D model (see Fig 7-18c), will be managed with a symphyseal autogenous bone graft. *(h)* The hex timing index is positioned for seating of the temporary cylinders. *(i)* The cylinders are seated, and the hex timing is transferred from the anatomic bone model to the mouth. *(j)* Temporary abutments have been placed and bone augmentation completed. *(k)* Radiographic evaluation of implant placement and abutment seating. *(l, m)* The provisional restoration has been adjusted as needed to provide passive fit and seated with temporary cement.

PHASE VII Definitive Restoration and Supportive Maintenance

After an appropriate healing period, the definitive prosthesis is placed (Figs 7-26a and 7-26b). The patient is monitored and provided with supportive maintenance for the new restoration.

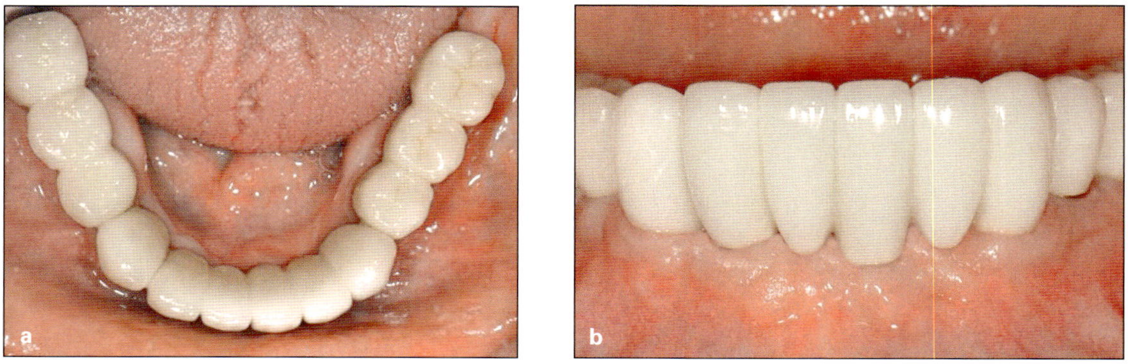

Figs 7-26a and 7-26b Note the proportions of the teeth in the definitive restoration from occlusal and frontal views. These dimensions are the same as the preoperative diagnostic waxup from which the scan appliance was fabricated. This outcome thus reflects the accurate identification and resolution of diagnostic inquiries (clinical, radiographic, and physical) in this patient's treatment pathway. It also demonstrates how the surgical guide serves as a conduit in the accurate transfer of the patient's virtual implant treatment plan to the patient's mouth during implant surgery.

Summary

With the advent of CT, a voluminous amount of diagnostic, surgical, and prosthetic information is available to collaborating practitioners prior to the start of active patient treatment. An algorithmic approach to managing diagnosis and planning as well as surgical execution creates an opportunity to more effectively manage critical information.

The pathway can be conceptualized as consisting of two major stages: assessment (phases I to IV) and active treatment (phases V to VII). Assessment consists of data collection, development of suitable scanning appliances, a proper CT study, interpretation of the CT study, development of the treatment plan, and consultation with the patient. The diagnostic, radiographic, and physical inquiries addressed at various points along the pathway focus attention on issues that can influence the treatment outcome, and the eight-step approach to CT treatment planning facilitates fabrication of a surgical guide that ensures that all proposed implant sites will support the outcome analysis determined by the scanning appliance. At the end of the assessment phase, the patient, implant surgeon, and restorative dentist clearly understand all risks and benefits and have evaluated treatment implications in an atmosphere of disclosure. In the active treatment phase, the treatment plan is incorporated into the design and fabrication of a surgical guide that will deliver the intended outcome, the surgery is performed, and the restoration is provided with appropriate follow-up and maintenance.

Development of new imaging technology and treatment procedures will not diminish the value of this systematized approach to information analysis as diagnosis and treatment planning will remain the cornerstone of patient care. In the next chapter the treatment pathway is demonstrated through the presentation of clinical cases.

Acknowledgments

The author would like to express a special thank you to prosthodontists Marco Padilla, DMD, MS, and Steven Rhodes, DDS, for their restorative collaboration, treatment, and assistance in developing this pathway.

References

1. Mecall R, Rosenfeld A. Use of prosthesis-generated tomographic information for diagnosis and surgical treatment planning. In: Rothman SLG (ed). Dental Applications of Computerized Tomography. Chicago: Quintessence, 1998: Chapter 9, 177–236.
2. Rosenfeld A, Mandelaris G, Tardieu P. Prosthetically directed implant software to ensure precise placement and predictable prosthetic outcomes. Part I. Diagnostics, imaging, and collaborative accountability. Int J Periodontics Restorative Dent 2006;26:215–221.
3. Turbyfill W. The art and science of complete denture prosthodontics. Bogart, Georgia, January 2007.
4. Spears F. State of the art esthetics. Presented at the Seattle Institute for Advanced Education, Seattle, 2007
5. Mecall R, Rosenfeld A. The influence of residual ridge resorption patterns on implant fixture placement and tooth position. Part II. Presurgical determination of prosthesis type and prosthetic design. Int J Periodontics Restorative Dent 1996;16:322–337.
6. Rosenfeld A, Mecall R. Using computerized tomography to develop realistic treatment objectives for the implant team. In: Nevins M, Mellonig JT (eds). Implant Therapy: Clinical Approaches and Evidence of Success. Chicago: Quintessence, 1998:37–42.

8

CLINICAL CASES

George A. Mandelaris, DDS, MS
Alan L. Rosenfeld, DDS, FACD
Philippe B. Tardieu, DDS

This chapter presents 14 clinical cases to demonstrate the treatment process using SimPlant, as detailed in chapter 7. Each case is introduced with background information, pertinent dental history, and the needs and concerns of the patient. Patient diagnoses, case type, and diagnostic inquiries are then determined, and critical actions are highlighted. The critical action represents the most influential treatment steps required to achieve the treatment outcome. Only case 4 required emergency-based planning.

Case 1 Maxillary Partial Edentulism

A 58-year-old woman presented with the chief complaint of unstable, generalized, advanced periodontitis. Her medical history was significant for controlled cardiovascular disease. She was a cigarette smoker with a 20-pack/year history. Her dental history included progressive attachment loss around her posterior natural dentition with poor long-term prognosis. The patient's needs and concerns were to have a stable-fitting implant-supported prosthesis that would be maintainable long term.

Diagnoses

- Generalized advanced chronic periodontitis
- Class I skeletal occlusion
- Bilateral sinus pneumatization

Case type: 4

- Predominantly vertical with some horizontal bone loss

Diagnostic inquiries

Clinical

- Optimal final tooth position
- Maxillomandibuar relationship and occlusion

Radiographic

- Degree of sinus proximity
- Extent of vertical and horizontal bone loss
- Overall health of the maxillary sinuses
- Patency of osteomeatal complex

Physical

- None

Critical actions

- Accurate diagnostic waxup reflecting desired final outcome
- Transfer of diagnostic waxup information to a scanning appliance 2 to 3 months postextraction
- CT-based treatment planning
- Preoperative prosthetic outcome determination: Fixed implant-supported prosthesis

PHASE I Initial Diagnostics

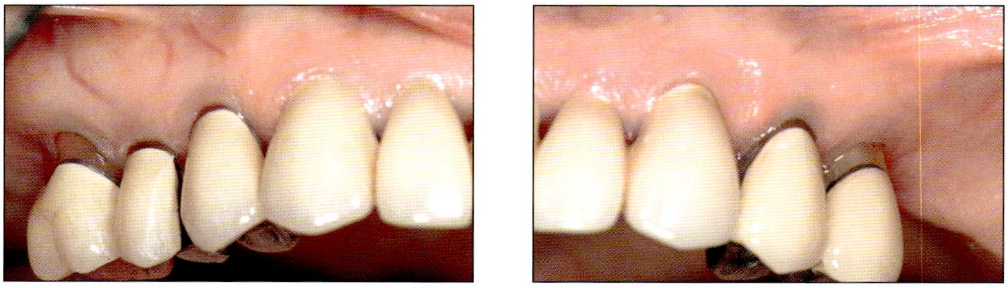

Pretreatment facial views.

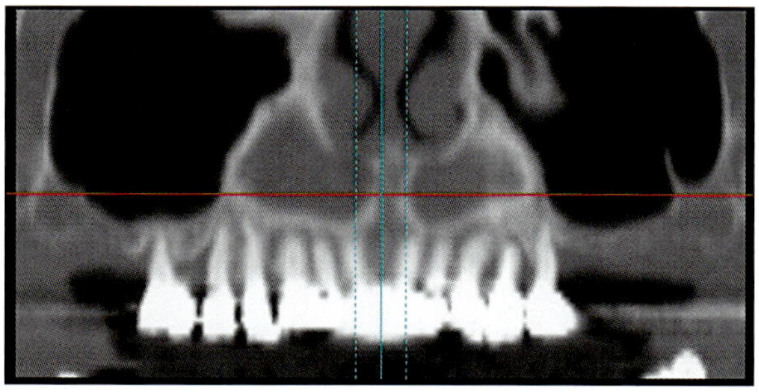

Initial panoramic CT scan used to diagnose, plan, and execute bilateral sinus bone grafting as well as extraction and socket grafting of all maxillary premolars and right first molar.

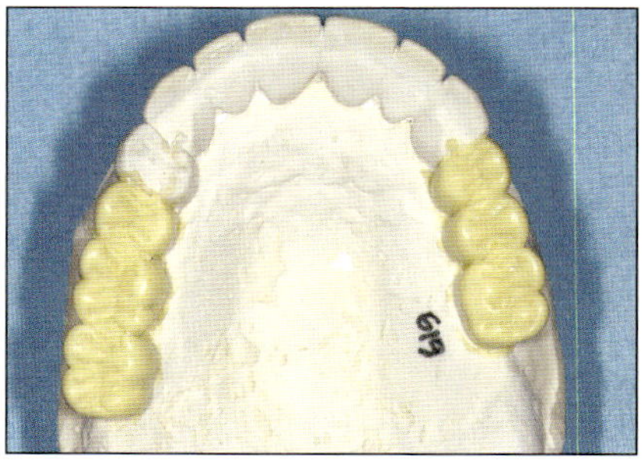

Postextraction diagnostic waxup to determine optimal final tooth positions.

PHASE II Scanning Appliance Fabrication

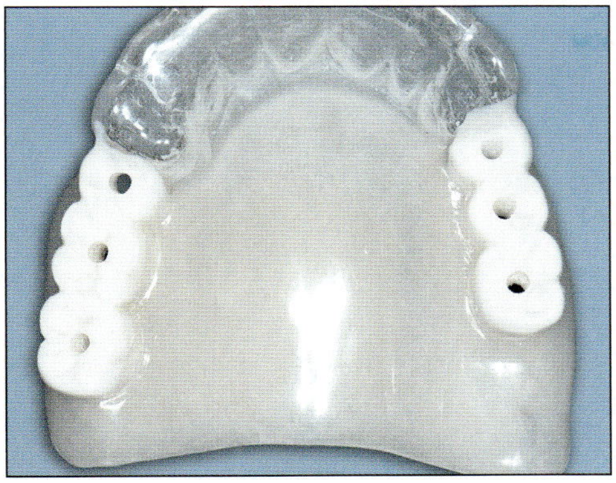

ScannoGuide representing optimal tooth positions.

PHASE III CT Scan and SimPlant Conversion

CT scans are taken, and the resulting DICOM files are processed into the SimPlant format. Masks of specific anatomic structures are created.

PHASE IV Eight-Step Treatment-Planning Process

Panoramic CT 9 months after sinus bone grafting with ScannoGuide in place.

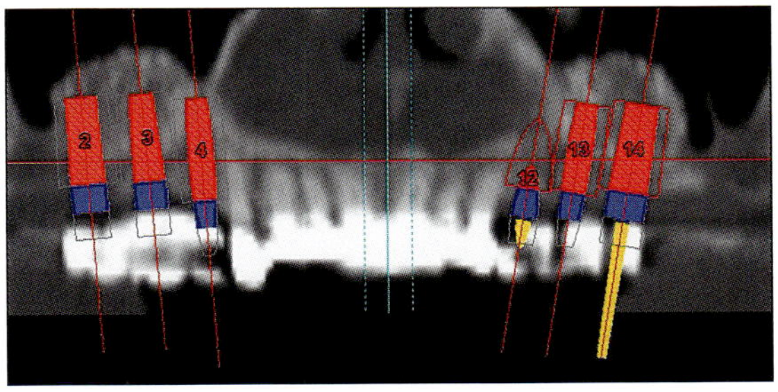

Maxillary 3D reconstruction and planning using SimPlant.

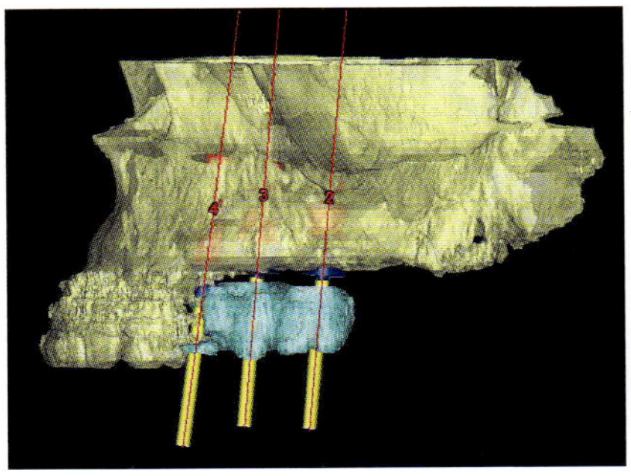

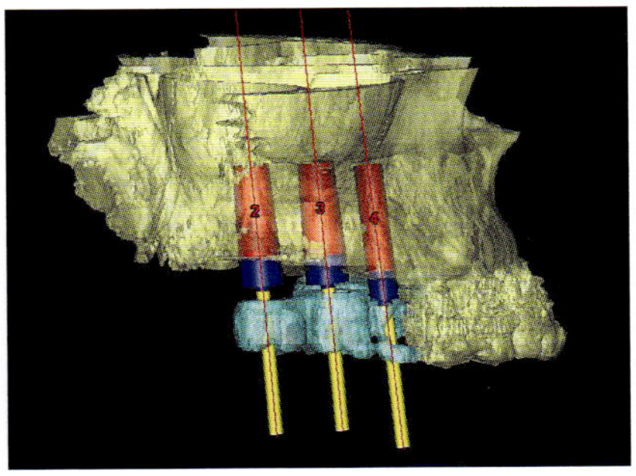

Superior view of 3D CT reconstruction demonstrating sinus bone graft augmentation *(red arrows)*.

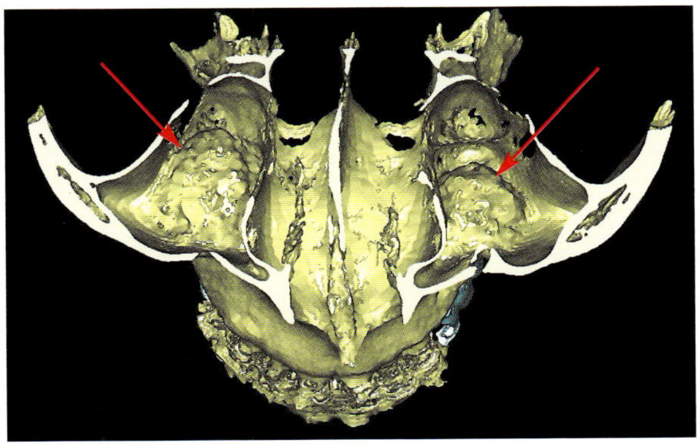

PHASE V Medical Modeling

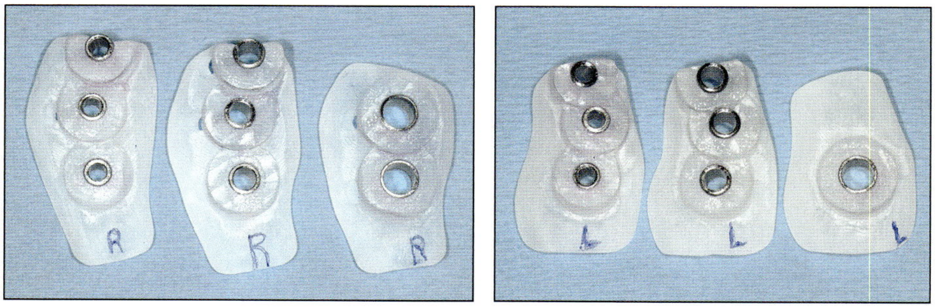

Bone-supported SurgiGuides.

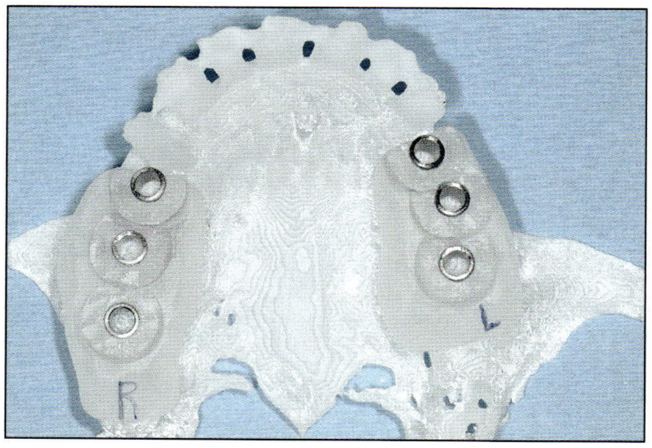

Medical model of maxilla with 3-mm SurgiGuides in place.

PHASE VI Surgery

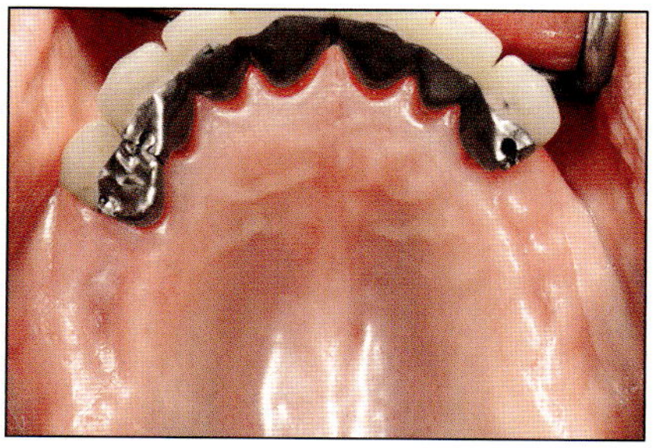

Clinical presentation before implant surgery.

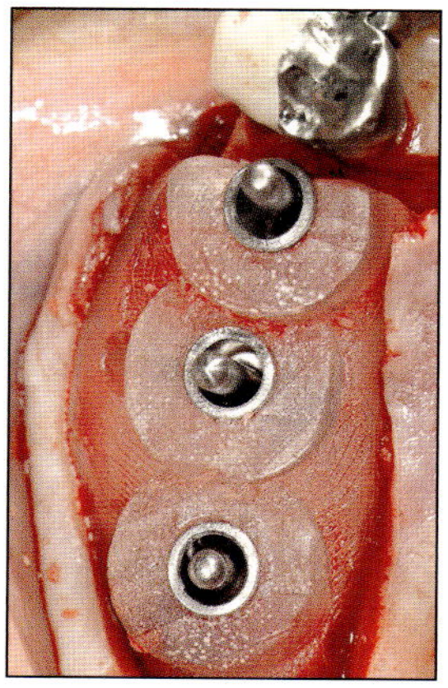

3-mm SurgiGuides.

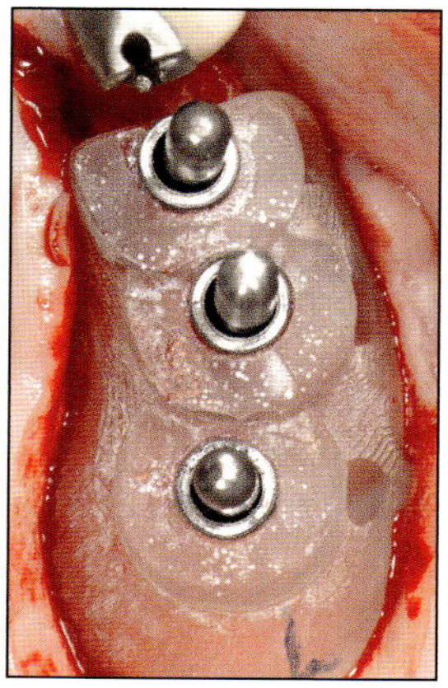

2-mm SurgiGuides.

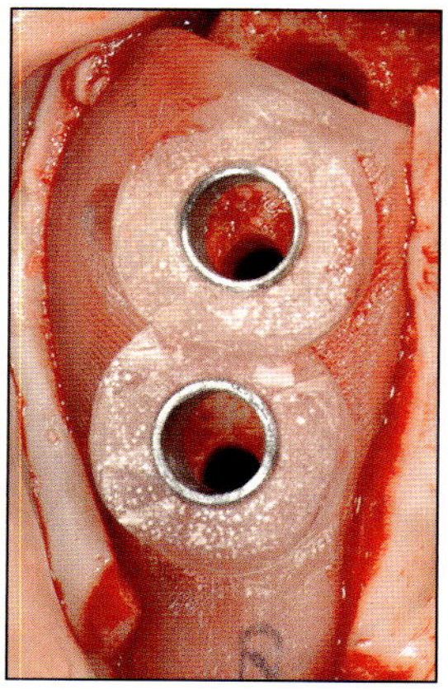

4.3-mm SurgiGuides.

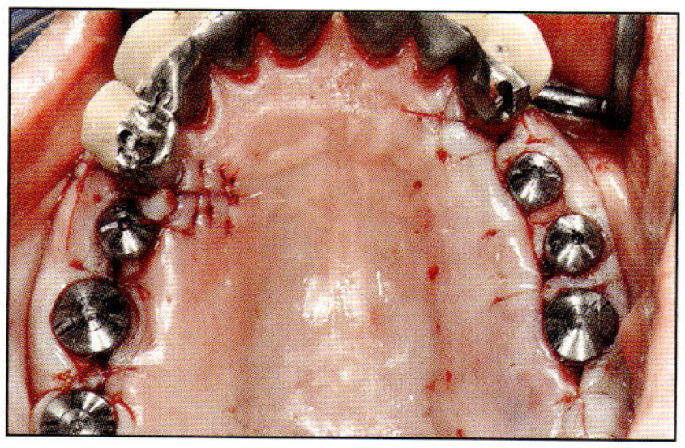

Clinical presentation following one-stage implant placement with healing abutments in place.

PHASE VII

Definitive Restoration and Supportive Maintenance

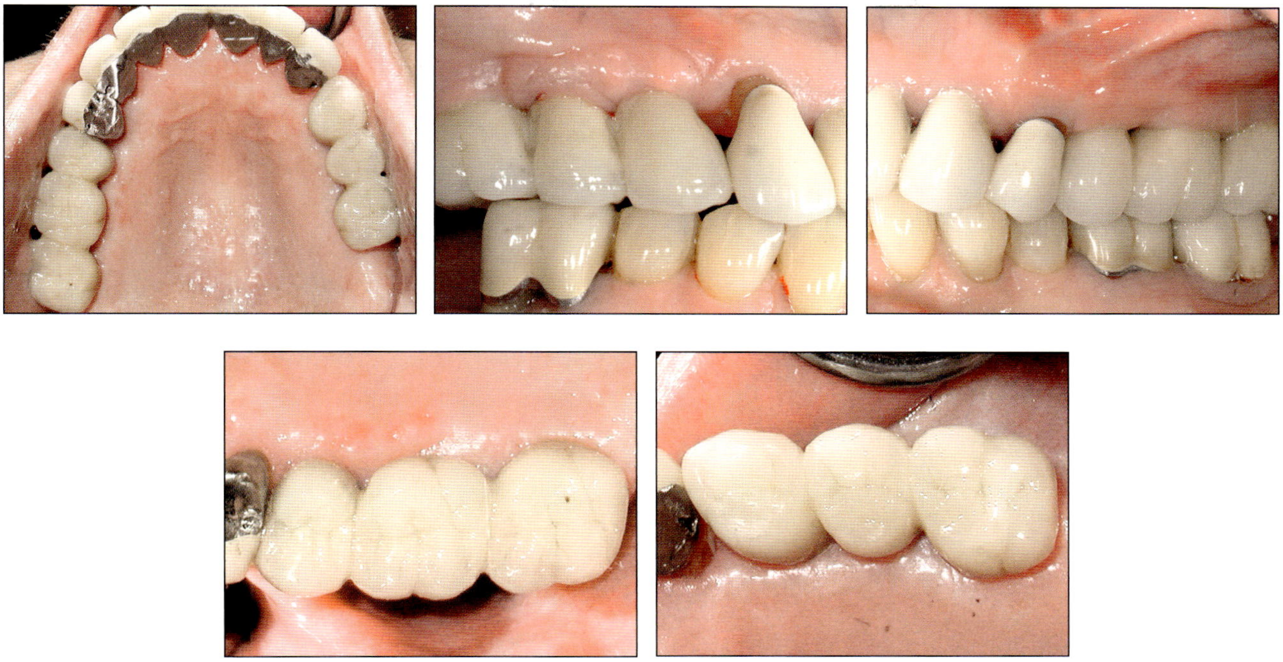

Clinical views of the definitive implant-supported fixed prostheses. (Restoration by Dr Stan Drab, Wheaton, IL.)

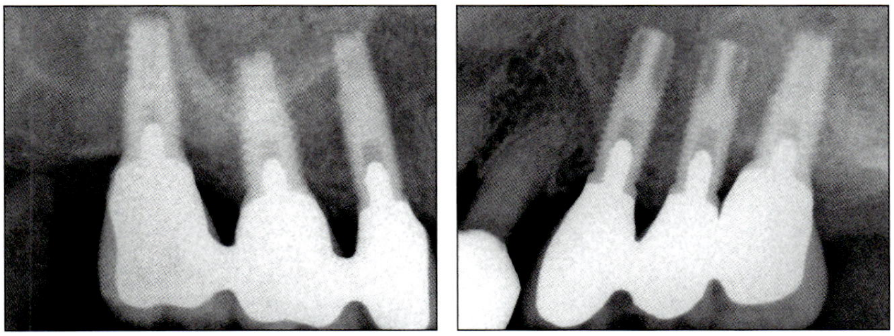

Radiographs of definitive prostheses.

Case 2 Mandibular Complete Edentulism

A 64-year-old man presented with the chief complaint of an ill-fitting and painful mandibular denture. He had been completely edentulous for 10 years. His medical history revealed controlled cardiovascular disease as the only significant finding. The patient's needs and concerns were to have a nonremovable implant-supported prosthesis.

Diagnoses

- Bilateral mental nerve dehiscence
- Class III skeletal malocclusion
- Advanced disuse atrophy of the edentulous mandible

Case type: 5

- Significant vertical and horizontal bone loss

Diagnostic inquiries

Clinical

- Optimal final tooth position
- Maxillomandibular relationship and occlusion

Radiographic

- Degree of sinus proximity
- Extent of vertical and horizontal bone loss
- Overall health of the maxillary sinuses
- Patency of osteomeatal complex

Physical

- None

Critical actions

- Trial tooth setup to determine proper maxillomandibular relationships for fabrication of accurate scanning appliance
- CT-based treatment planning
- Surgical dress rehearsal using stereolithographic model
- Preoperative prosthetic outcome determination: Fixed buccolingual cantilever prosthesis

PHASE I Initial Diagnostics

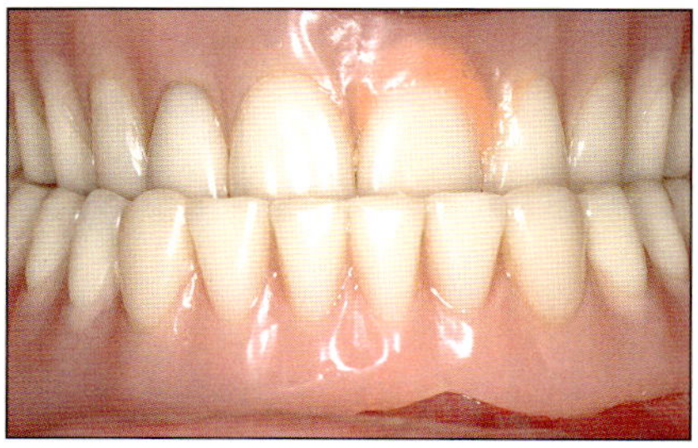
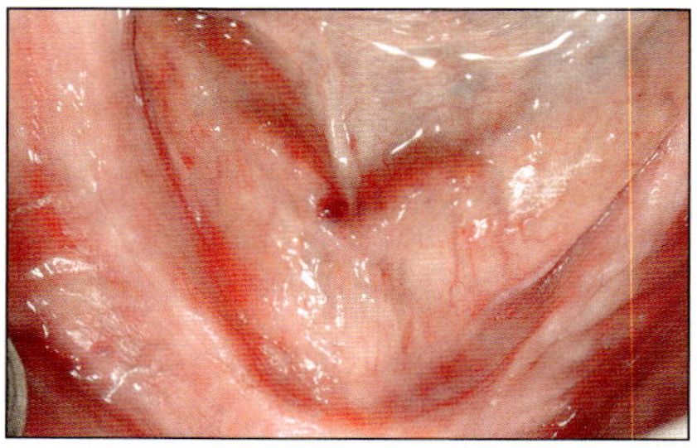

Initial presentation.

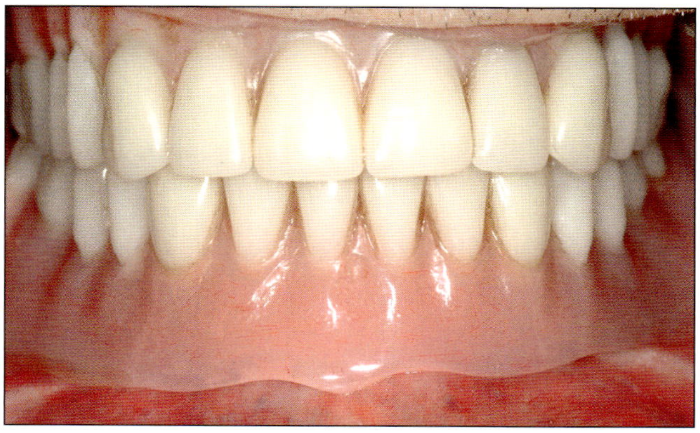

Newly constructed accurate dentures.

PHASE II Scanning Appliance Fabrication

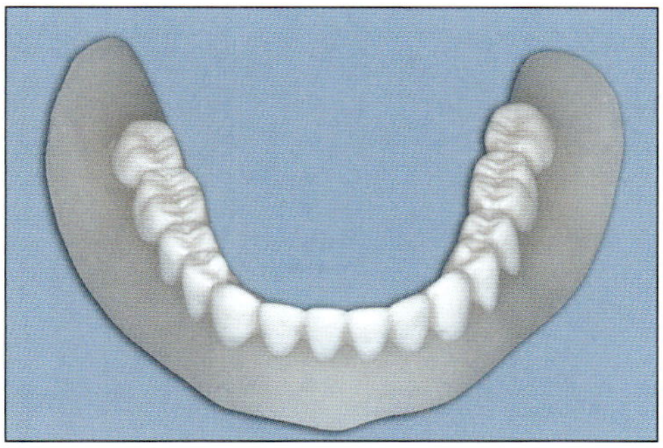

ScannoGuide reflecting new denture dimensions.

PHASE III CT Scan and SimPlant Conversion

CT scans are taken, and the resulting DICOM files are processed into the SimPlant format. Masks of specific anatomic structures are created.

PHASE IV Eight-Step Treatment-Planning Process

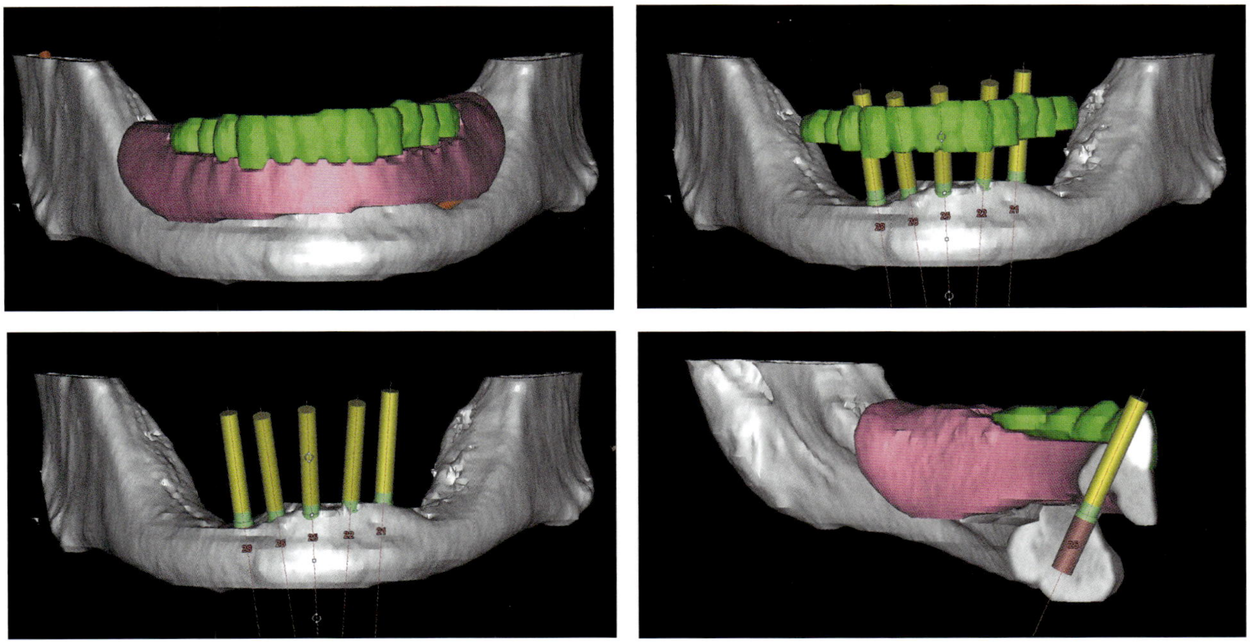

SimPlant planning. Masks of the mandible, denture base *(pink)*, denture teeth *(green)*, and proposed implant positions *(yellow)* can be seen.

PHASE V Medical Modeling

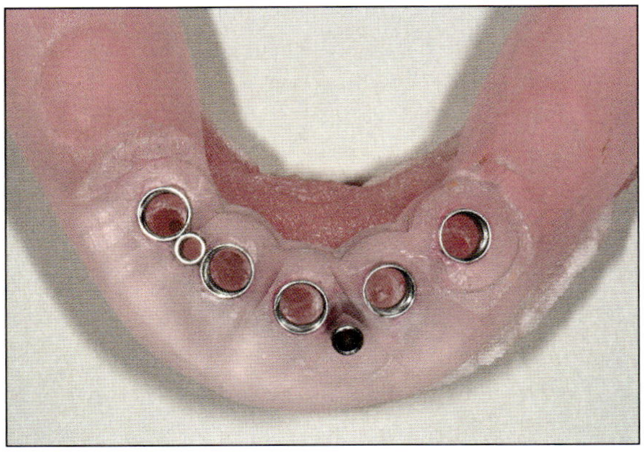

Mucosal SAFE SurgiGuide selected for surgery.

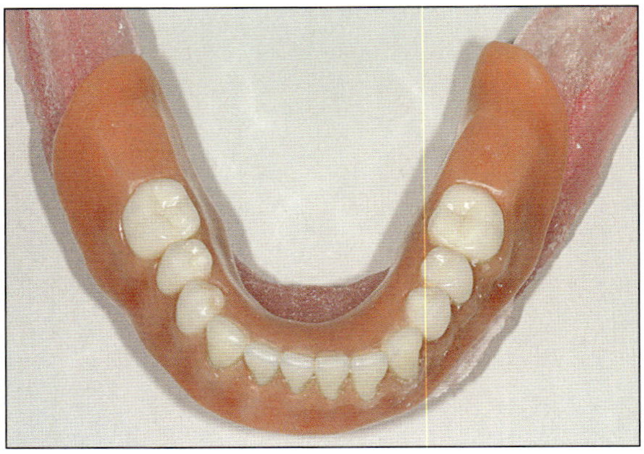

Denture seated on mucosal stereolithographic model.

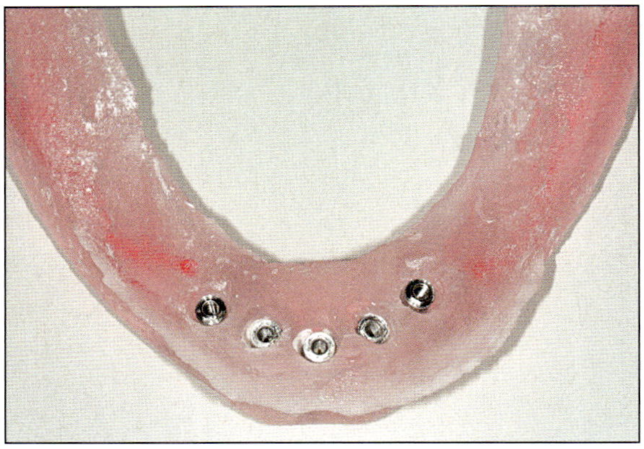

Implant analogues in place on mucosal model.

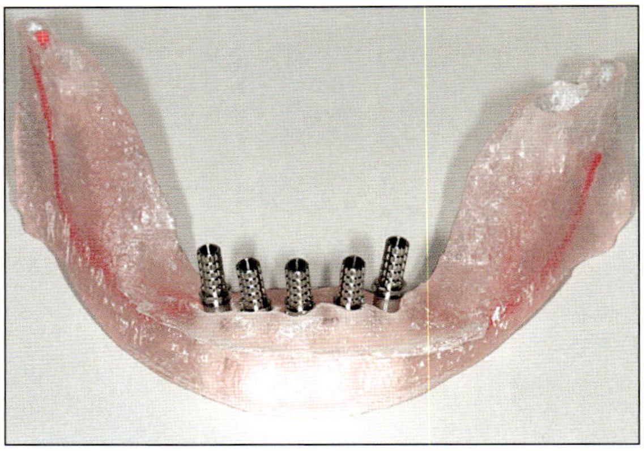

Abutments and temporary cylinders fixed to implant analogues in mucosal model. Note colorization of inferior alveolar nerves incorporated in mandibular model.

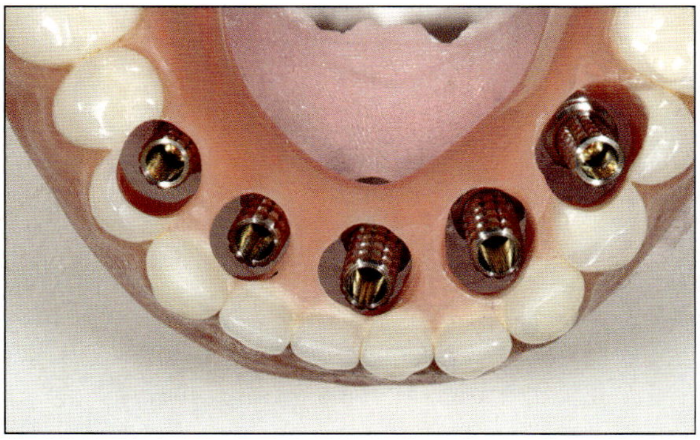

Mandibular denture converted to immediate-load prosthesis.

PHASE VI Surgery

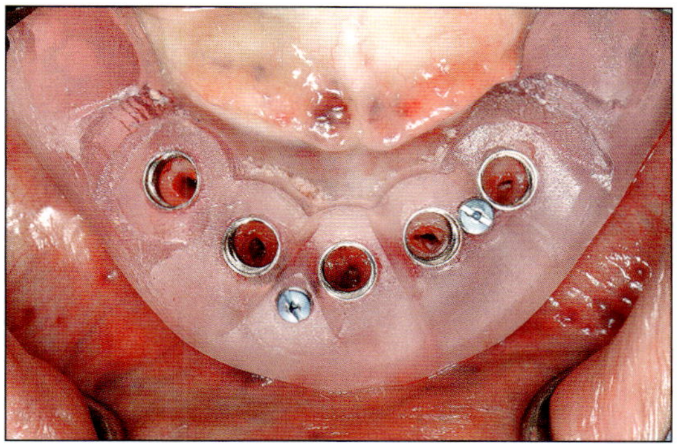

Mucosal SAFE SurgiGuide and two fixation pins in place.

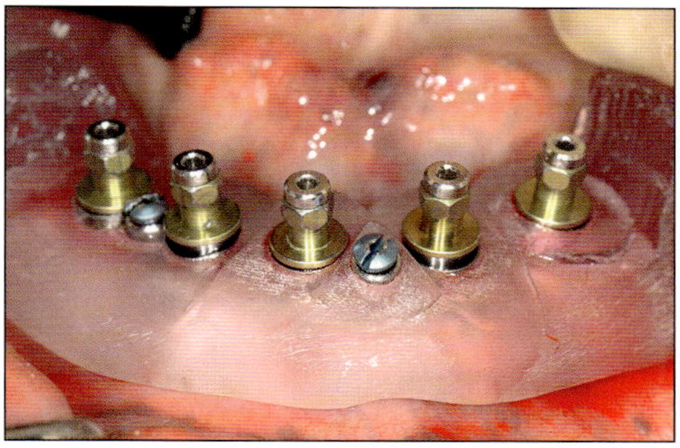

Implants placed using the SAFE delivery mounts.

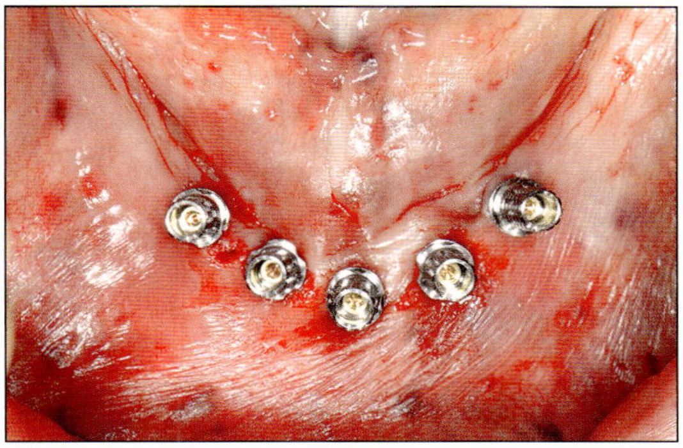

Completion of flapless implant surgery.

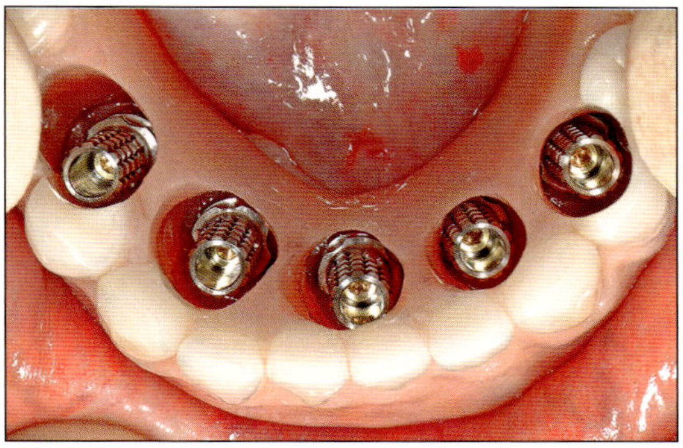

Preoperatively modified denture seated on the mandible, ready for conversion to immediate-load prosthesis.

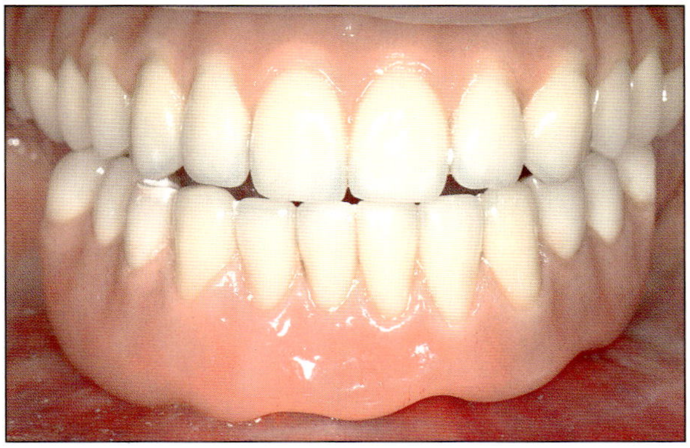

Completed immediate-load prosthesis. Note that the patient is in a protruded position as a result of local anesthesia.

PHASE VI

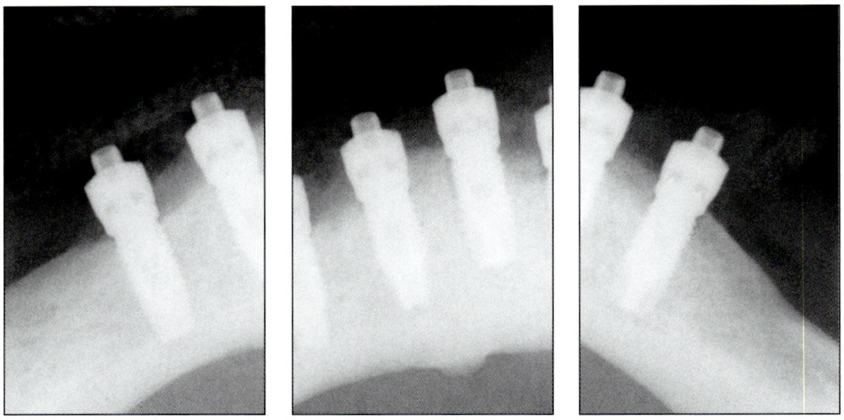

Radiographs obtained immediately following surgery.

PHASE VII

Definitive Restoration and Supportive Maintenance

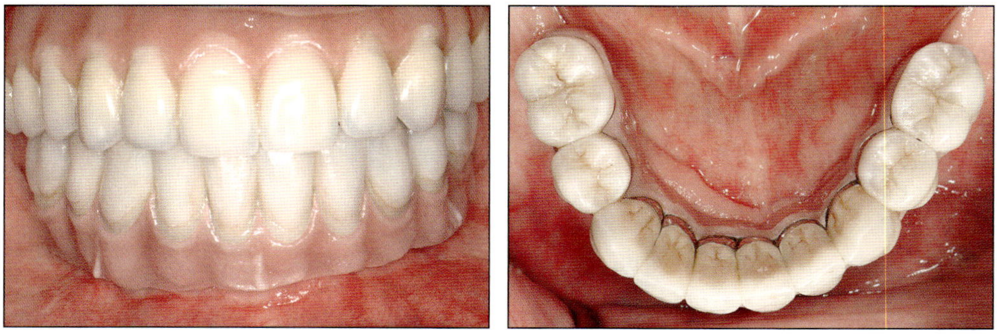

Definitive prosthesis in place. (Restoration by Dr Brian Vence, West Dundee, IL. Laboratory technician: David Guelde, CDT, Clarkston, MI.)

Case 3 Advanced Generalized Caries and Chronic Periodontitis

A 73-year-old man presented with the chief complaint of generalized advanced caries and an inability to eat comfortably. His medical history was complex. He had xerostomia due to the many medications he was taking. His dental history revealed caries-related tooth loss and progressive periodontitis, which was compromising his ability to maintain a stable prosthesis for any predictable period of time. The patient's needs and concerns were to have a stable-fitting implant-supported prosthesis that would be maintainable long term and allow him to eat comfortably.

Diagnoses

- Generalized early chronic periodontitis
- Class I maxillomandibular relationship
- Generalized caries
- Medication-induced xerostomia

Case type: 5

- Significant vertical and horizontal bone loss

Diagnostic inquiries

Clinical

- Influence of skeletal patterns on prosthesis design
- Influence of patient hygiene ability on prosthesis design

Radiographic

- Nerve proximity
- Extent of posterior atrophy
- Bone availability
- Bone quality

Physical

- Chronic obstructive pulmonary disease

Critical actions

- Extraction of maxillary dentition and placement of immediate maxillary denture for analysis of the mandibular arch
- Fabrication of an accurate mandibular denture, used to make a differential barium gradient scanning appliance 3 months after extractions
- Surgical dress rehearsal of mandibular immediate-load surgery using stereolithographic model
- Preoperative prosthetic outcome determination: Removable implant-supported prosthesis

PHASE I Initial Diagnostics

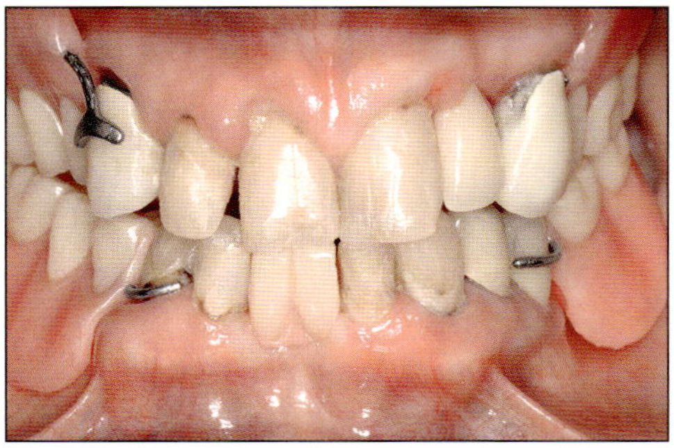

Pretreatment frontal view.

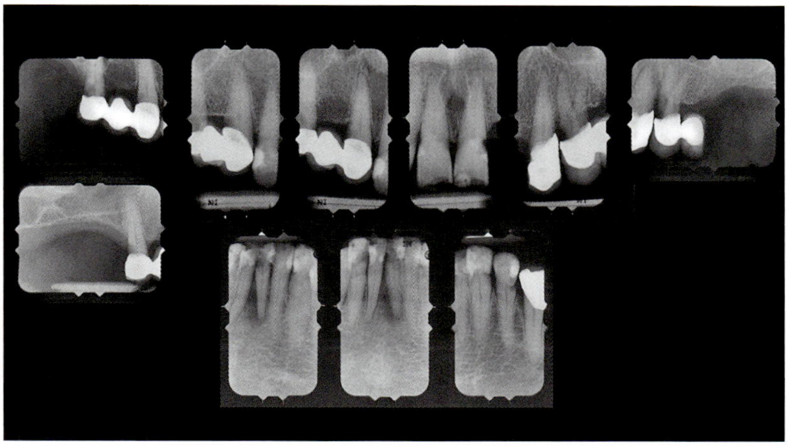

Pretreatment radiographs.

PHASE II

Scanning Appliance Fabrication

A third-generation scanning appliance, replicating the new partial denture, was created.

PHASE III

CT Scan and SimPlant Conversion

CT scans are taken, and the resulting DICOM files are processed into the SimPlant format. Masks of specific anatomic structures are created.

PHASE IV

Eight-Step Treatment-Planning Process

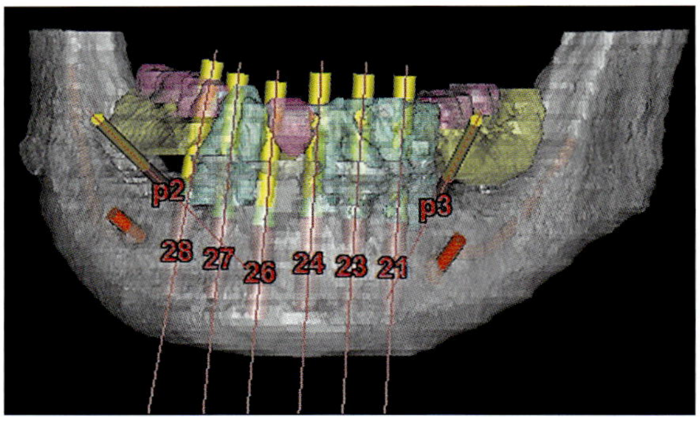

3D view of CT scan of the mandible with scanning appliance in place. The implants are planned apical to the existing tooth roots.

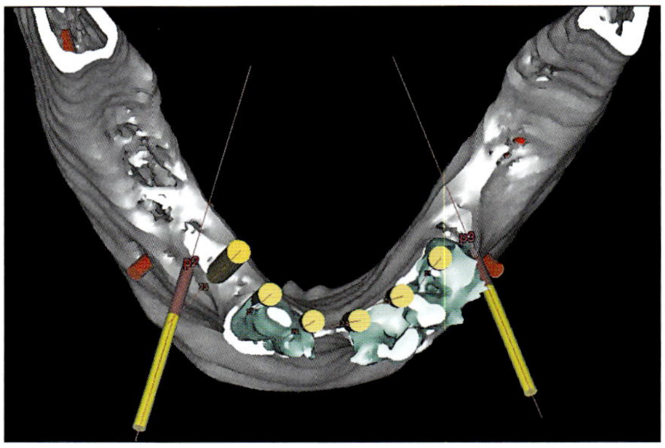

Occlusal view with masks of the denture base and teeth removed. Lateral fixation pins are planned to stabilize the guide.

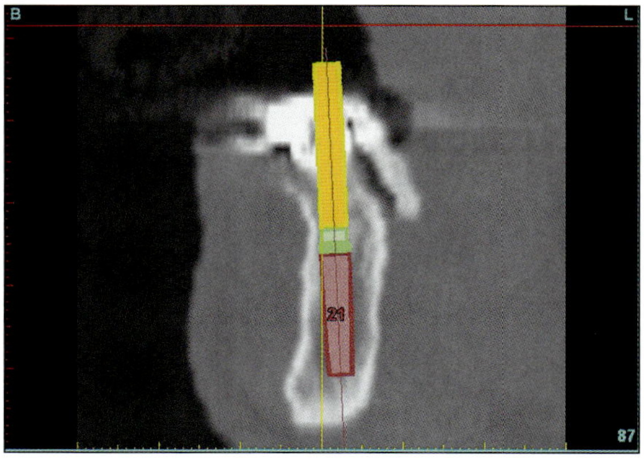

Cross-sectional view of the mandibular right central incisor.

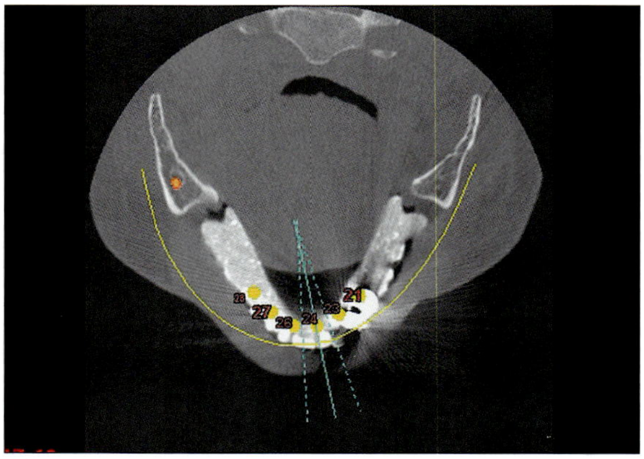

Axial view. The average bone quality at the planned implant sites was 454 Hounsfield units (type 3 to 4).

PHASE IV

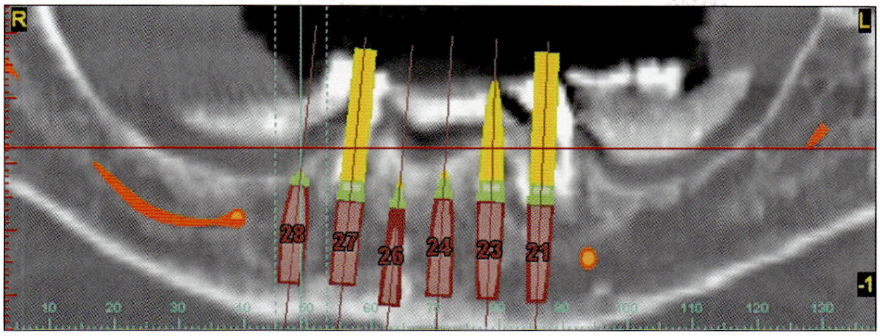

Panoramic view of the treatment plan.

PHASE V

Medical Modeling

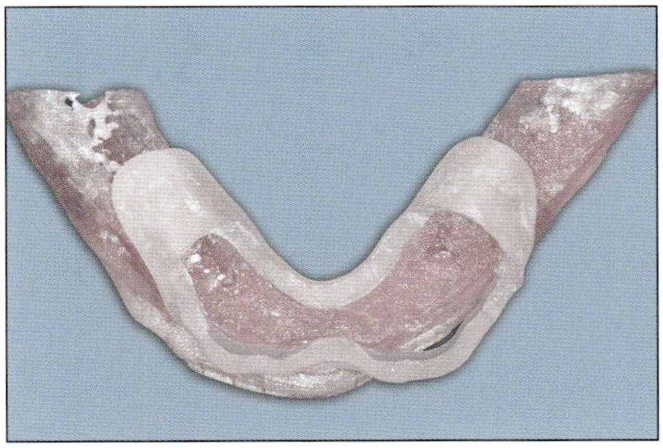

Mandibular model with bone reduction guide in place.

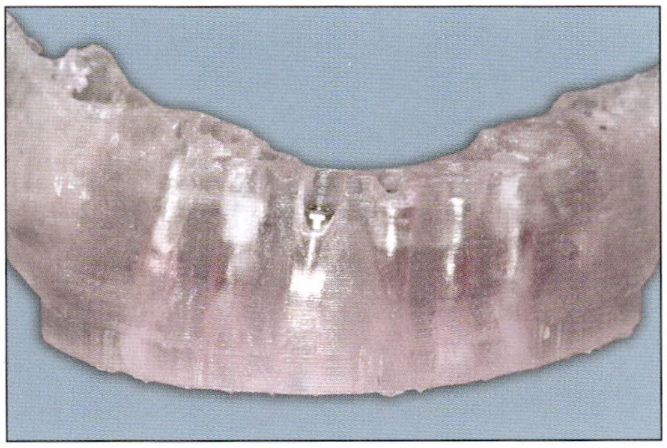

Model after bone reduction.

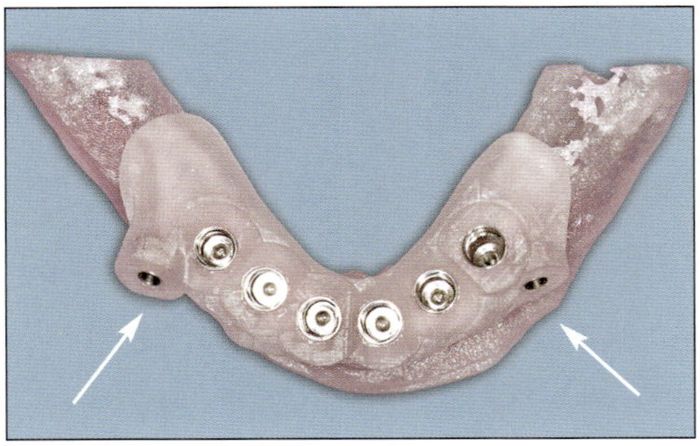

Lateral bone fixation positions *(white arrows)*.

PHASE VI

Surgery

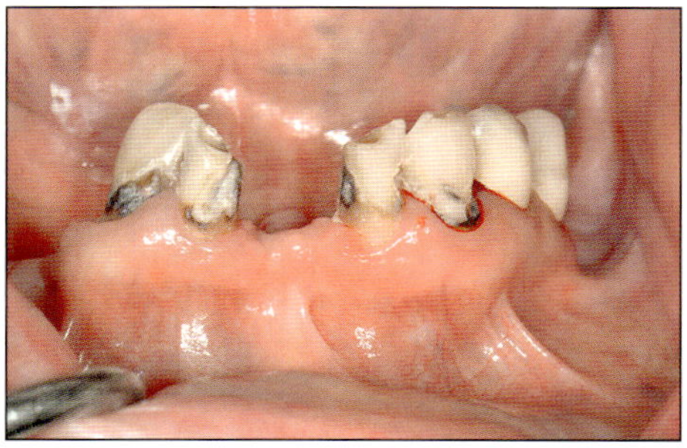

Initial view.

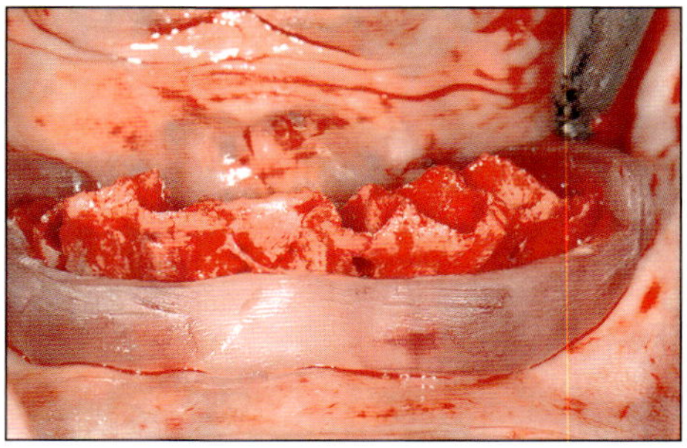

Clinical view following atraumatic extractions, open flap surgery, and bone reduction.

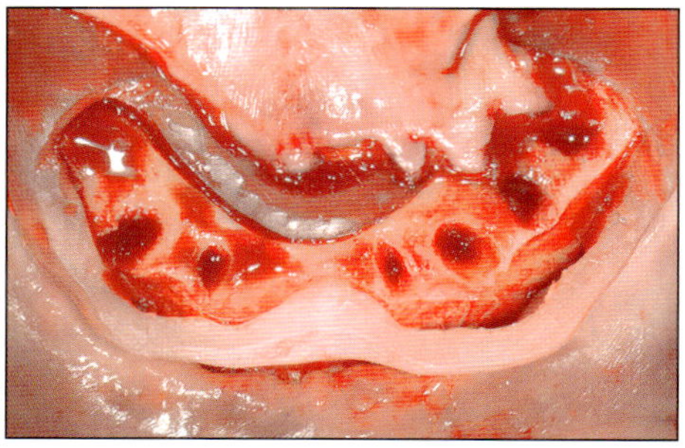

Precision osteoplasty has been performed.

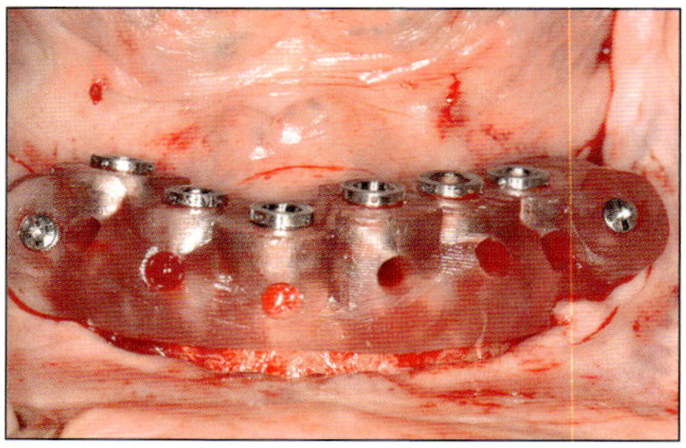

Bone-supported SAFE SurgiGuide fixed in place.

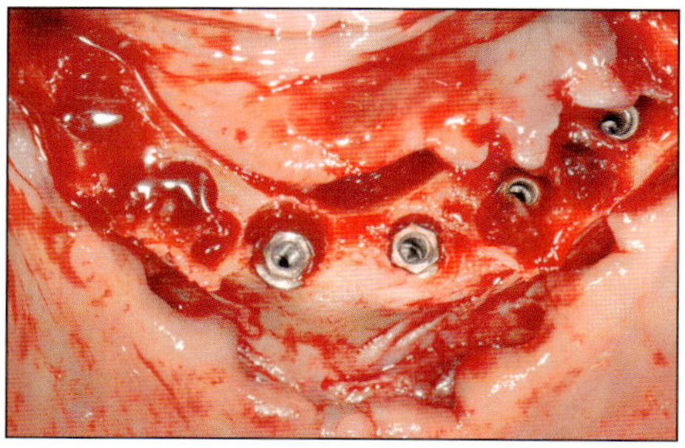

Placement of implants completed.

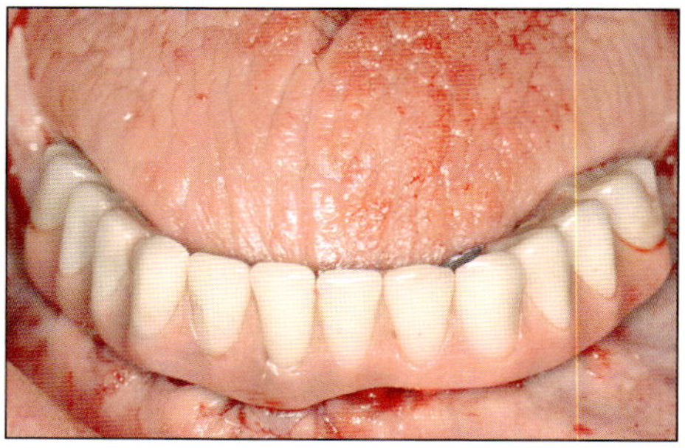

Immediate-load prosthesis completed.

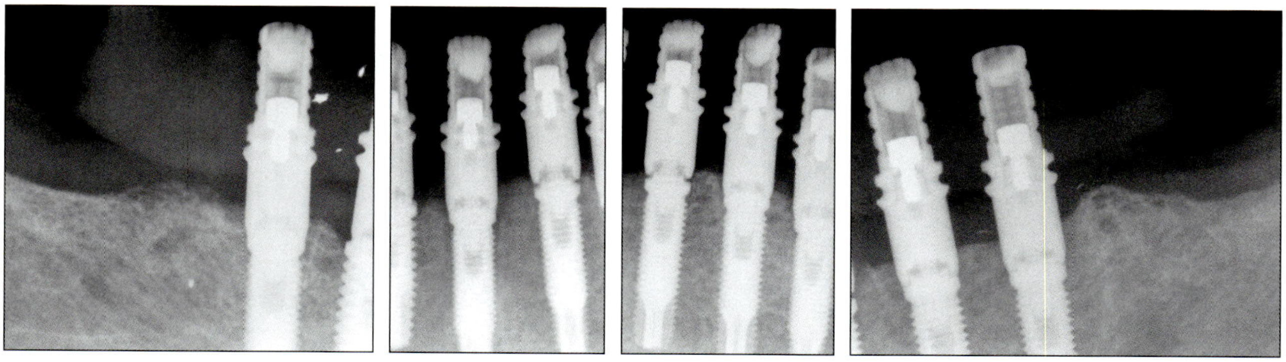

Radiographs immediately following surgery.

PHASE VII

Definitive Restoration and Supportive Maintenance

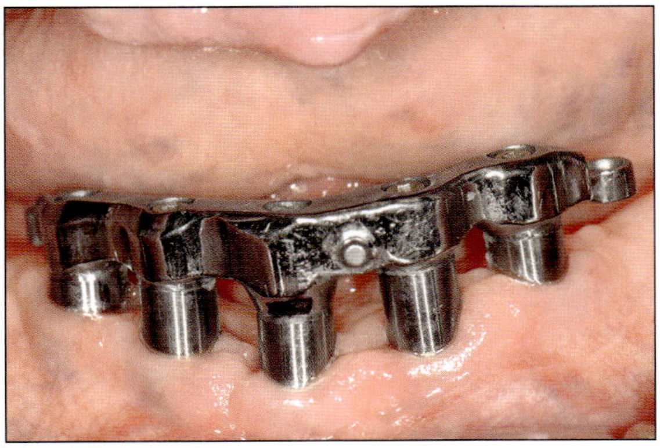

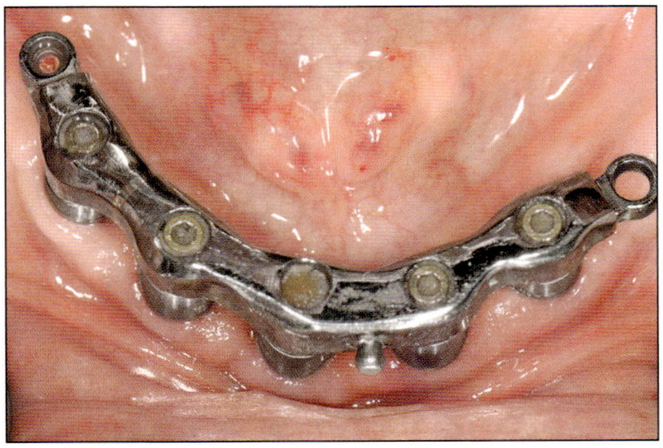

Bar connector and definitive removable implant-supported fixed prosthesis. (Restoration by Dr Brad Weiss, Evanston, IL.)

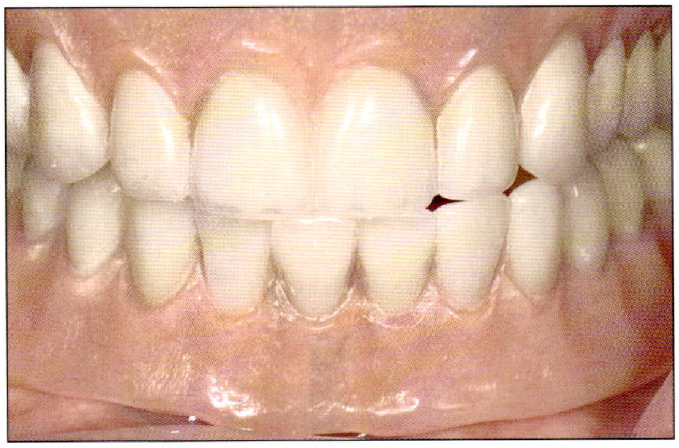

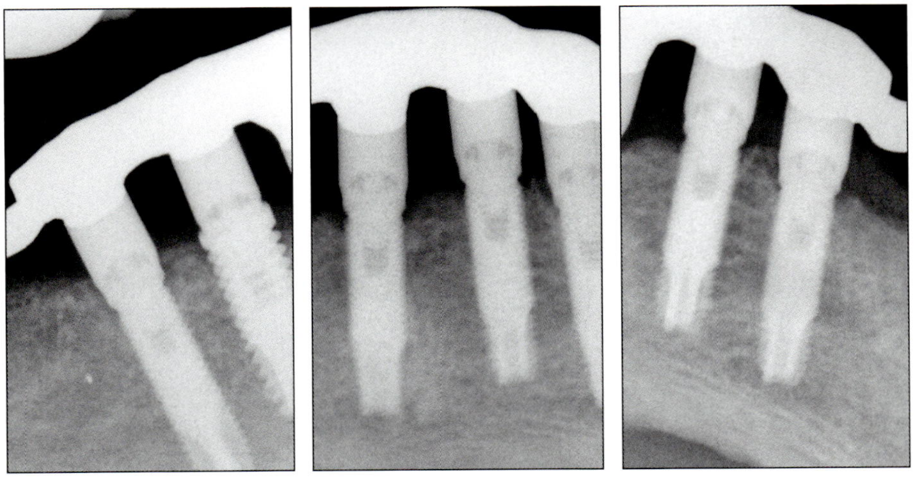

Final radiographs.

Case 4 Maxillary Anterior Trauma

A 76-year-old woman presented with the chief complaint of loose maxillary anterior teeth. She had recently fallen and traumatized the anterior maxilla and associated dentition. Pain on clinical mobility and suppurative exudate were noted at the maxillary right central and lateral incisors on examination. Her medical history was significant for controlled cardiovascular disease as well as mitral valve prolapse with regurgitation. The patient's needs and concerns were to have a stable-fitting implant-supported prosthesis that would be maintainable long term and be as similar to her natural dentition as possible.

Diagnoses

- Maxillary right anterior alveolar fracture
- Partial avulsion of maxillary right incisors
- Enamel fracture of all incisors
- Class I maxillomandibular relationship

Case type: 3
- Horizontal bone loss in the form of fractured alveoli

Diagnostic inquiries

Clinical
- Extent of alveolar bone loss and fracture
- Infection/exudate at the maxillary right incisors

Radiographic
- Extent of maxillary bone fractures
- Position of nasopalatine foramen and canal
- Position of nasal sinus

Physical
- None

Critical actions

- Immediate treatment of infection
- Preservation and/or augmentation of alveoli following extraction of hopeless teeth
- Diagnosis and prognosis of maxillary left incisors
- Fabrication of an accurate scanning appliance representing accurate final tooth position
- CT-based treatment planning
- Preoperative prosthetic outcome determination: Fixed implant-supported prosthesis

PHASE I Initial Diagnostics

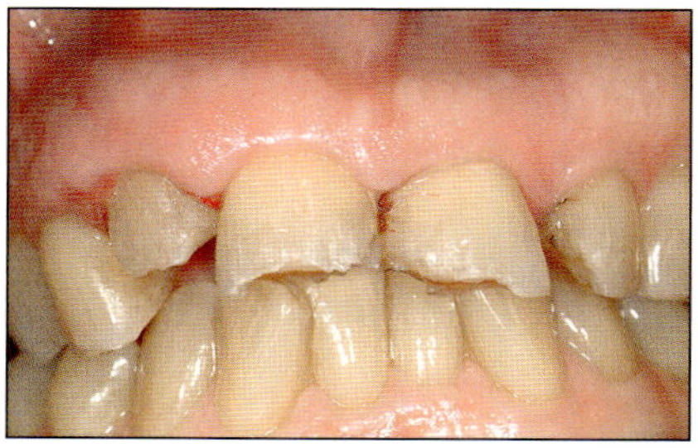
Initial presentation. Note the fractured and nonrestorable maxillary right incisors.

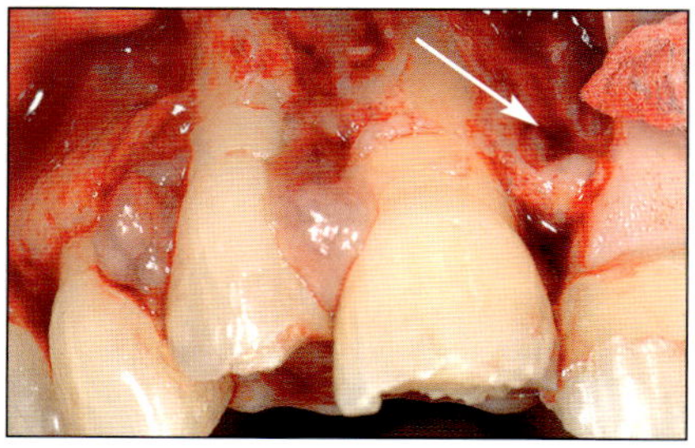
Emergency-based open flap surgery. Note the interseptal bone fracture between the maxillary central incisors *(arrow)*.

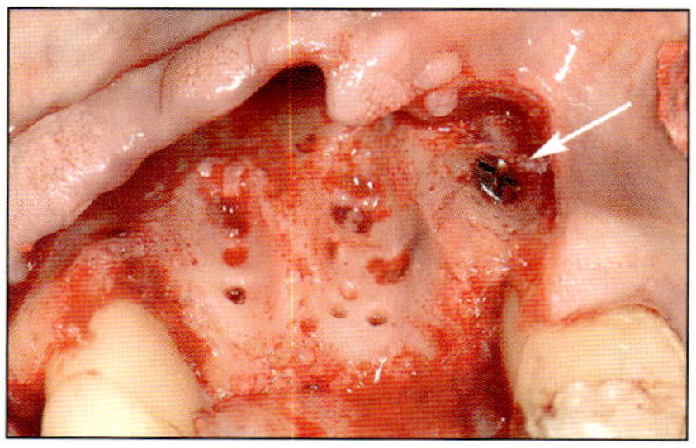
Following extraction of hopeless teeth and stabilization of the fractured interseptal bone. Note the bone fixation screw *(arrow)*.

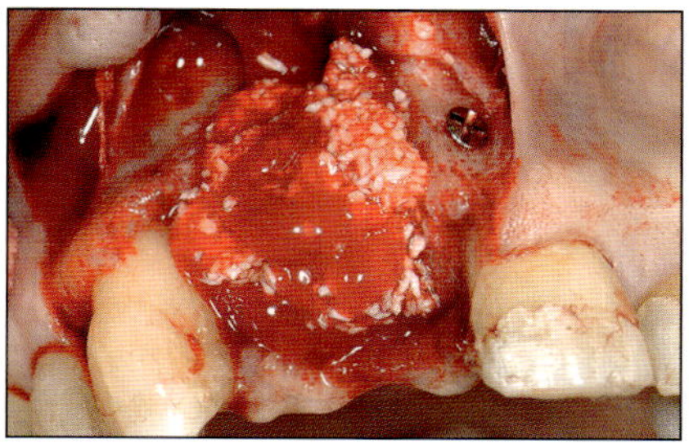

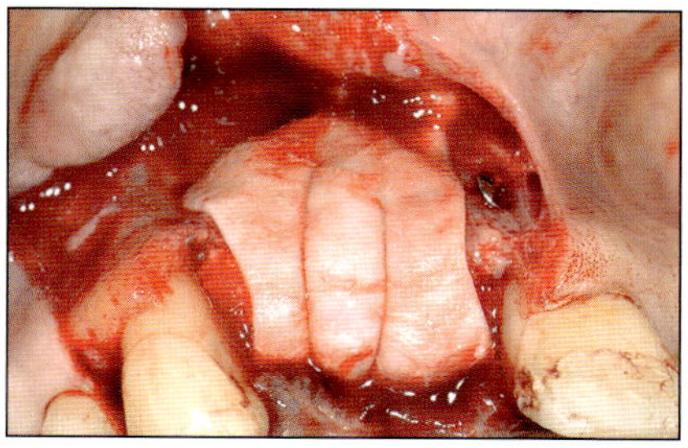
Guided bone regeneration is accomplished in the maxillary right incisor area via particulate composite bone grafting and placement of a membrane.

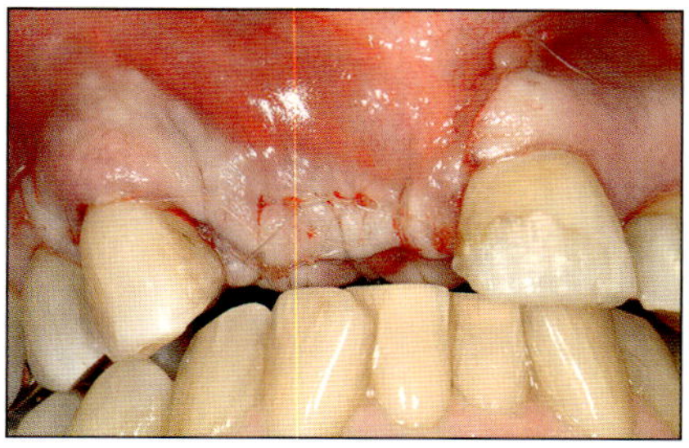
Following suturing.

PHASE II Scanning Appliance Fabrication

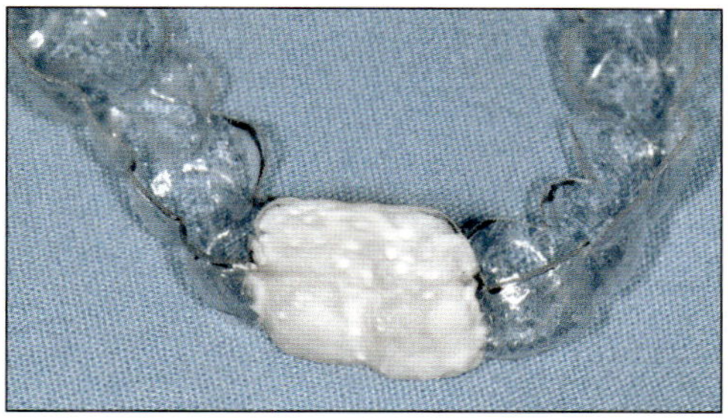

Second-generation scanning appliance reflecting accurate tooth position based on the diagnostic waxup.

PHASE III CT Scan and SimPlant Conversion

CT scans are taken, and the resulting DICOM files are processed into the SimPlant format. Masks of specific anatomic structures are created.

PHASE IV Eight-Step Treatment-Planning Process

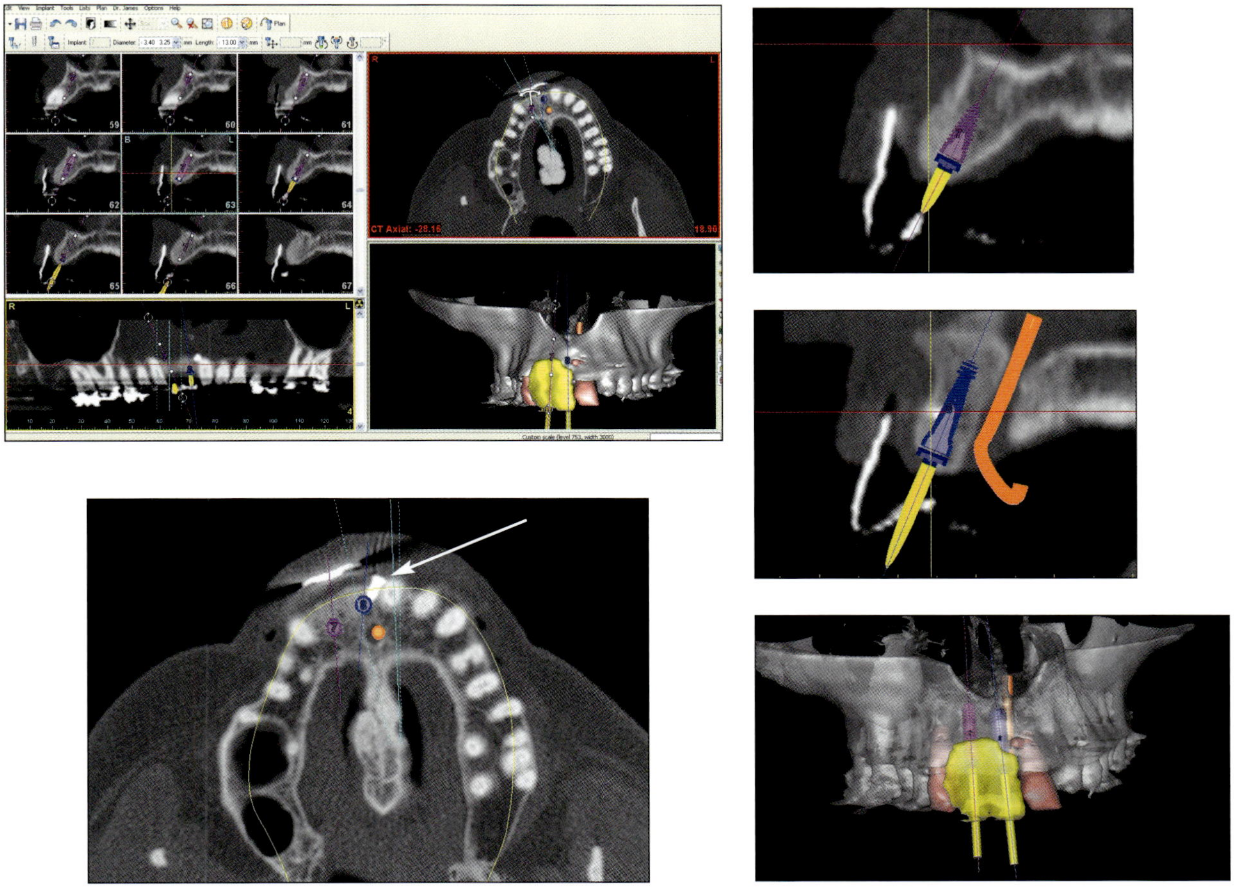

Preoperative planning for implant placement. Note the presence of the bone fixation screw *(arrow)*, which was used to stabilize the fractured bone segment at the emergency surgery.

PHASE V Medical Modeling

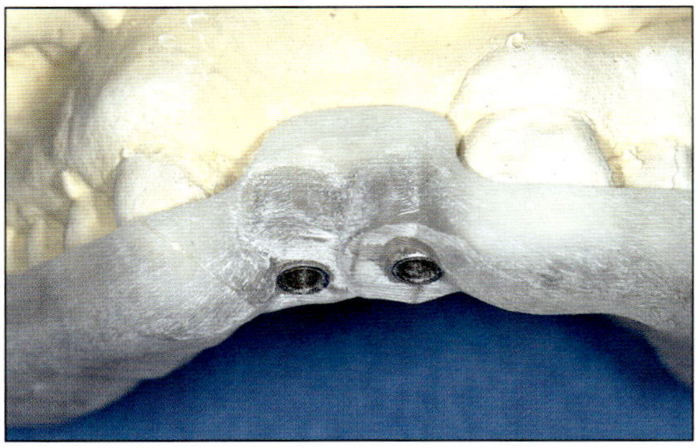

Tooth-supported SurgiGuide selected for surgery.

PHASE VI Surgery

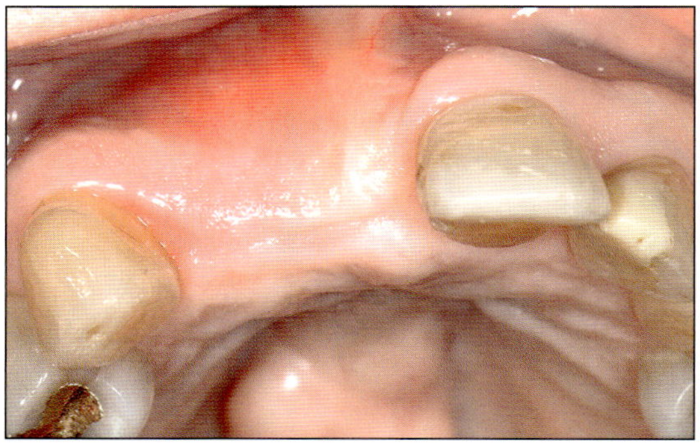

Clinical occlusal view prior to implant placement, 6 months following emergency surgery. The tissues have healed following guided bone regeneration procedures.

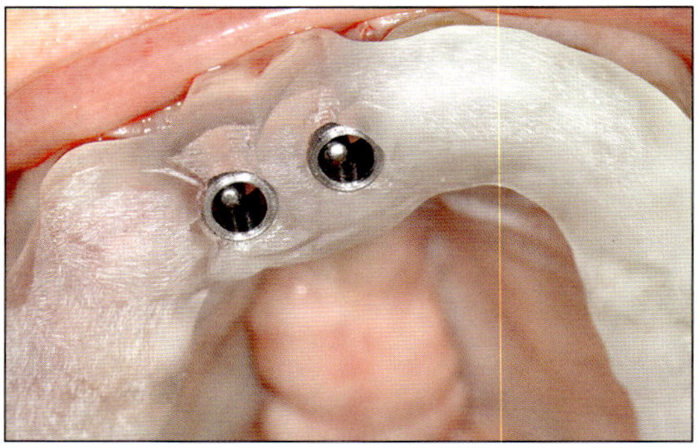

SurgiGuide in place at the 3-mm osteotomy site level. The guide pins are in place, verifying the 3D position of the guide.

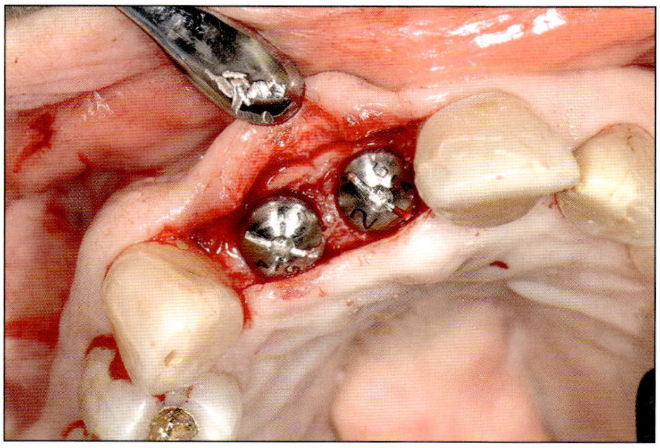

The implants have been placed using a one-stage surgical approach.

PHASE VII

Definitive Restoration and Supportive Maintenance

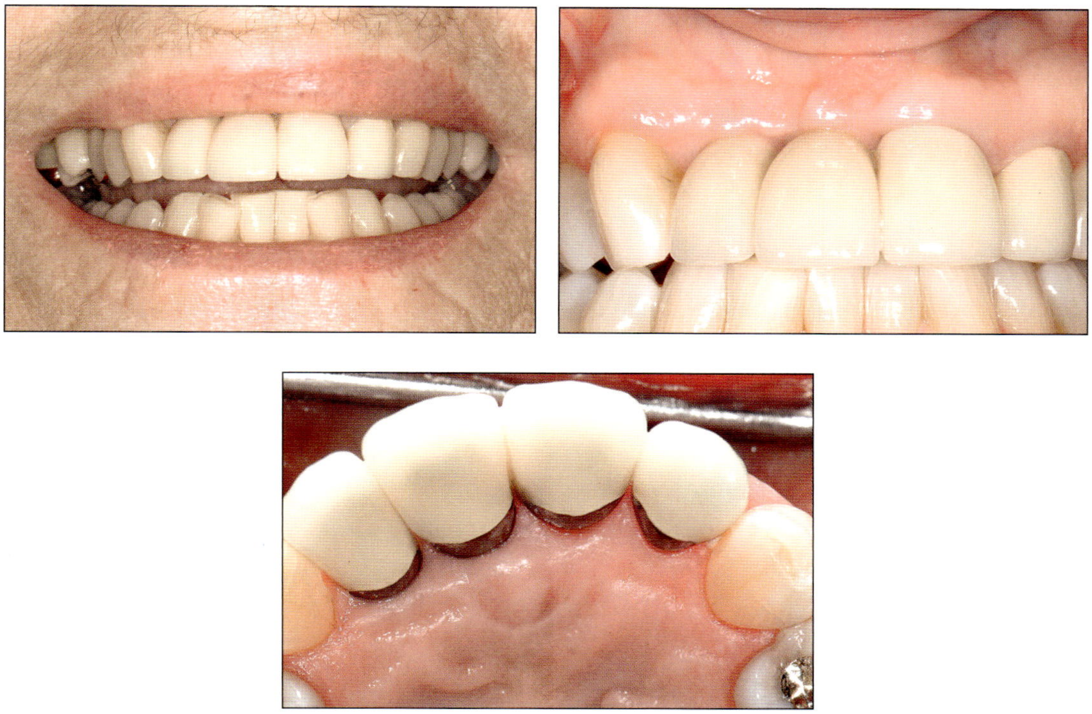

Clinical views of the definitive implant-supported fixed prosthesis. (Restoration by Dr Michael Criscione, Skokie, IL.)

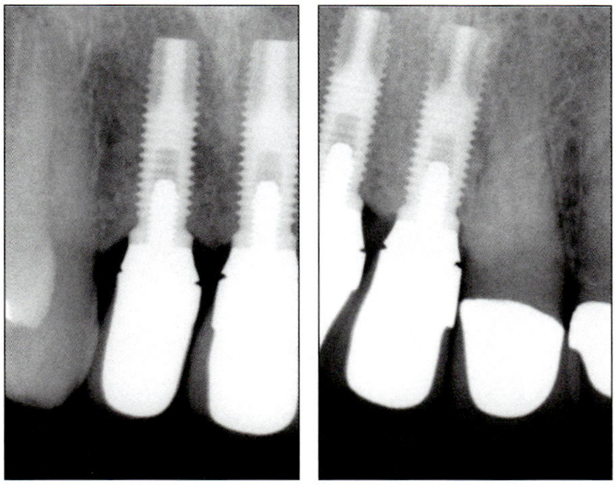

Radiographs of the implants and definitive prosthesis.

Case 5 Mandibular Complete Edentulism

A 68-year-old woman presented with the chief complaint of loose dentures, which impaired her ability to eat comfortably and made her feel self-conscious. Her medical history revealed asthma and controlled cardiovascular disease. She was a smoker with a 40-pack/year history. Her dental history revealed that she had been completely edentulous for 2 years due to progressive periodontitis, a condition she had for 30 years. In addition, unsuccessful implant placement 2 years previously resulted in preprosthetic implant failure, and she was extremely afraid of having the same experience. The patient's needs and concerns were to have a stable prosthesis that would restore esthetics and function without pain.

Diagnoses

- Bilateral mental nerve dehiscence
- Class I skeletal occlusion
- Abnormal disuse atrophy of the edentulous mandible
- Advanced posterior residual ridge resorption

Case type: 5

- Significant vertical and horizontal bone loss

Diagnostic inquiries

Clinical

- Accurate denture verified
- Accurate scanning appliance fabricated

Radiographic

- Nerve dehiscence
- 10 mm of unusable bone height in the anterior mandible based on severe buccolingual bone position discrepancy
- Advanced bilateral posterior disuse atrophy

Physical

- None

Critical actions

- Creation of accurate mandibular denture, which will be duplicated to fabricate a scanning appliance
- CT-based treatment planning
- Surgical dress rehearsal using stereolithographic medical model
- Preoperative prosthetic outcome determination: Removable or fixed implant-supported prosthesis (patient desired flexibility between the two options prior to definitive prosthetic phase)

PHASE I Initial Diagnostics

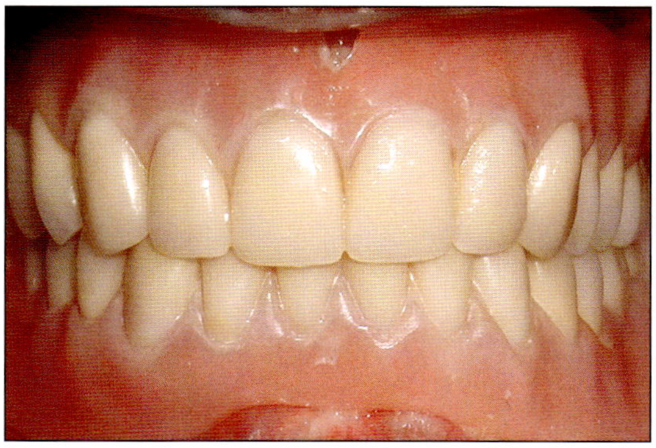

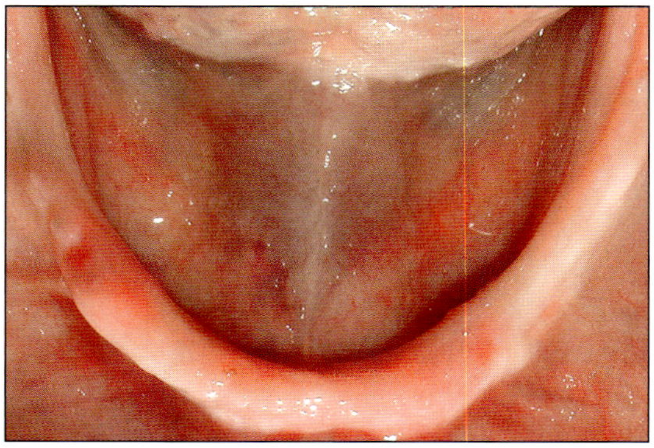

Pretreatment frontal and occlusal views.

PHASE II Scanning Appliance Fabrication

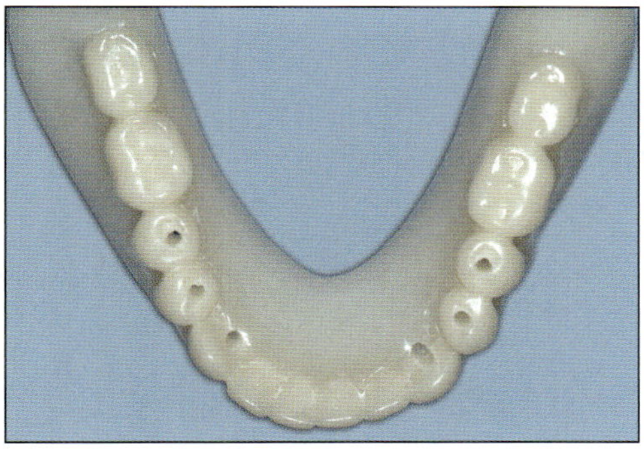

Scanning appliance based on accurate denture setup.

PHASE III CT Scan and SimPlant Conversion

CT scans are taken, and the resulting DICOM files are processed into the SimPlant format. Masks of specific anatomic structures are created.

PHASE IV Eight-Step Treatment-Planning Process

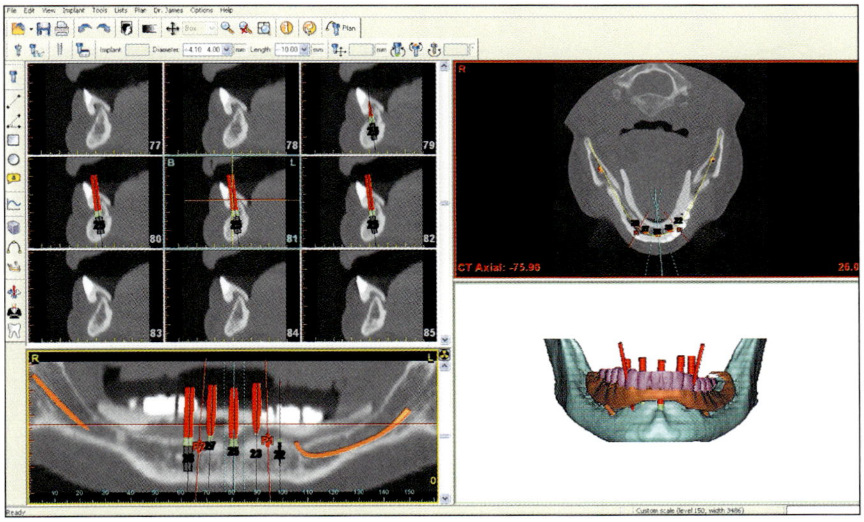

Overview of SimPlant plan, based on CT scans of the mandible with the scanning appliance in place.

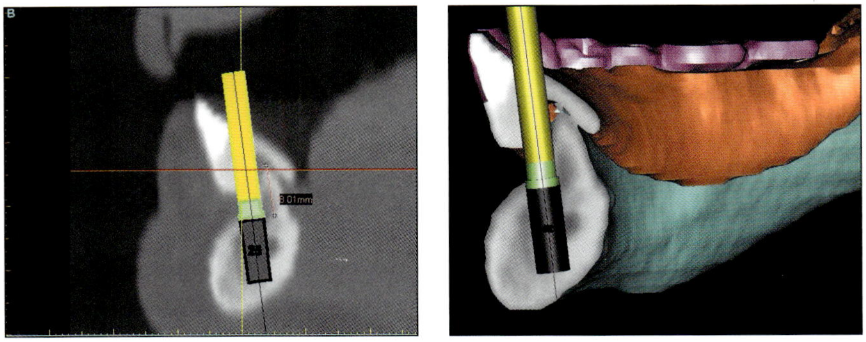

The buccolingual bone height discrepancy is revealed, and it is determined that an open flap surgical approach will be needed.

PHASE IV

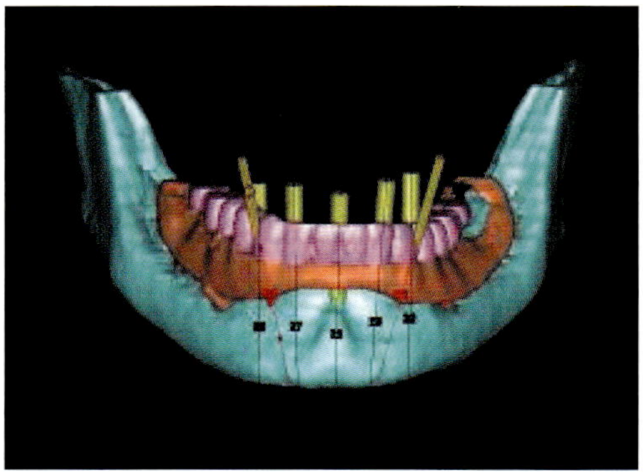
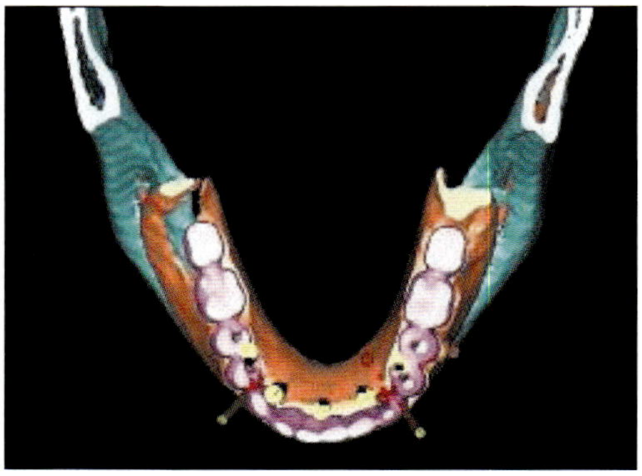

All masks have been incorporated: bone, denture base, teeth, implants, and nerves.

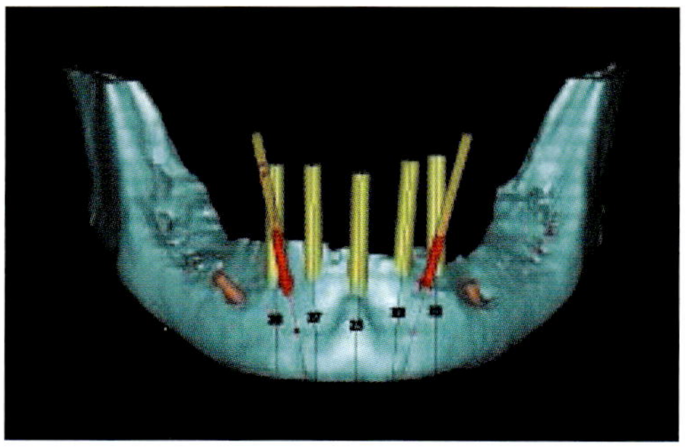

Note the planned stabilization pins *(red)*.

PHASE V Medical Modeling

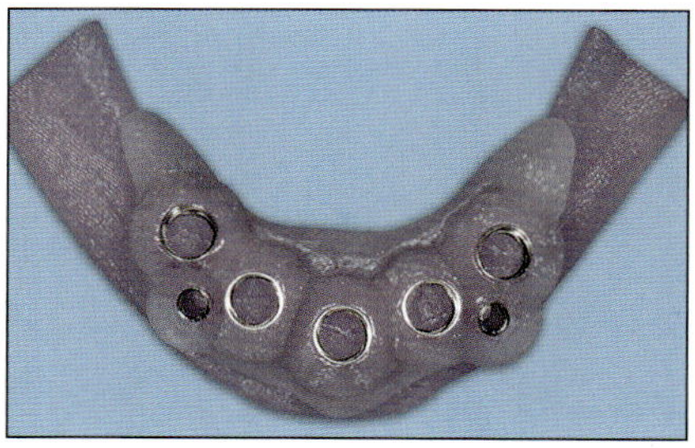

Bone-supported SAFE SurgiGuide selected for surgery.

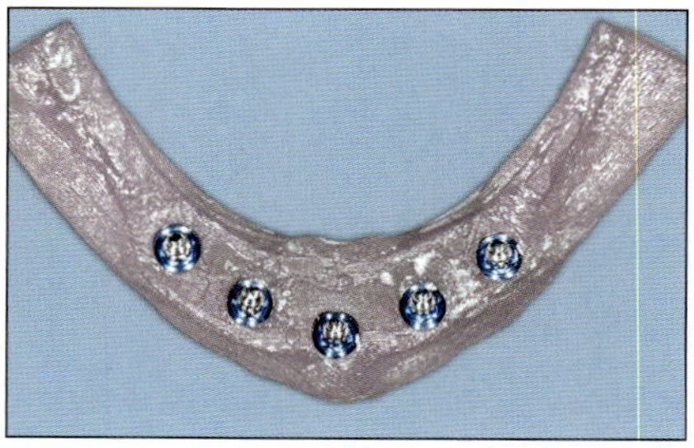

Medical model with implant analogues in place.

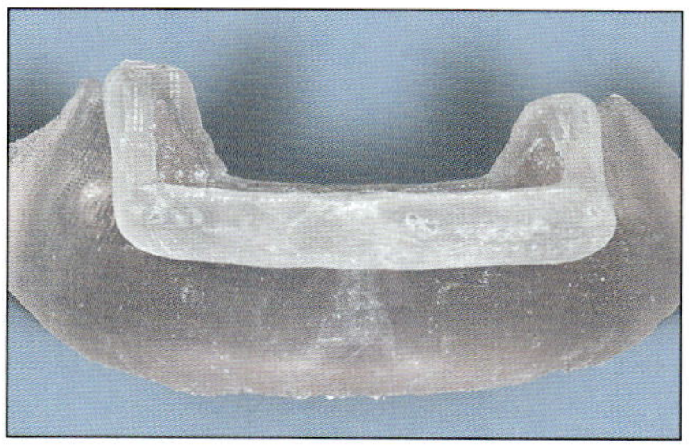

Bone reduction guide.

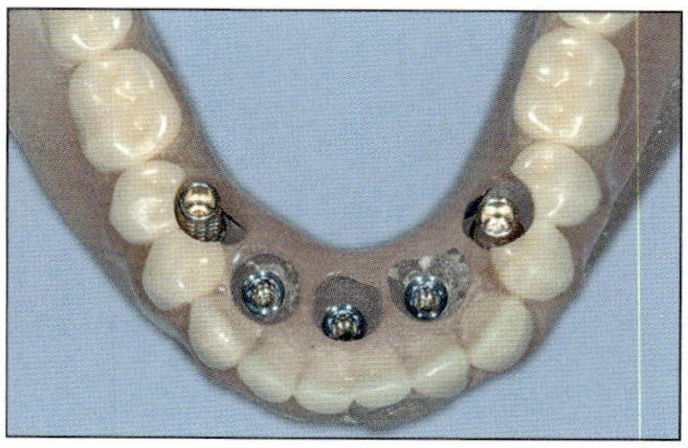

The denture planned for immediate loading, following modification on the medical model during the surgical dress rehearsal.

PHASE VI

Surgery

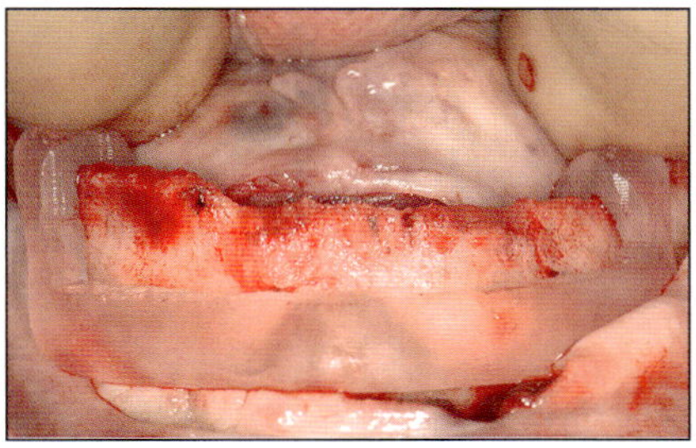

Initiation of open flap surgery. The bone reduction guide is in place.

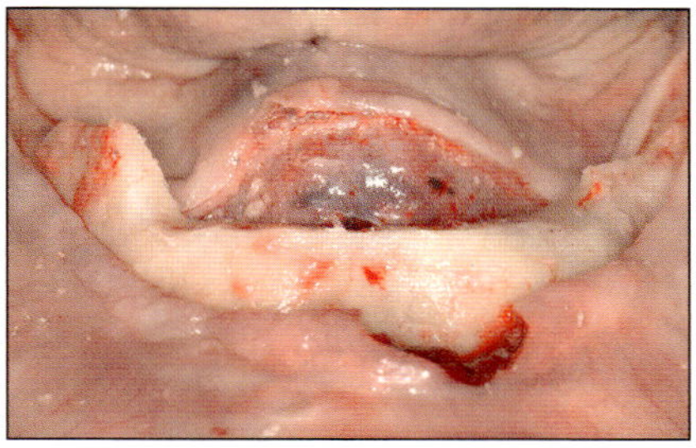

Precision osteoplasty has been performed to reduce the buccolingual bone height discrepancy.

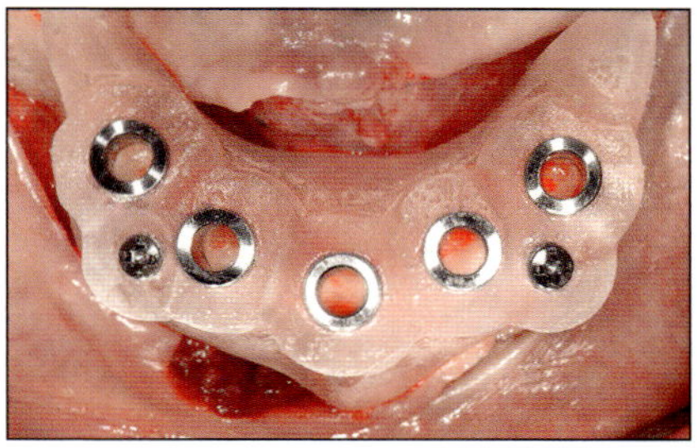

SAFE SurgiGuide fixed in place with two stabilization pins.

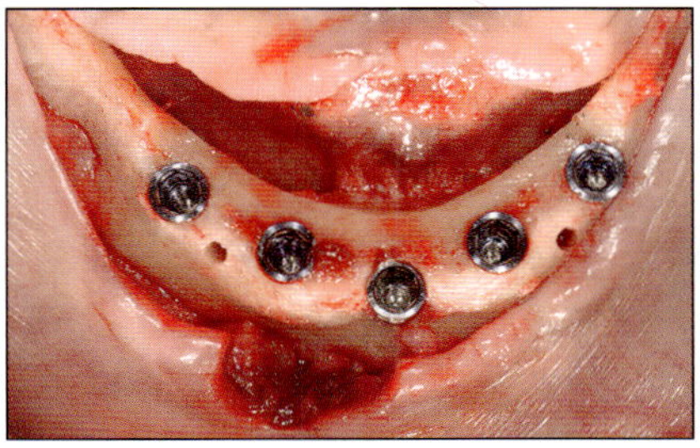

Implants placed.

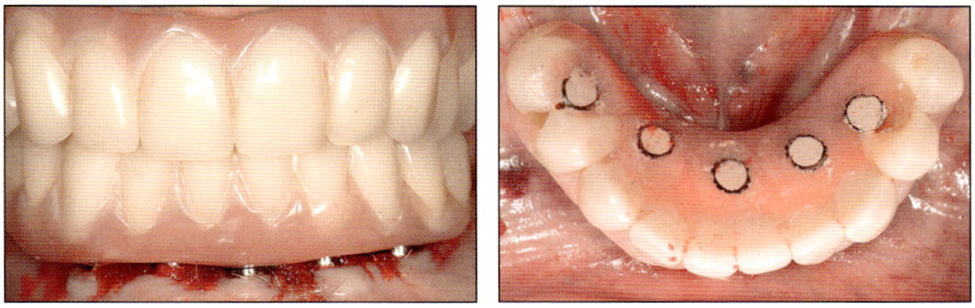

Prosthesis following immediate loading.

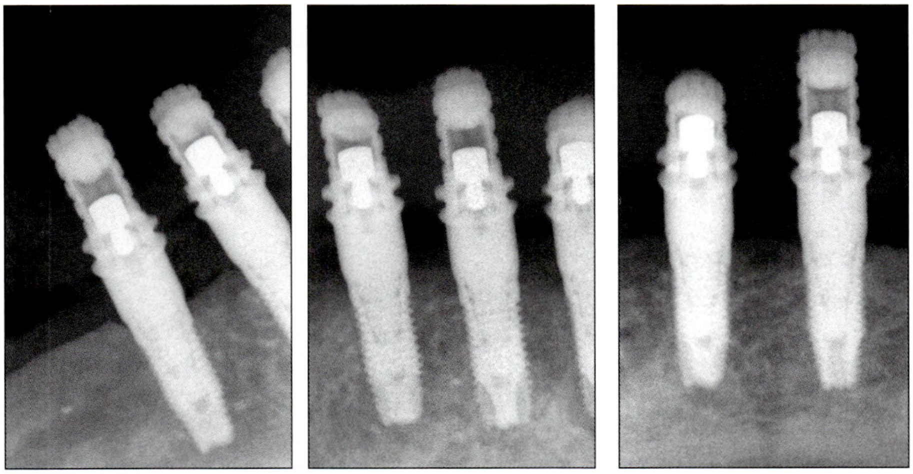

Radiographic view immediately following surgery.

PHASE VII

Definitive Restoration and Supportive Maintenance

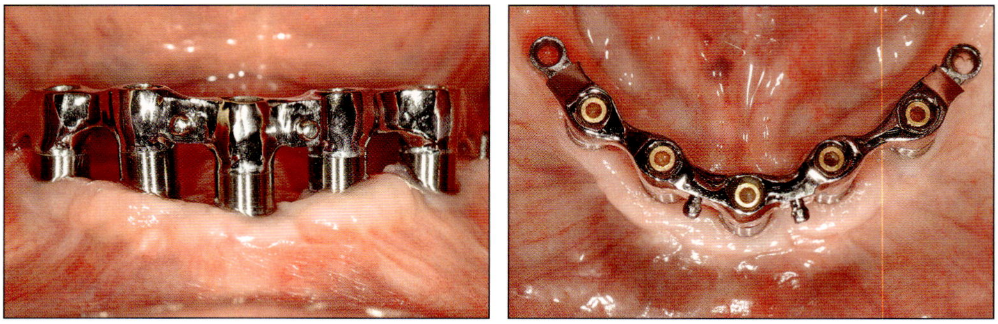

Connector bar in place for definitive restoration.

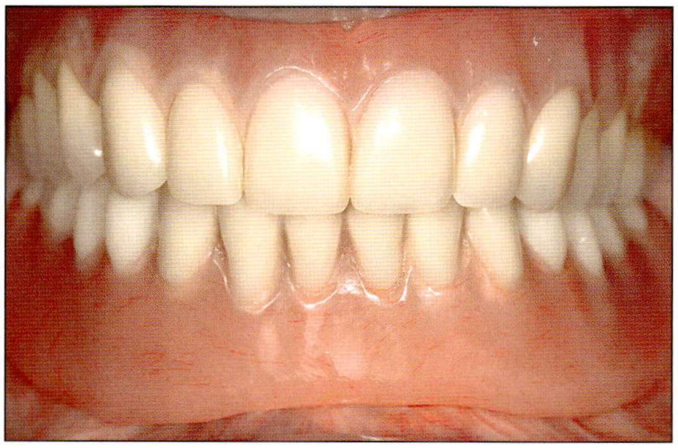

Definitive implant-supported removable prosthesis. (Restoration by Dr Stan Drab, Wheaton, IL.)

Case 6 Advanced Posterior Mandibular Atrophy

A 91-year-old woman presented with the chief complaint of a fractured, nonrestorable, and abscessed mandibular right canine. Her medical history revealed a recently diagnosed gastric ulcer, requiring cessation of anticoagulants.

The patient's needs and concerns were to have a stable-fitting, implant-supported prosthesis that would be maintainable long term and allow her to enjoy eating comfortably again.

Diagnoses

- Mucogingival deficiency of the mandibular right canine
- Wear and compensatory eruption of the mandibular anterior teeth
- Advanced disuse atrophy of the edentulous mandible
- Advanced posterior residual ridge resorption

Case type: 5

- Significant vertical and horizontal bone loss

Diagnostic inquiries

Clinical

- Periodontally compromised teeth
- Influence of resorption patterns on existing native bone
- Nerve proximity

Radiographic

- Bilateral nerve dehiscence
- Unusable mandibular bone height superior to the apices of natural teeth

Physical

- Physiologic changes associated with aging
- Cardiovascular disease
- Management of anxiety associated with oral surgery

Critical actions

- CT-based treatment planning
- Preoperative prosthetic outcome determination: Cantilevered fixed implant-supported prosthesis

PHASE I Initial Diagnostics

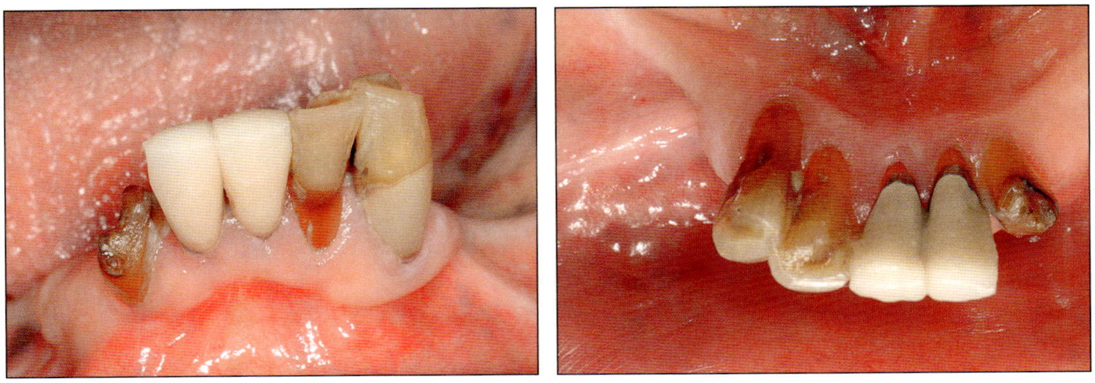

Pretreatment frontal and occlusal views.

PHASE II Scanning Appliance Fabrication

No scanning appliance was fabricated. The patient's remaining natural dentition was used to determine the labiolingual tooth position.

PHASE III CT Scan and SimPlant Conversion

CT scans are taken, and the resulting DICOM files are processed into the SimPlant format. Masks of specific anatomic structures are created.

PHASE IV Eight-Step Treatment-Planning Process

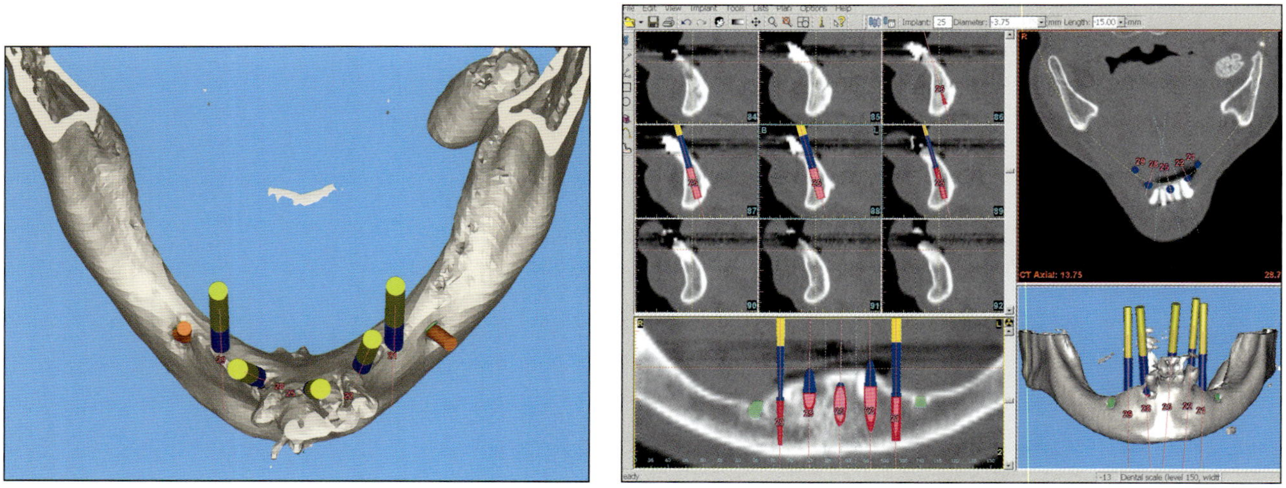

3D implant planning in SimPlant based on CT scans of the mandible.

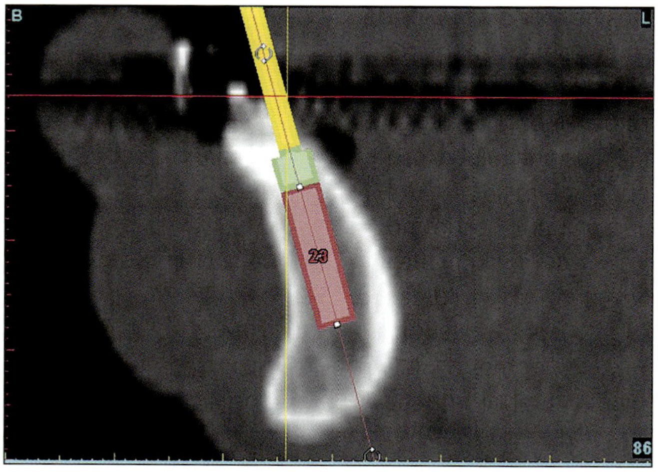

Cross-sectional image. Note the implant position compared to that of natural tooth.

PHASE V Medical Modeling

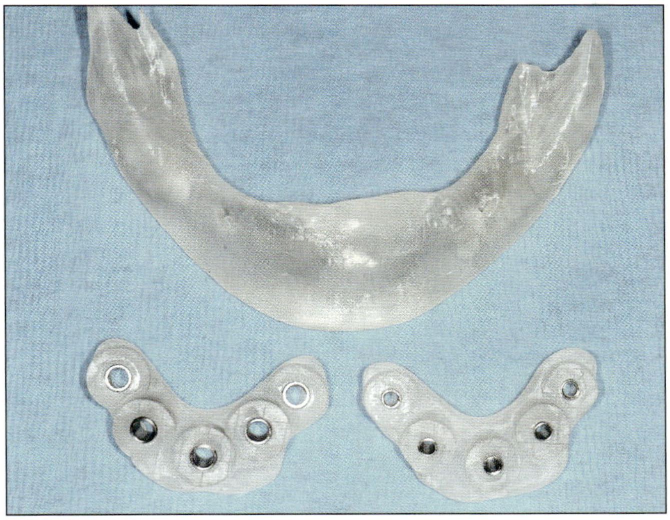

Bone-supported SurgiGuides were selected for surgery; 2-mm and 3-mm guides are shown *(bottom)*. Computerized extractions were performed on the stereolithographic medical model *(top)*.

PHASE VI Surgery

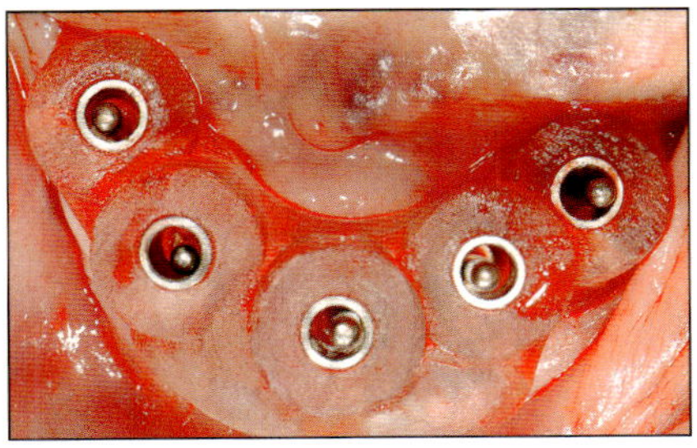

3-mm SurgiGuide in place. Extractions have been performed and the osteotomy sites have been prepared.

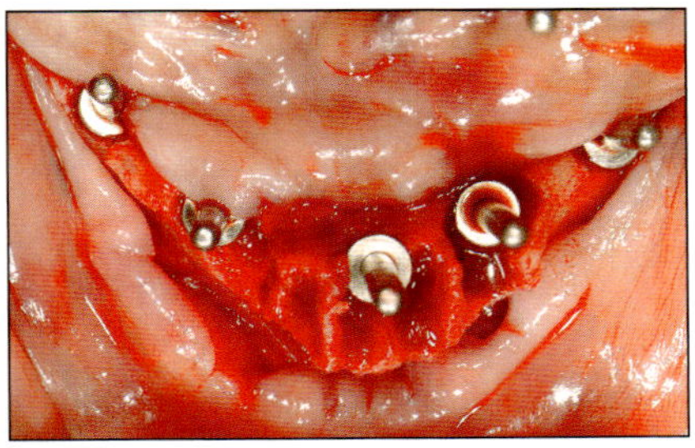

The SurgiGuide has been removed, and the guide pins are in place. Note the position and configuration of the extraction sites compared with the osteotomy sites.

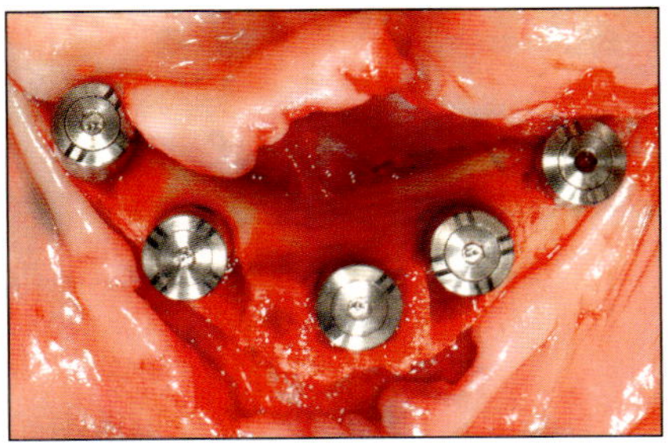

Osteoplasty has been performed, and the implants and healing abutments have been placed.

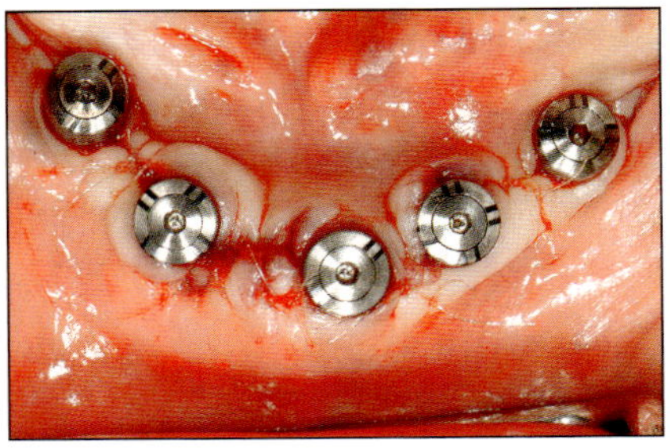

Sutures have been placed, and the one-stage surgical protocol has been completed.

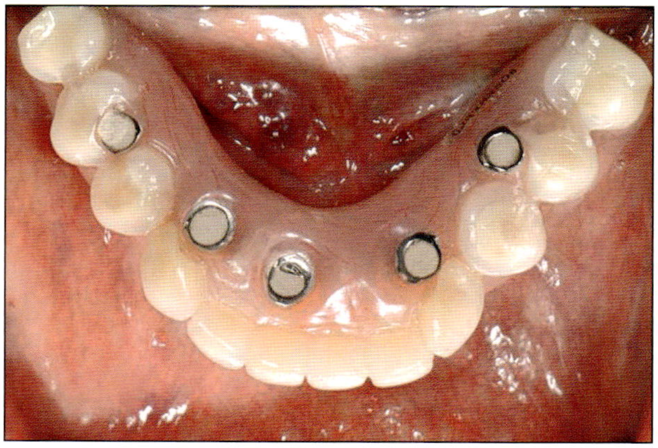

Definitive cantilevered implant-supported fixed prosthesis. (Restoration by Dr Ken Milin, Winnetka, IL.)

Case 7 Maxillary Complete Edentulism

A 59-year-old woman presented with the chief complaint of having a removable denture. A review of her dental history showed that the patient had been completely edentulous for 42 years. Tooth loss occurred when the patient was a teenager and was not of periodontal origin. Her medical history was noncontributory. Conventional open flap surgery was refused by this patient because of perceived pain related to surgery.

Fear and anxiety associated with dental implant surgery had prevented her from receiving treatment in the past. Her desires were to achieve a stable-fitting, fixed implant-supported prosthesis without having to go through open flap surgery. The patient's needs and concerns were to have a functioning stable prosthesis that would restore perioral form, function, and overall self-esteem without pain.

Diagnoses

- Bilateral sinus pneumatization
- Class I maxillomandibular relationship
- Advanced disuse atrophy of the edentulous maxilla

Case type: 5

- Significant vertical and horizontal bone loss

Diagnostic inquiries

Clinical

- Accurate denture

Radiographic

- Bilateral sinus pneumatization
- Limited ridge width

Physical

- Extreme fear and anxiety associated with surgery

Critical actions

- Fabrication of an accurate maxillary ScannoGuide based on patient's maxillary denture
- Ability to fabricate a mucosa-supported SurgiGuide to allow for flapless implant surgery
- Surgical dress rehearsal using stereolithographic medical model
- Preoperative discussion that select implants will be in embrasure positions in the definitive fixed metal-ceramic prosthesis because of bone availability
- Preoperative prosthetic outcome determination: Fixed implant-supported prosthesis

PHASE I Initial Diagnostics

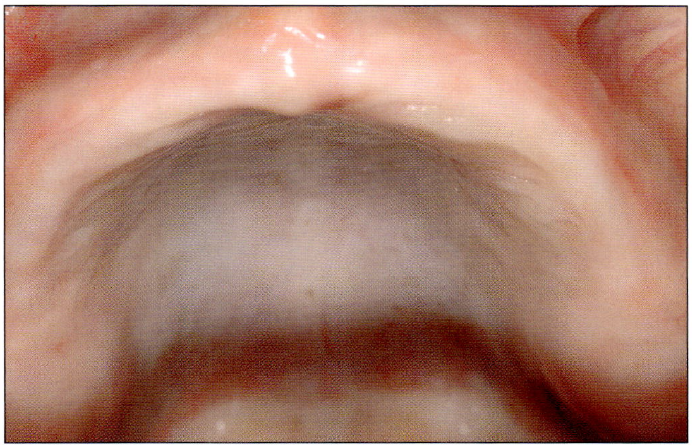

Pretreatment view of maxillary arch.

PHASE II Scanning Appliance Fabrication

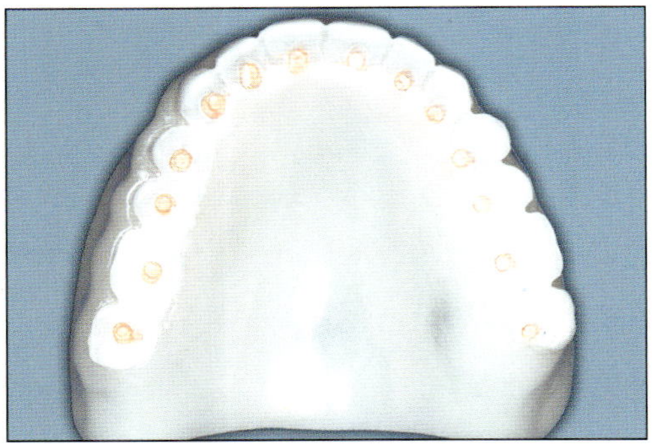

ScannoGuide reflecting the accurate denture.

PHASE III CT Scan and SimPlant Conversion

CT scans are taken, and the resulting DICOM files are processed into the SimPlant format. Masks of specific anatomic structures are created.

PHASE IV Eight-Step Treatment-Planning Process

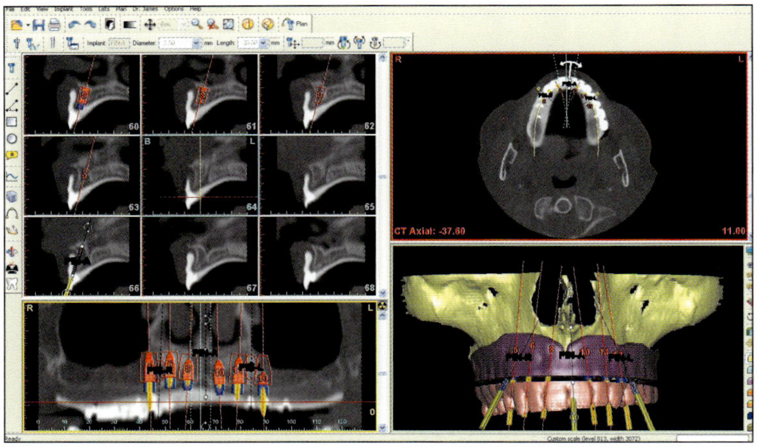

Overview of CT scan and plan of the maxilla.

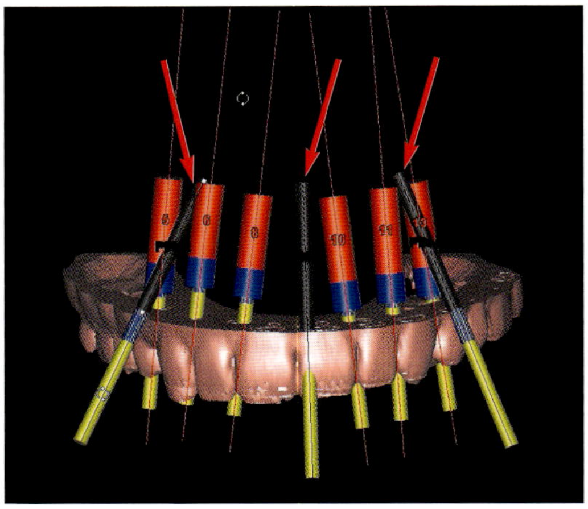

3D implant plan with fixation screws in place *(red arrows).*

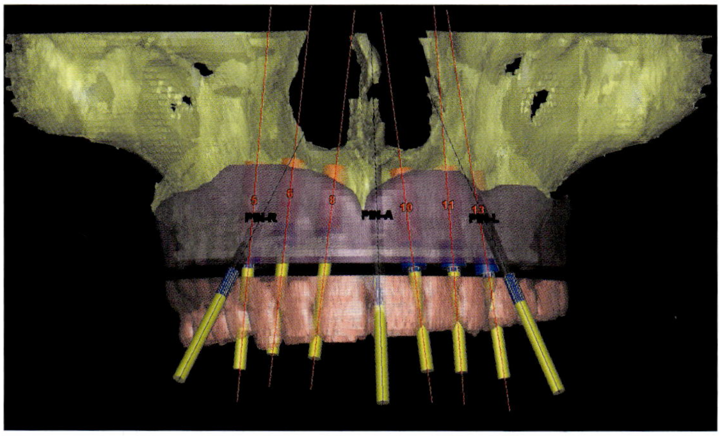

Transparent 3D implant plan with masks visible.

PHASE V Medical Modeling

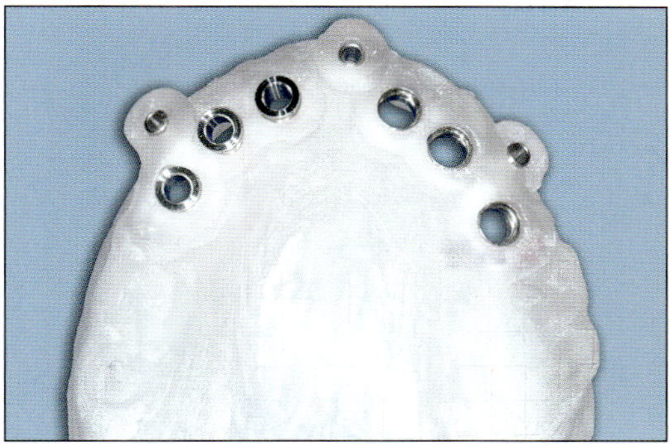

Mucosa-supported SAFE SurgiGuide selected for flapless surgery.

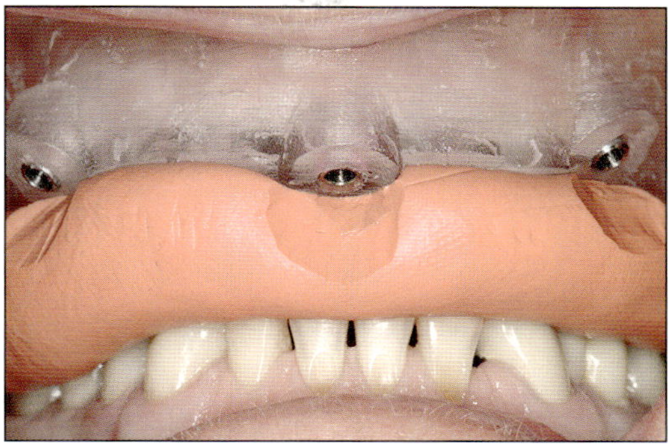

Mucosa-supported SAFE SurgiGuide stability verified preoperatively with occlusal registration.

PHASE VI Surgery

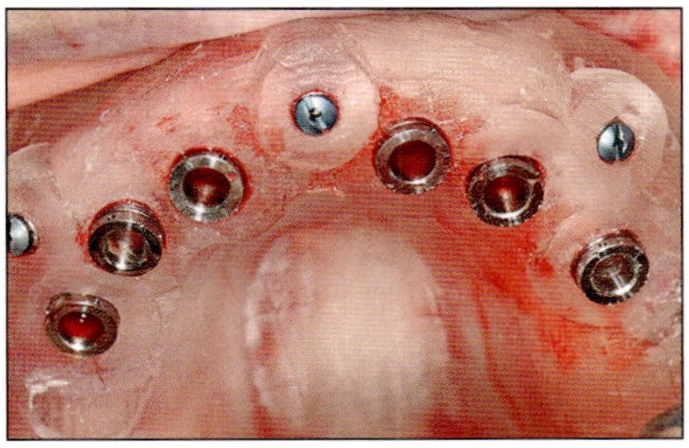

Mucosa-supported SurgiGuide affixed with three screws.

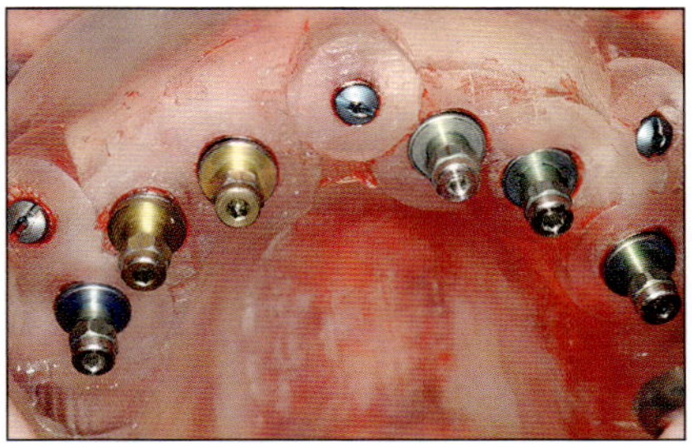

Implants placed through SAFE SurgiGuide using preselected specialized delivery mounts.

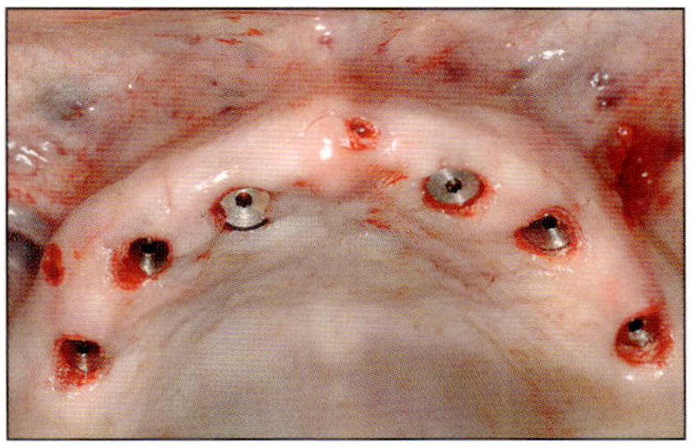

Completion of surgery.

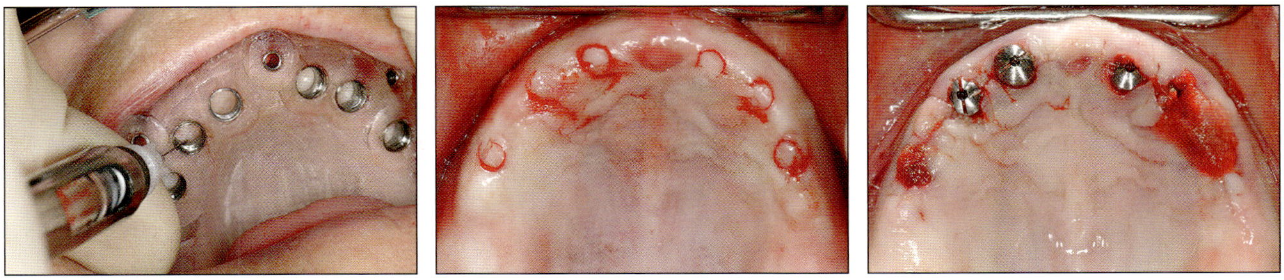

SAFE SurgiGuide used for minimally invasive uncovering of implants at stage 2 surgery.

PHASE VII Definitive Restoration and Supportive Maintenance

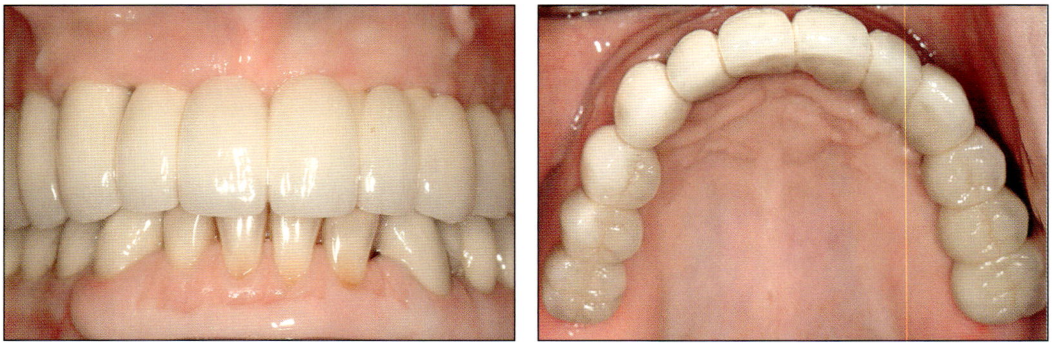

Definitive maxillary fixed prosthesis. (Restoration by Dr Robert Radin, Palatine, IL; laboratory technician: Leonard Sabo, CDT, Skokie, IL.)

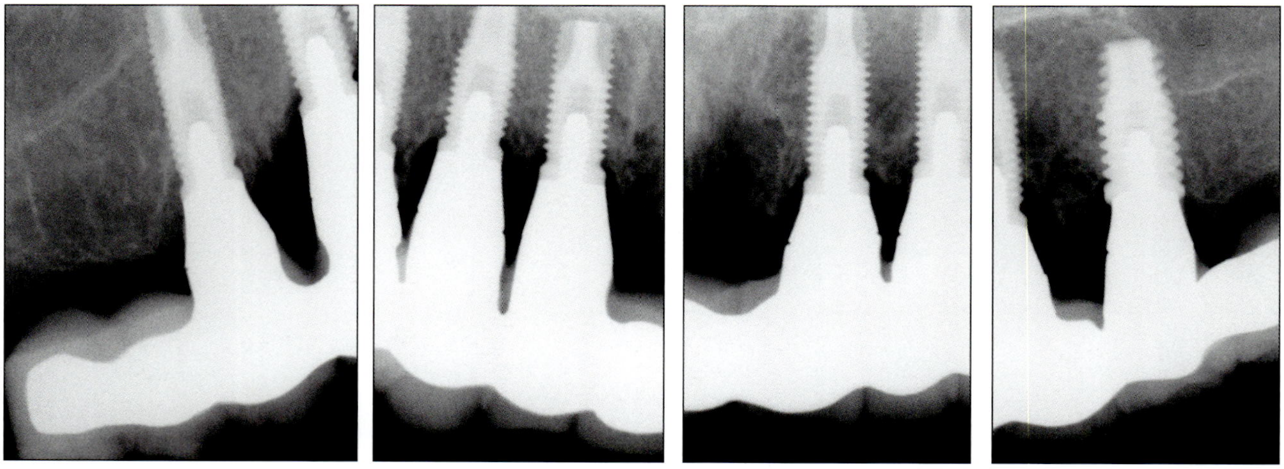

Final periapical radiographs.

Case 8 Mandibular Complete Edentulism

A 69-year-old woman presented with the chief complaint of unstable, generalized, advanced, chronic periodontitis. A review of her pertinent medical history revealed controlled cardiovascular disease and hypothyroidism. A review of her dental history revealed that the patient had been struggling with caries-related tooth loss and progressive periodontitis, and this was compromising her ability to maintain a stable prosthesis for any predictable period of time. The patient's needs and concerns were the achievement of a functioning stable prosthesis that would restore perioral form and function with predictability as her most significant concern.

Diagnoses

- Generalized advanced chronic periodontitis
- Class II division I malocclusion
- Generalized caries

Case type: 5

- Significant vertical and horizontal bone loss

Diagnostic inquiries

Clinical

- Accurate denture postextraction
- 10 mm of unusable bone height (anterior)

Radiographic

- Nerve proximity
- Extent of posterior atrophy
- Bone quality

Physical

- None

Critical actions

- Fabrication of an accurate mandibular denture into a differential barium-gradient ScannoGuide 3 months after extractions
- Surgical dress rehearsal of immediate-load surgery using stereolithographic medical model
- Preoperative prosthetic outcome determination: Fixed implant-supported prosthesis

PHASE I Initial Diagnostics

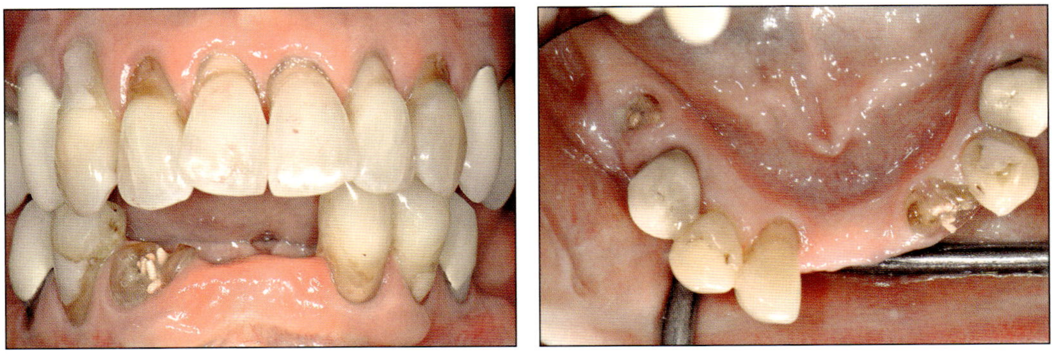

Pretreatment frontal and occlusal views.

PHASE II Scanning Appliance Fabrication

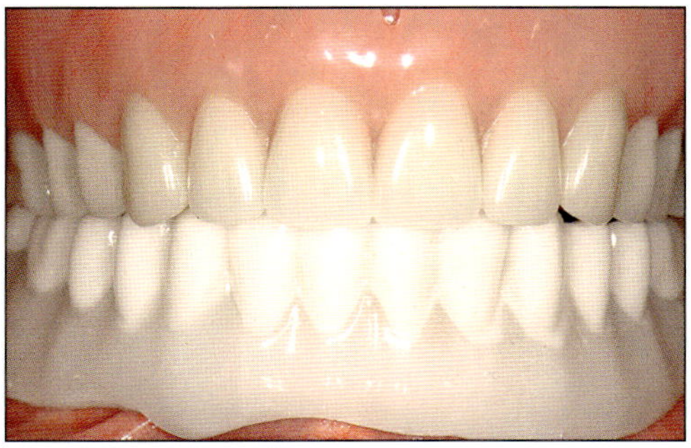

ScannoGuide reflecting accurate mandibular denture position.

PHASE III CT Scan and SimPlant Conversion

CT scans are taken, and the resulting DICOM files are processed into the SimPlant format. Masks of specific anatomic structures are created.

PHASE IV Eight-Step Treatment-Planning Process

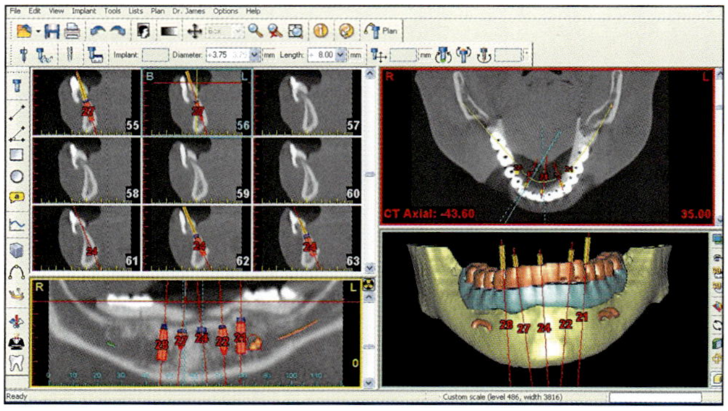

CT scan of the mandible with accurate ScannoGuide.

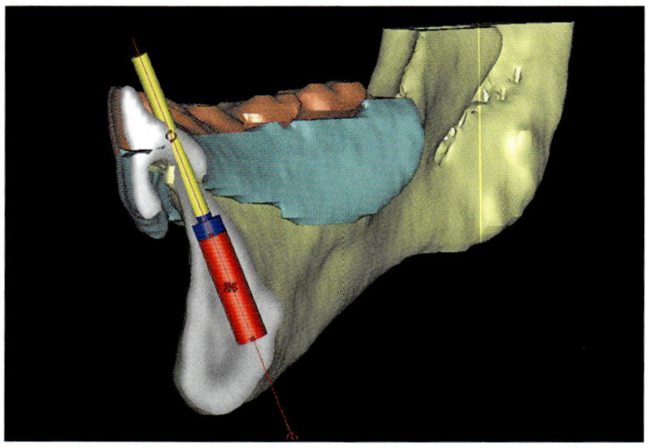

Determining unusable bone height.

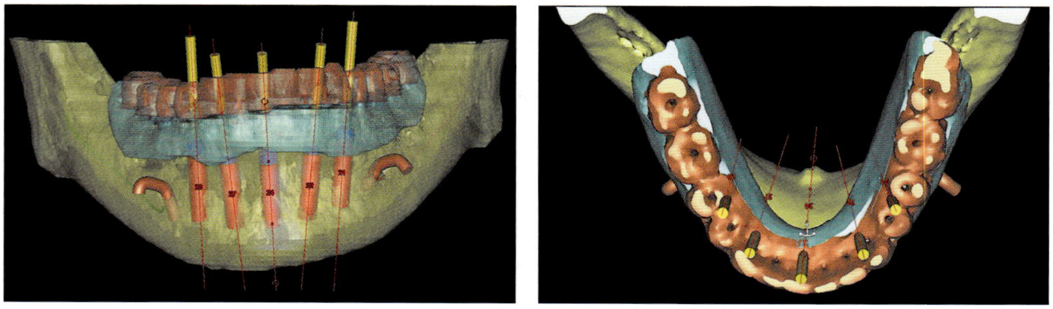

Collaboratively based 3D implant treatment plan.

PHASE V

Medical Modeling

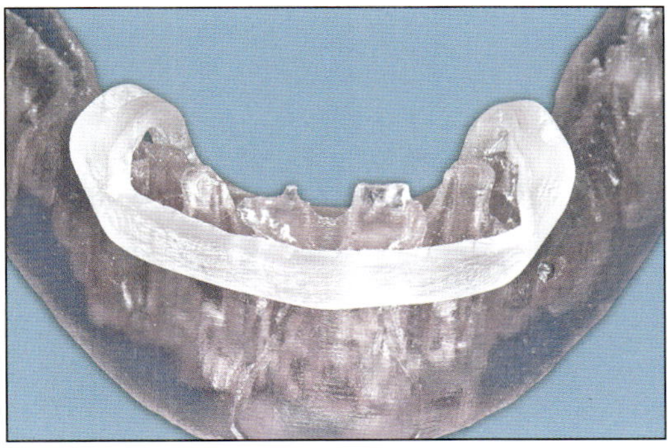

Medical model with bone reduction guide in place.

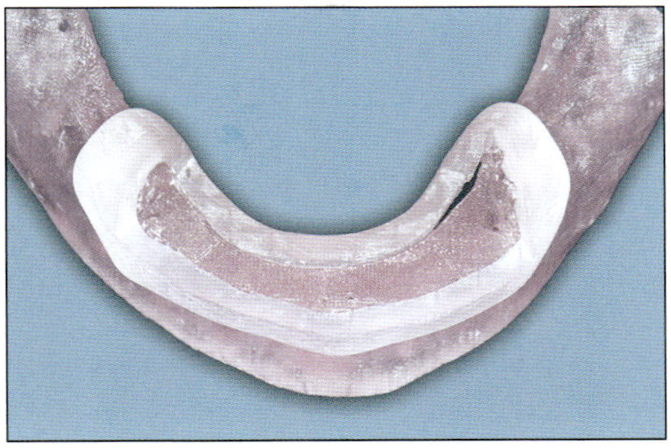

Medical model following bone reduction.

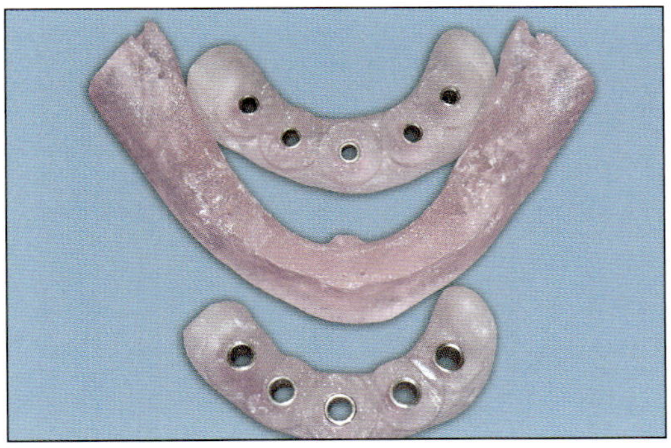

Bone-supported SurgiGuides selected for surgery: 2 mm *(top)* and 3 mm *(bottom)*.

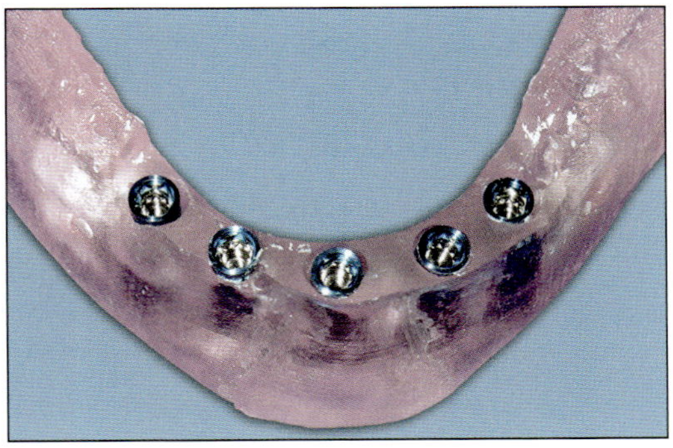

Medical model with implant analogues in place post–bone reduction.

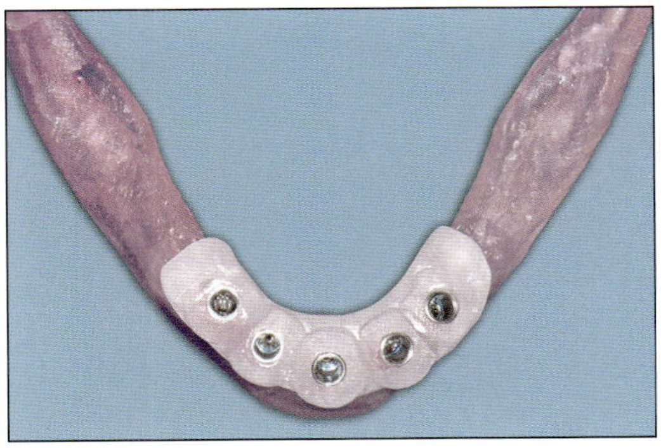

Medical model with implant analogues in place and 3-mm SurgiGuide in position.

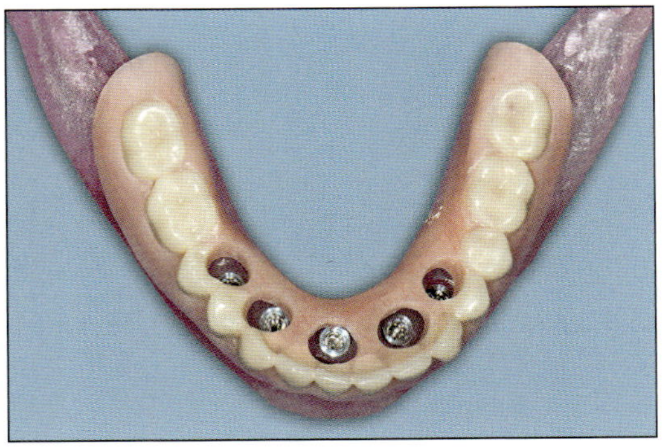

Denture modified on medical model. Surgical dress rehearsal completed.

PHASE VI Surgery

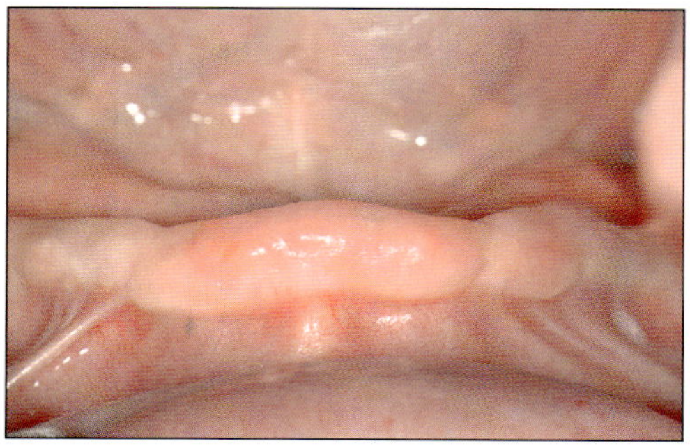

Preoperative view.

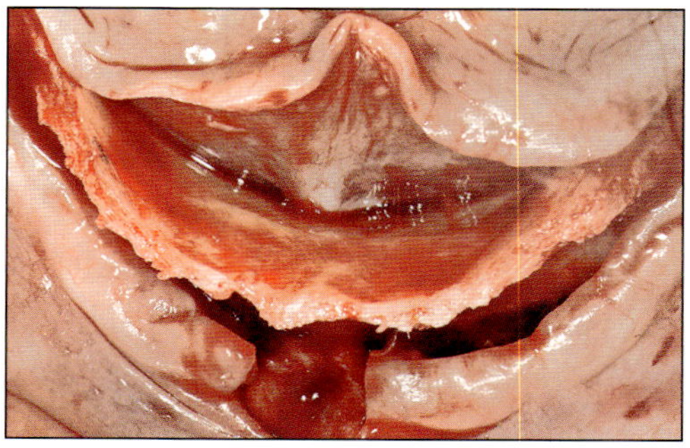

Intraoperative inspection of anatomy.

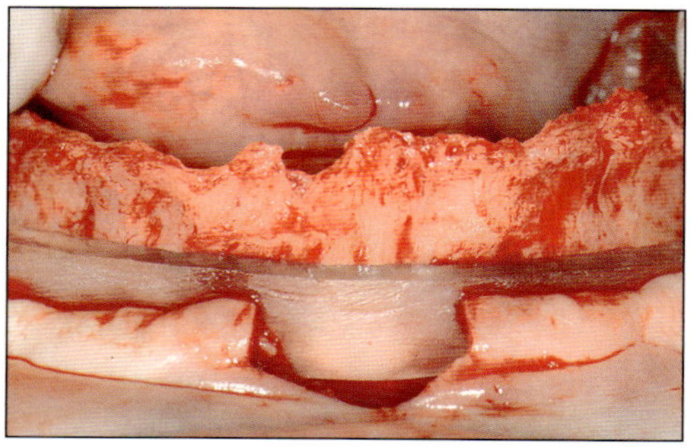

Bone reduction guide in place for precision osteoplasty.

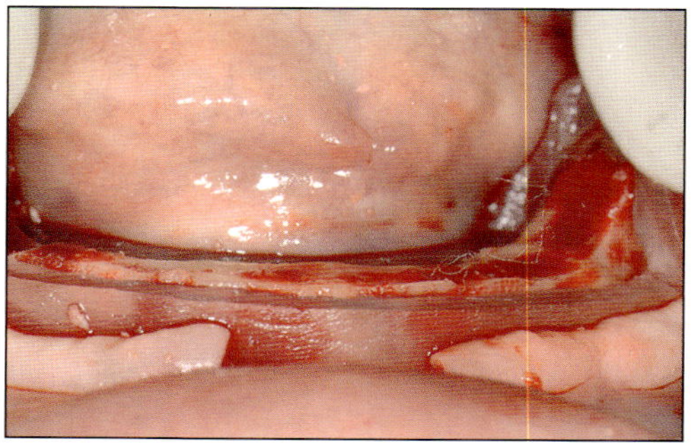

Postoperative view following the precision osteoplasty.

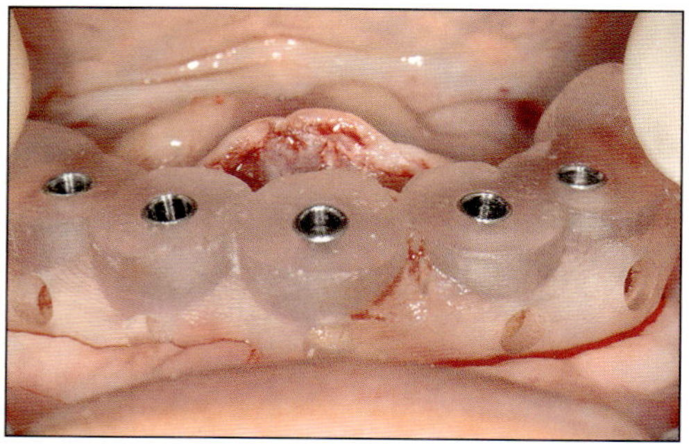

Bone-supported SurgiGuide in place (2 mm level).

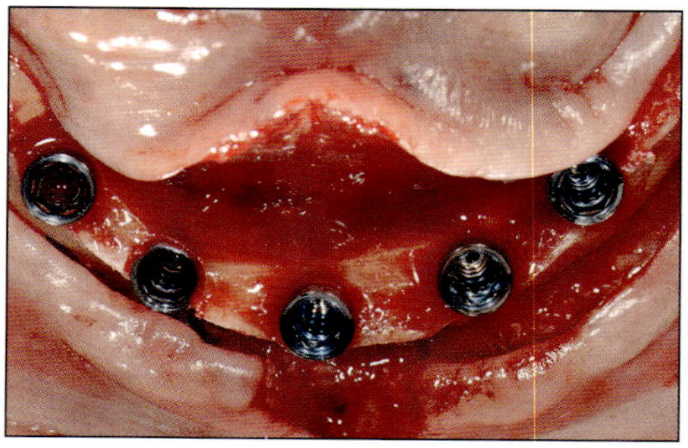

Implants placed.

PHASE VI

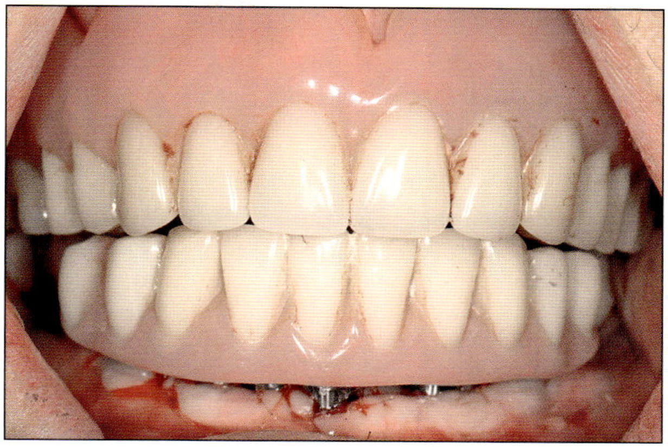

Immediate-load prosthesis completed.

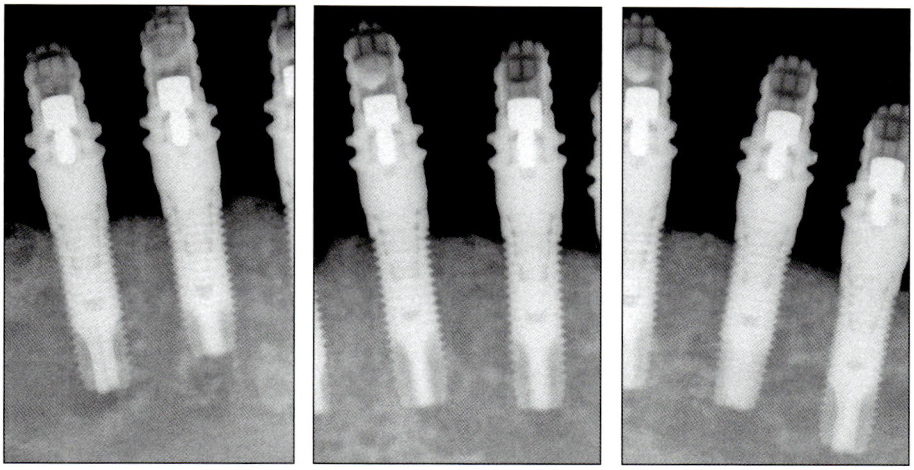

Periapical radiographs taken 4 months post–immediate loading.

PHASE VII Definitive Restoration and Supportive Maintenance

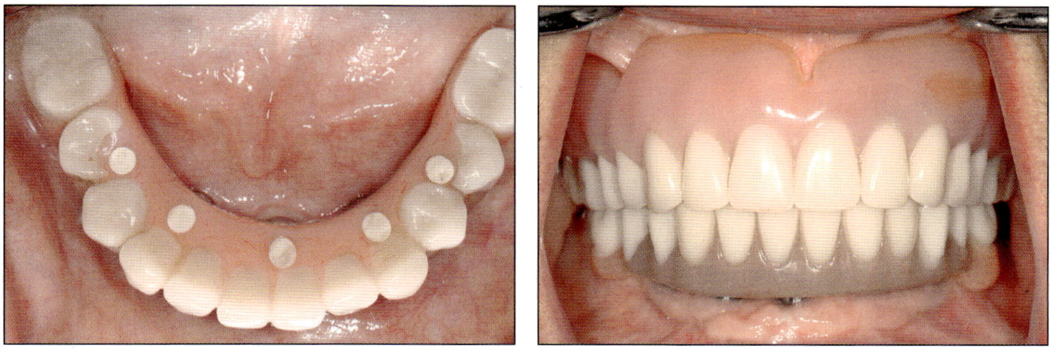

Definitive implant-supported fixed prosthesis. (Restoration by Dr Dan Nykaza, Evanston, IL; laboratory technician: Leonard Sabo, CDT, Skokie, IL.)

Case 9 Maxillary Anterior Implant Reconstruction

A 59-year-old woman presented with the chief complaint of a failing maxillary anterior partial denture. A review of her pertinent medical history revealed cardiovascular disease and hypothyroidism. Her dental history showed that the patient had developed recurrent caries at her maxillary right central and left lateral incisors, which served as abutments for her denture. Following removal of the caries, the restorative prognosis was determined to be poor. The patient's needs and concerns were to have a stable-fitting, fixed implant-supported prosthesis that would be maintainable long-term.

Diagnoses

- Recurrent caries at the right central and left lateral incisors
- Class I occlusion
- Nonrestorable right central and left lateral incisors
- Healthy periodontium

Case type: 1

- Existing tooth position acceptable
- Gingival symmetry, volume, and color normal
- Bone height and width normal

Diagnostic inquiries

Clinical

- Final prosthetic outcome requirements
- Acceptable existing tooth position for planned implants

Radiographic

- Position of alveoli versus available maxillary bone
- Position of nasopalatine nerve, canal, and nasal sinuses

Physical

- None

Critical actions

- Fabrication of an accurate maxillary scanning appliance
- Surgical dress rehearsal of immediate implant surgery using stone cast
- Preoperative prosthetic outcome determination: Fixed implant-supported prosthesis

PHASE I

Initial Diagnostics

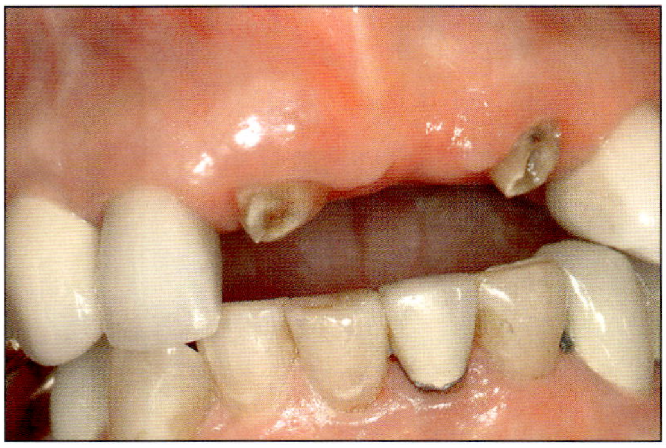

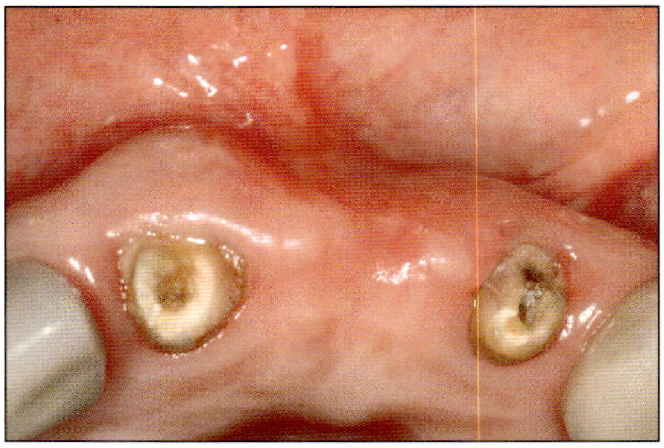

Pretreatment frontal and occlusal views.

PHASE II Scanning Appliance Fabrication

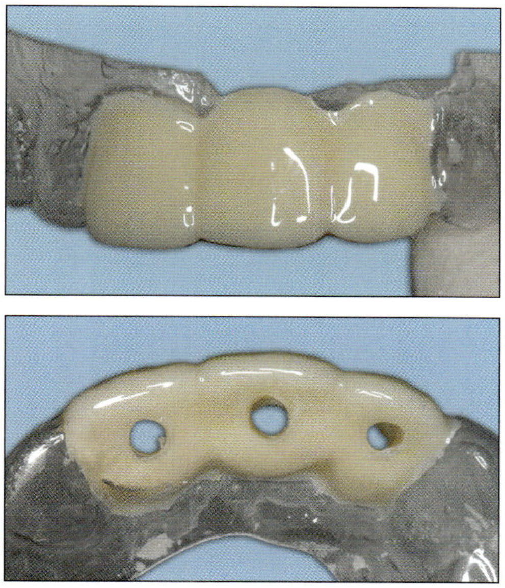

Second-generation scanning appliance reflecting accurate mandibular denture position.

PHASE III CT Scan and SimPlant Conversion

CT scans are taken, and the resulting DICOM files are processed into the Sim-Plant format. Masks of specific anatomic structures are created.

PHASE IV Eight-Step Treatment-Planning Process

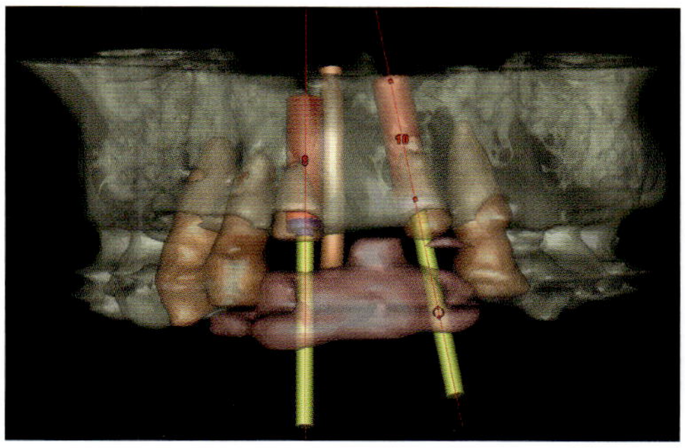

CT scan of the maxilla with accurate ScannoGuide. Collaboratively based 3D implant treatment plan.

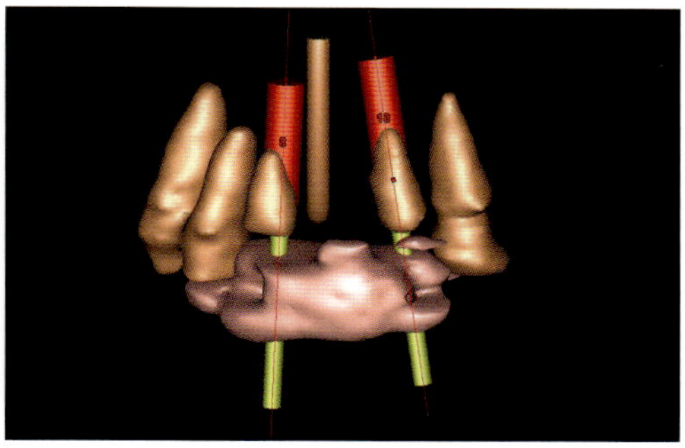

Mask of maxilla removed.

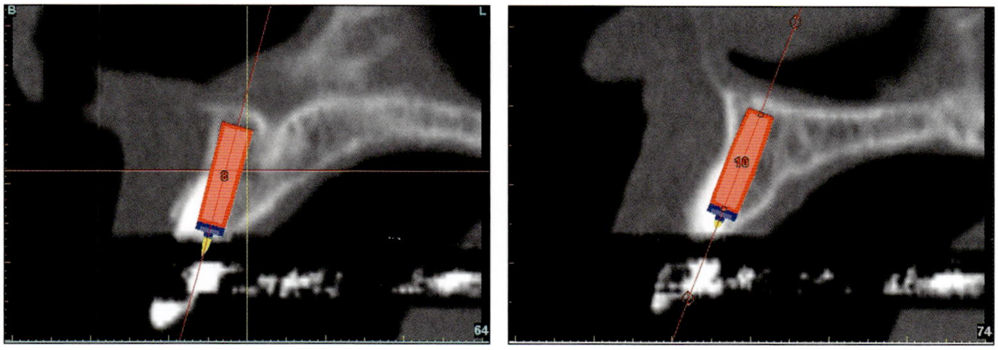

Cross-sectional views of the site of the maxillary right central and left lateral incisors.

PHASE V

Medical Modeling

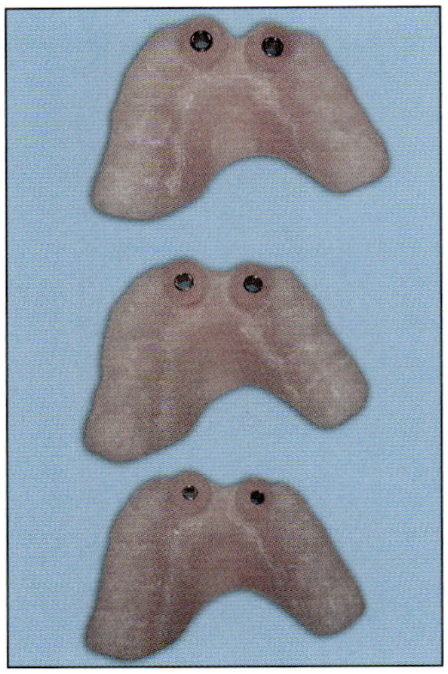

Tooth-supported SurgiGuides selected for surgery.

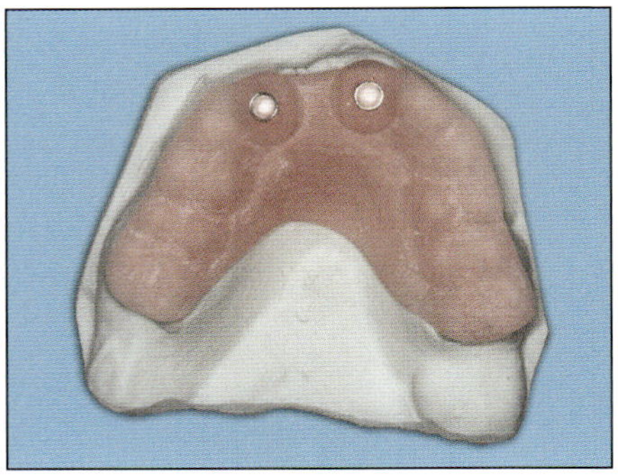

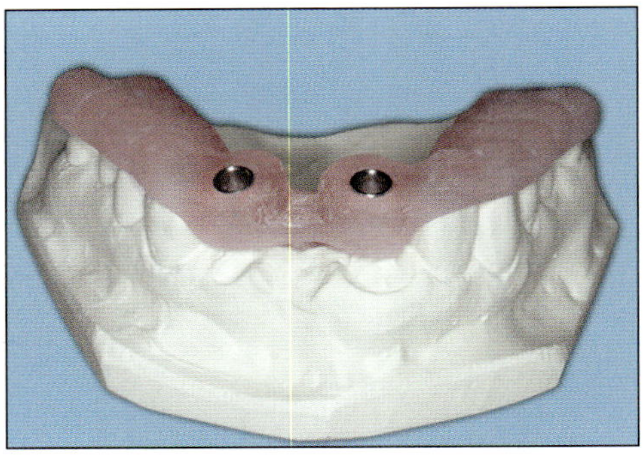

Tooth-supported SurgiGuide on accurate stone cast, allowing for dress rehearsal of osteotomy site preparation to be performed and reviewed preoperatively.

PHASE VI

Surgery

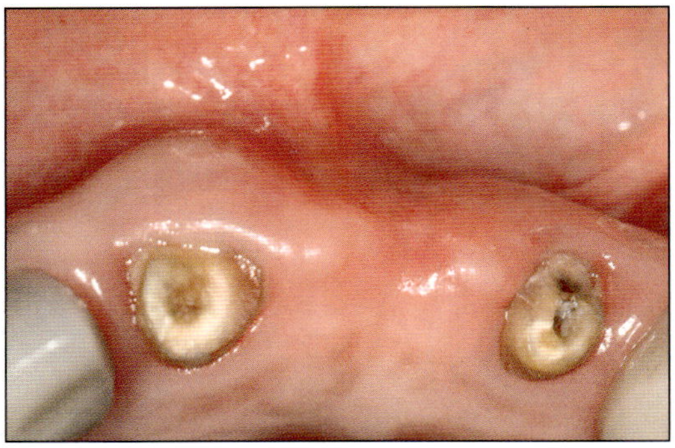

Preoperative occlusal view.

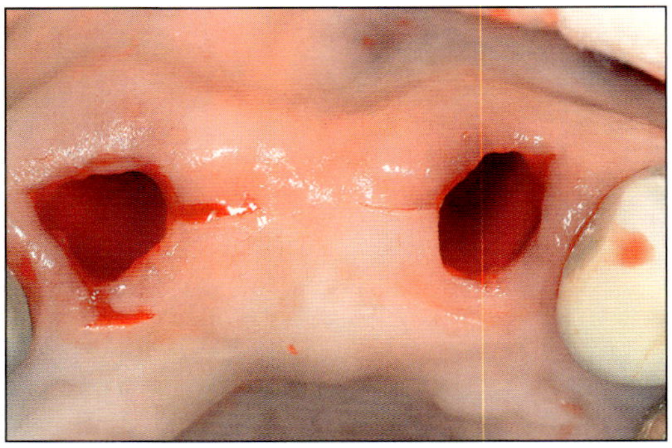

Atraumatic extraction of the right central and the left lateral incisors.

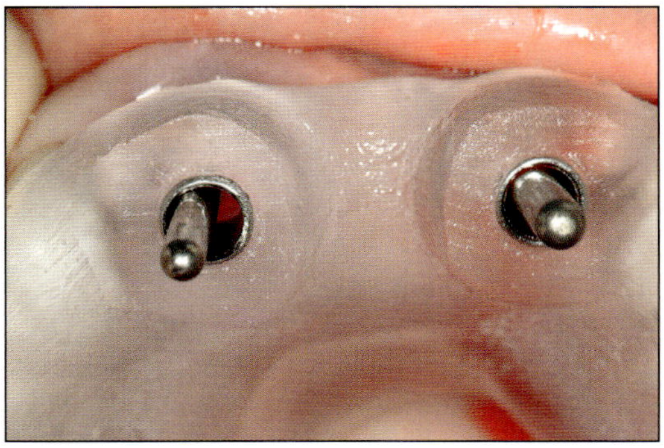

Flapless and precise osteotomy site preparation. The 2-mm SurgiGuide is in place.

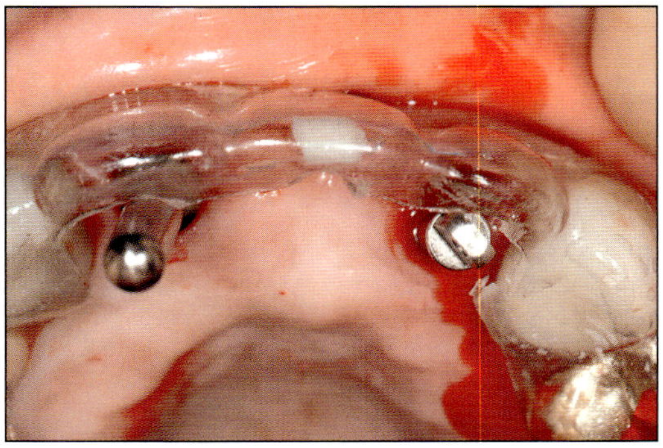

Traditional surgical guide for clinical verification of osteotomy site preparation with SurgiGuide compared to optimal final tooth position in space.

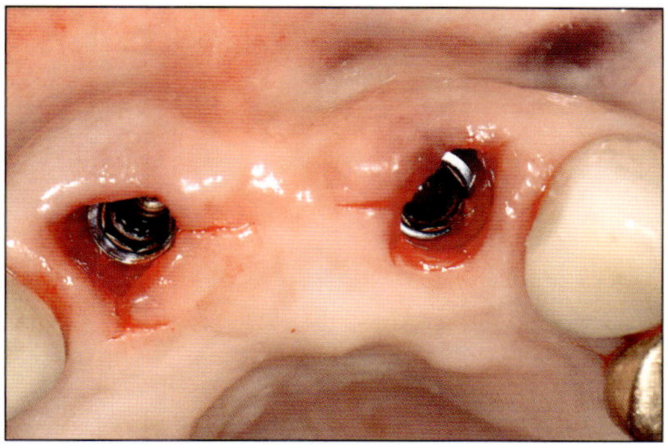

Implants placed.

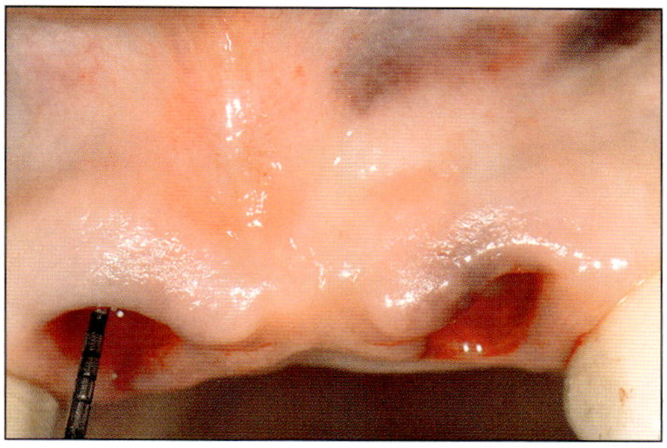

Vertical depth of platforms verified.

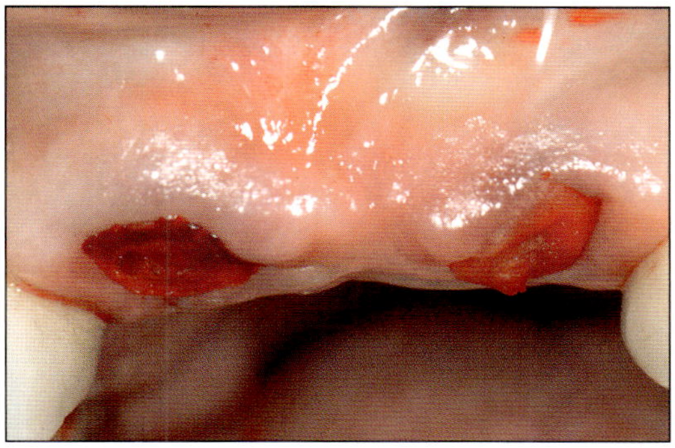

Bone grafting and membrane placement.

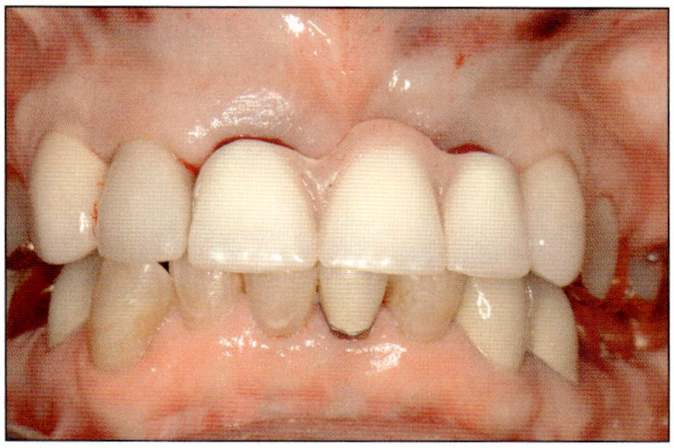

Removable prosthesis placed at the completion of surgery.

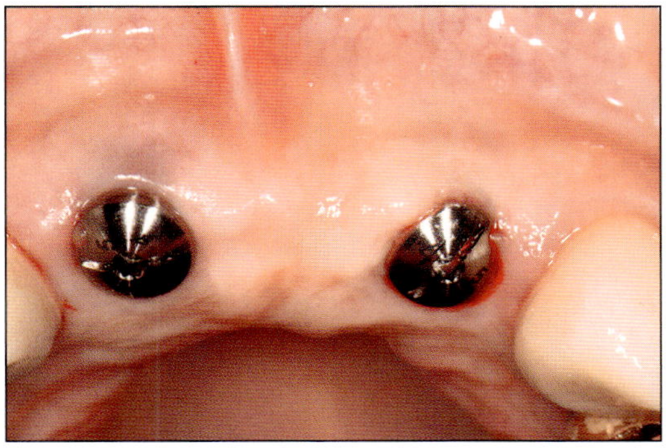

Flapless uncovering procedure 4 months postoperative.

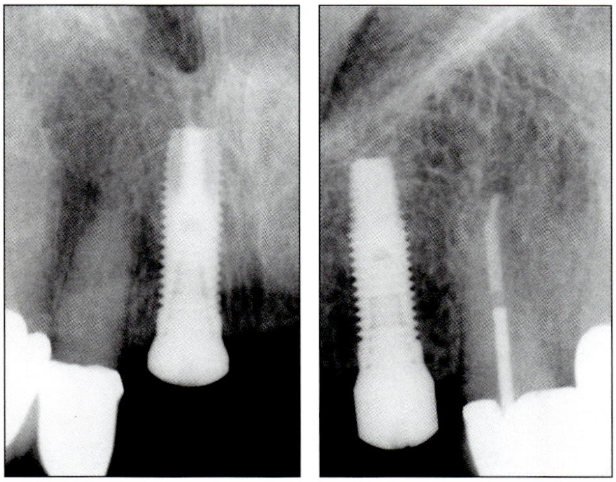

Radiographs at the time of the uncovering surgery verifying implant positioning as well as complete seating of the healing abutments.

PHASE VII
Definitive Restoration and Supportive Maintenance

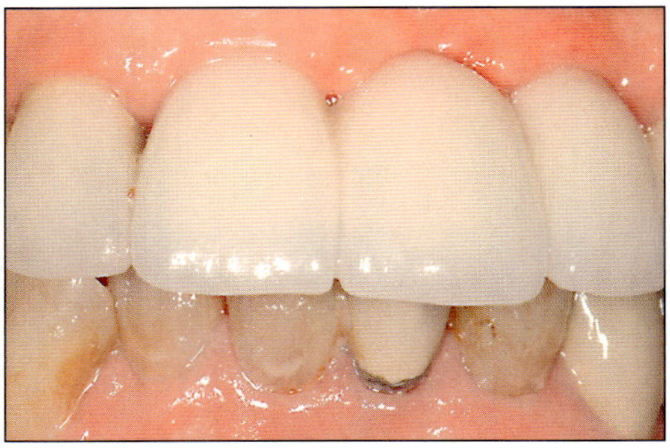

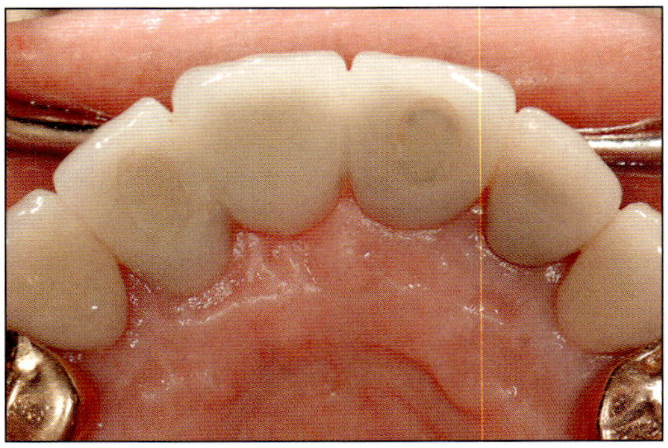

Facial and occlusal views of the implant-supported fixed prosthesis replacing the maxillary right and the two central incisors. (Restoration by Dr Ken Milin, Winnetka, IL.)

Case 10 Bilateral Maxillary Partial Edentulism

A 56-year-old man presented with the chief complaint of unstable recurrent and progressive periodontitis. His medical history revealed gastroesophageal reflux disease and emphysema. He was a former smoker with a 20-pack/year history. His dental history revealed progressive periodontitis with a high level of plaque despite periodontal surgery and compliance with maintenance care. The patient's needs and concerns were to have a stable-fitting, fixed, implant-supported prosthesis that would be maintainable long term.

Diagnoses

- Generalized advanced chronic periodontitis
- Class I occlusion
- Primary and secondary occlusal trauma
- Bruxism

Case type: 4

- Predominantly vertical and some horizontal bone loss

Diagnostic inquiries

Clinical

- Biomechanical and occlusal demands of prosthesis tested in the provisional

Radiographic

- Amount of available native bone height
- Bone quality
- Health of maxillary sinuses; patency of the osteomeatal complex

Physical

- None

Critical actions

- Fabrication of a provisional prosthesis that can be duplicated into a scanning appliance for identifying optimal tooth position following extraction and socket preservation
- CT scan review that would allow for collaboratively based treatment planning
- Preoperative prosthetic outcome determination: Fixed implant-supported prosthesis

PHASE I Initial Diagnostics

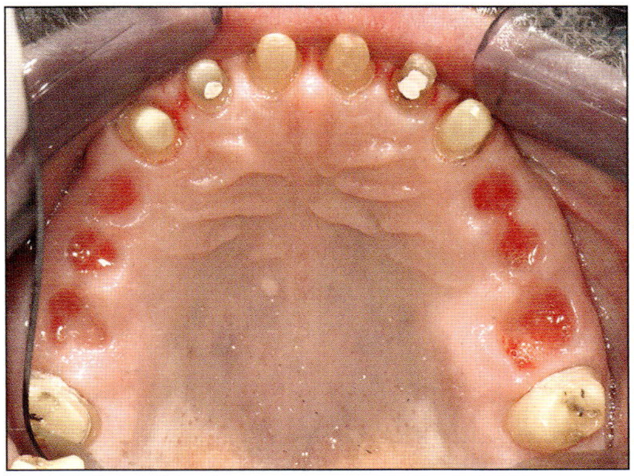

Occlusal view following socket grafting of the sites from maxillary first molar to first premolar bilaterally. Provisional maxillary prosthesis fabricated.

PHASE II Scanning Appliance Fabrication

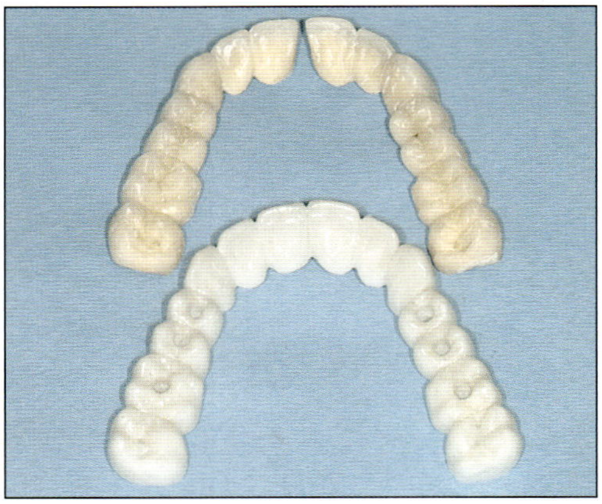

Provisional prosthesis *(top)*; 10% barium prosthesis *(bottom)* represents scanning appliance for CT scan, which is a duplicate of the provisional prosthesis.

PHASE III CT Scan and SimPlant Conversion

CT scans are taken, and the resulting DICOM files are processed into the SimPlant format. Masks of specific anatomic structures are created.

PHASE IV Eight-Step Treatment-Planning Process

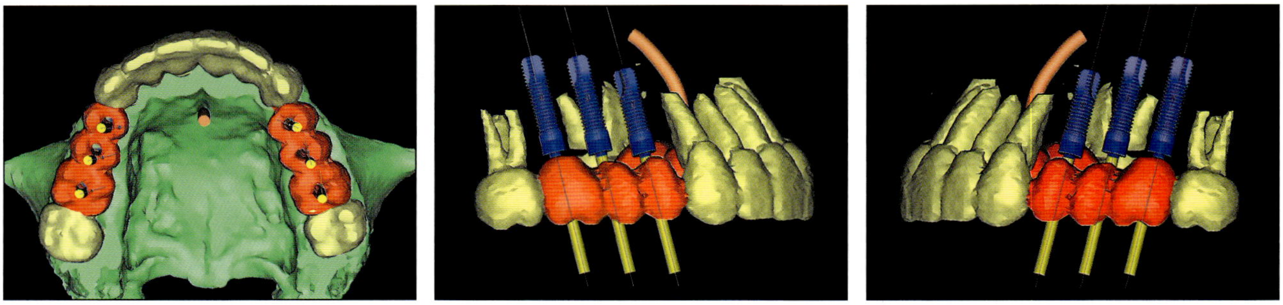

CT scan of the maxilla with 10% barium provisional in place. Collaboratively based 3D implant treatment plan.

PHASE V Medical Modeling

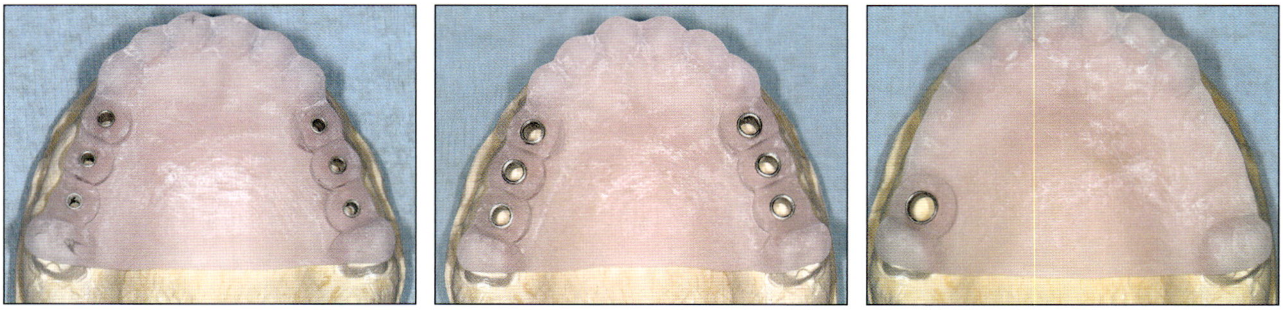

Tooth-supported SurgiGuides (2 mm, 3 mm, 4.3 mm) selected for surgery.

PHASE VI Surgery

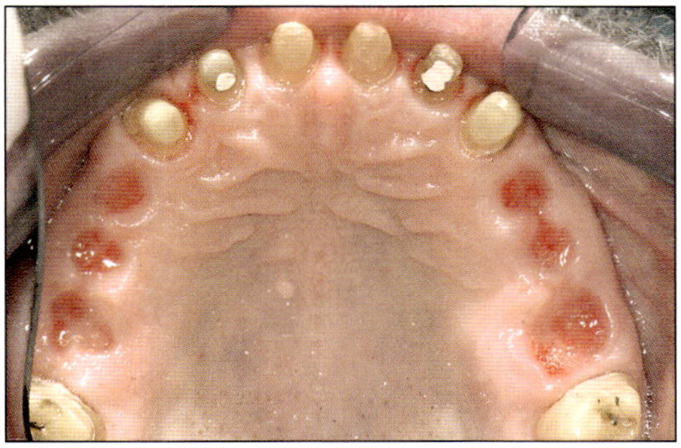

Pre-implant surgery view, 6 months after socket grafting.

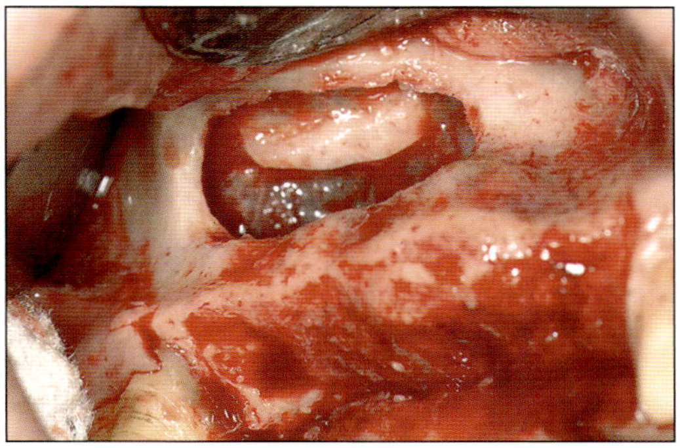

Antral approach to sinus grafting.

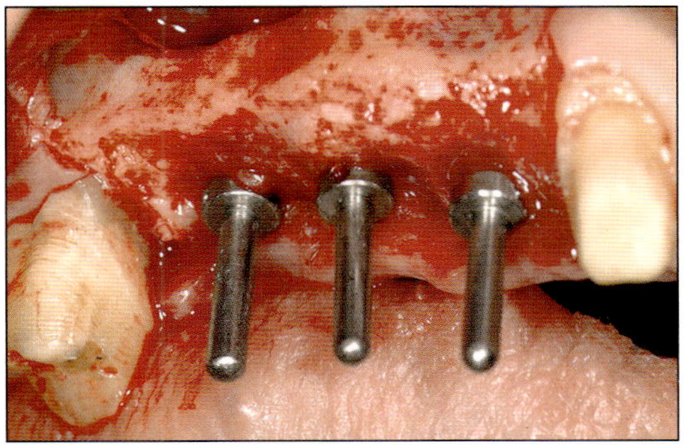

Osteotomy sites created following elevation of sinus membrane.

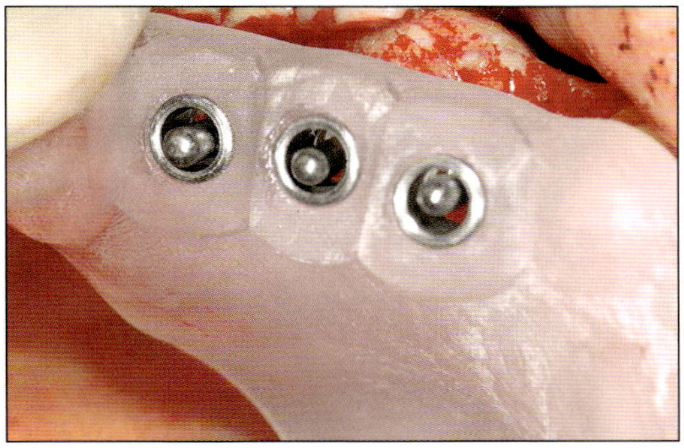

SurgiGuide in position with direction indicators in SurgiGuide-assisted osteotomy site demonstrating accurate preparation.

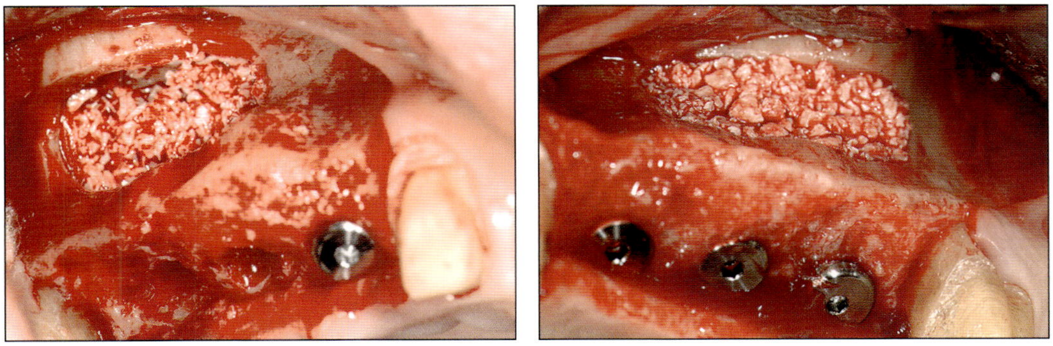

Implants placed and sinus bone grafting complete.

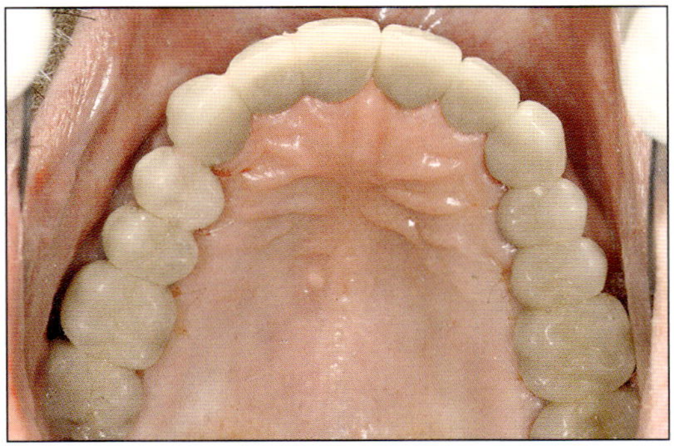

Sutures and provisional prosthesis cemented.

PHASE VI

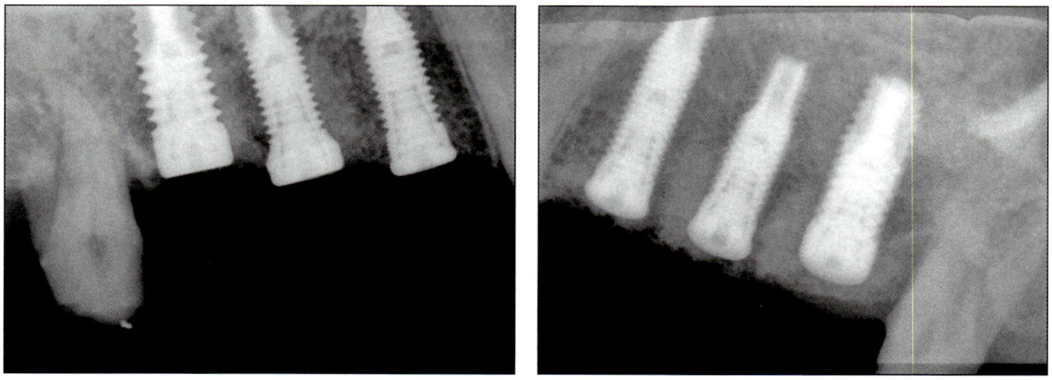

Immediate postoperative radiographs following simultaneous implant placement and bilateral sinus bone grafting.

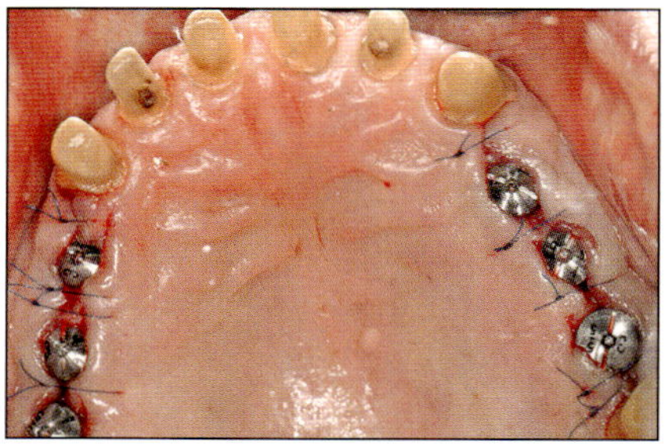

Uncovering of implants and placement of healing abutments.

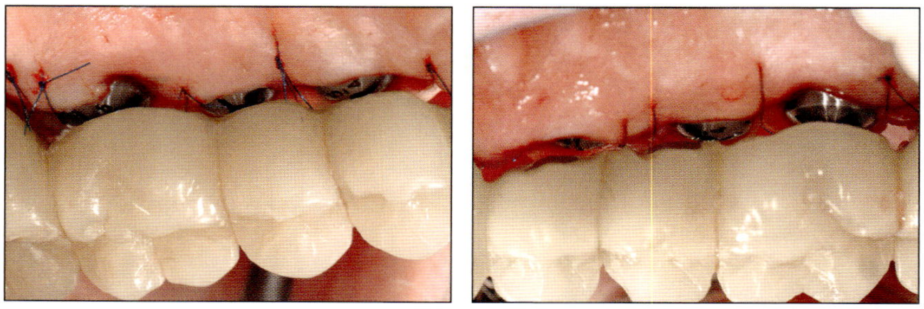

Sutures and provisional prostheses recemented.

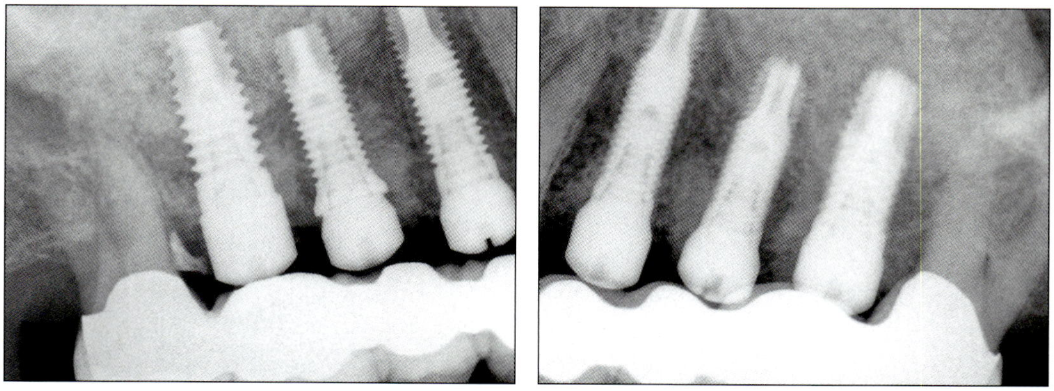

Radiographs following stage 2 implant surgery. Healing abutments seated.

PHASE VII
Definitive Restoration and Supportive Maintenance

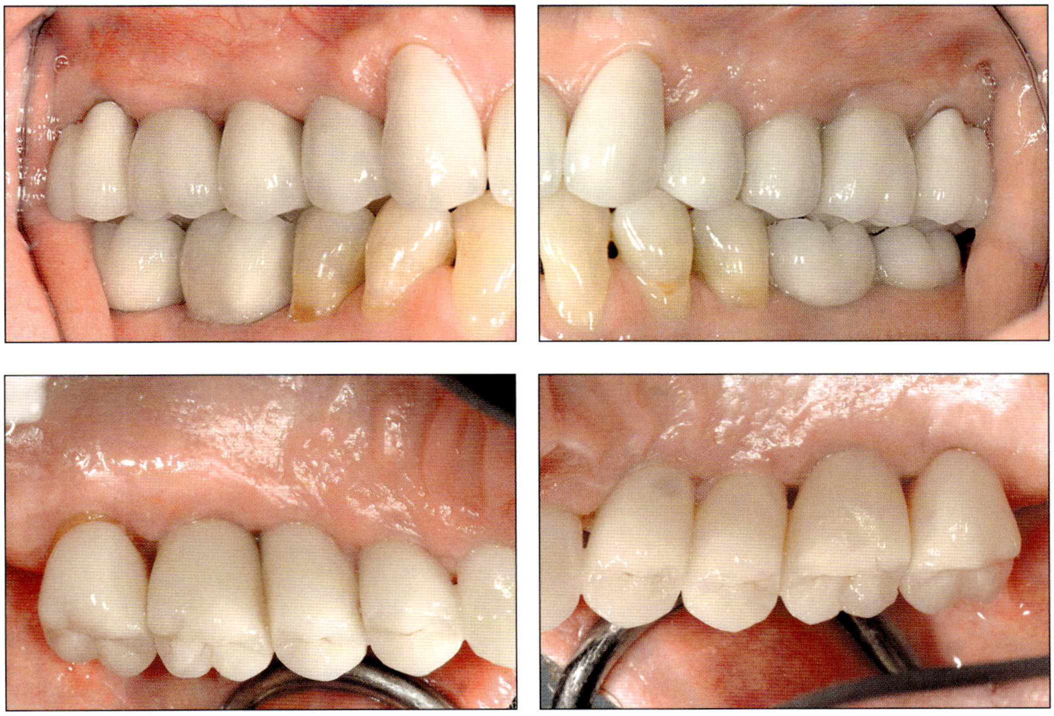

Definitive implant-supported fixed prostheses.

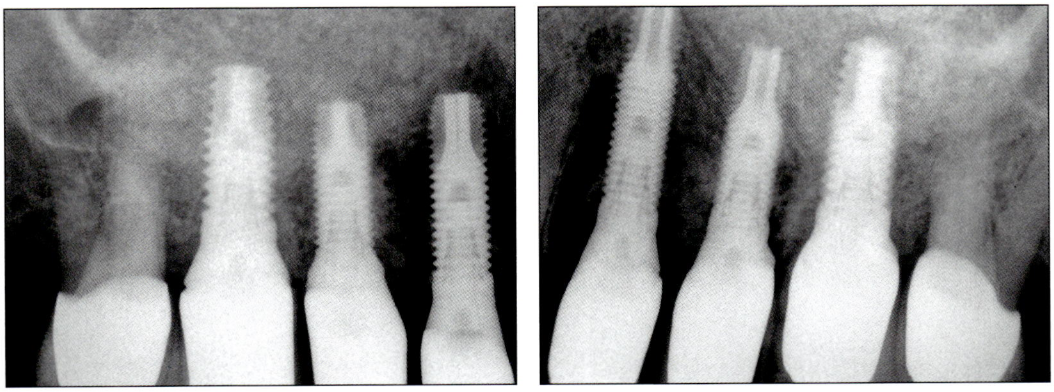

Postoperative radiographs. (Restoration by Dr Joseph Caruso, Chicago, IL.)

Case 11 Maxillary Anterior Implant Failure

A 48-year-old man presented with the chief complaint of a failing implant at the site of the maxillary right lateral incisor. His medical history revealed controlled insulin-dependent diabetes and current cigarette smoking. The patient's needs and concerns were to have a stable-fitting implant-supported prosthesis that would resolve the current infection and restore health to the anterior maxilla.

Diagnoses

- Failing implant at the site of the right lateral incisor.
- Class I occlusion
- Implant malpositioning at the site of the left lateral incisor

Case type: 3

- Predominantly horizontal bone loss with some vertical loss as well
- Less than optimal mesiodistal spacing as a result of the malposed left lateral incisor implant

Diagnostic inquiries

Clinical

- Diagnostic waxup to determine final outcome
- Manage malposed left lateral incisor implant and incorporate it into the definitive prosthesis

Radiographic

- Position of nasopalatine foramen and nerve
- 3D position of left lateral incisor implant in relation to proposed final outcome
- Available bone width and quality

Physical

- None

Critical actions

- Preservation of osteotomy at right lateral incisor site following implant removal
- Diagnostic waxup and accurate scanning appliance construction to allow for correct planning
- CT scan of the maxilla with scanning appliance in position to allow for 3D analysis of spatial positioning of left lateral incisor to be made and to determine which other sites are possible implant candidates to support final outcome
- Preoperative understanding of compromised future implant positioning with the existing position of left lateral incisor
- Preoperative prosthetic outcome determination: Fixed implant-supported prosthesis

PHASE I Initial Diagnostics

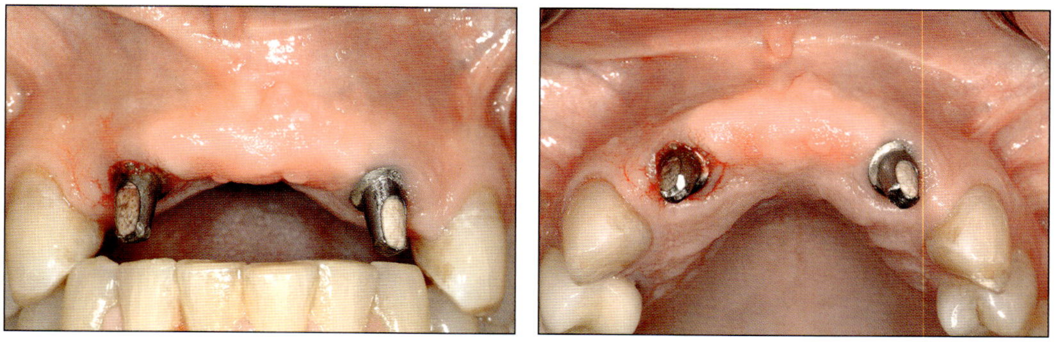

Pretreatment frontal and occlusal views.

PHASE I

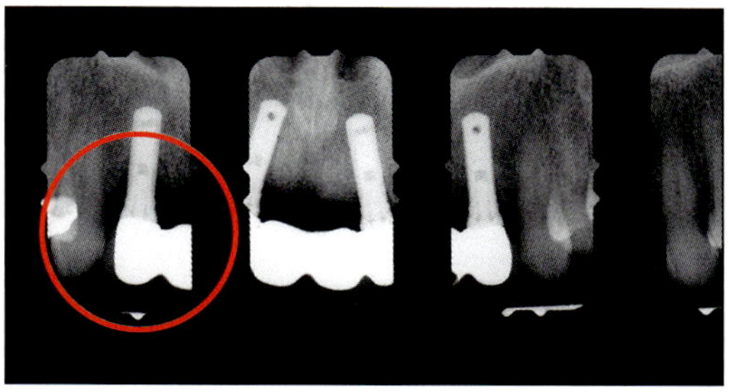

Initial radiographs. Red circle denotes failed implant.

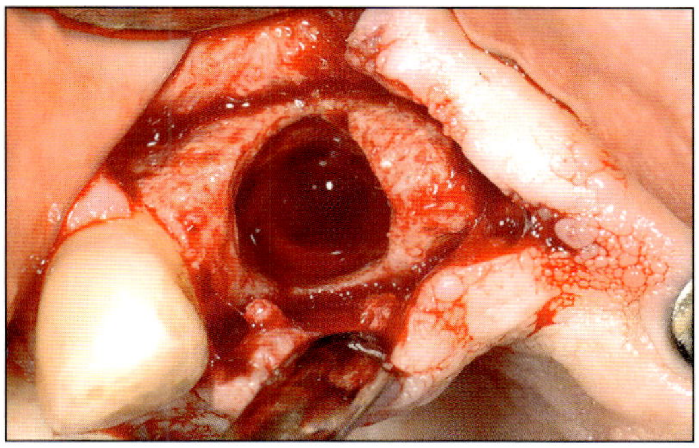

Extraction of failed implant at right lateral incisor site. Area bone grafted and osteotomy site preserved.

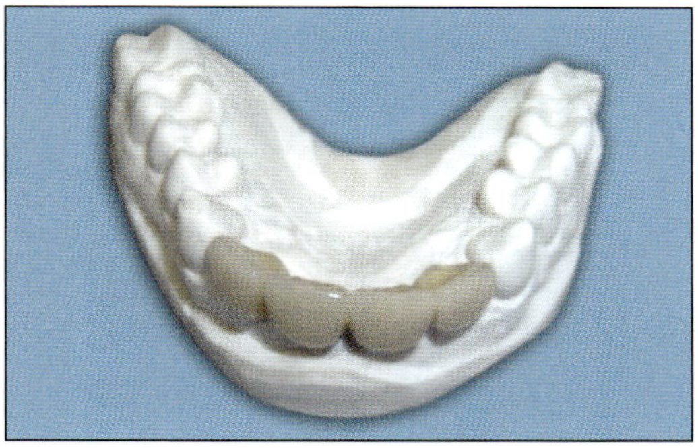

Diagnostic waxup of the anterior maxilla from the right lateral incisor to the left lateral incisor.

PHASE II Scanning Appliance Fabrication

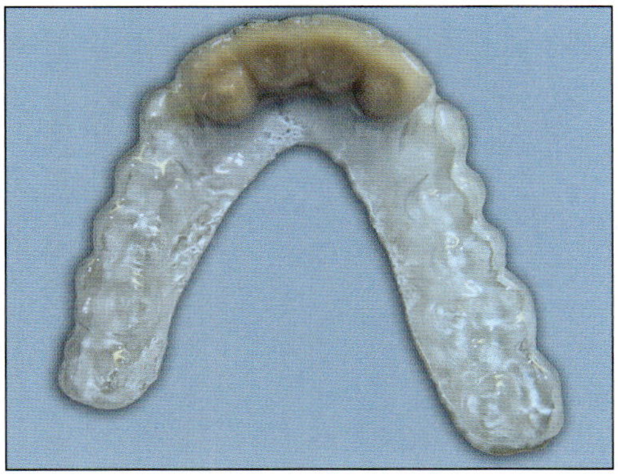

Second-generation scanning appliance reflecting desired prosthetic outcome of the area from the right lateral incisor to the left lateral incisor.

PHASE III CT Scan and SimPlant Conversion

CT scans are taken, and the resulting DICOM files are processed into the SimPlant format. Masks of specific anatomic structures are created.

PHASE IV Eight-Step Treatment-Planning Process

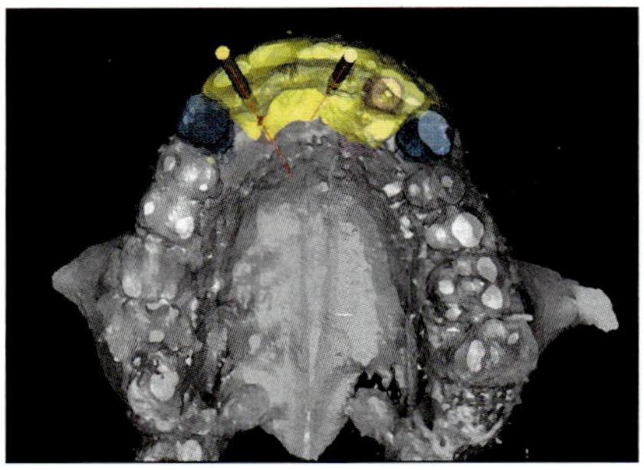

CT scan of the maxilla with the scanning appliance in place.

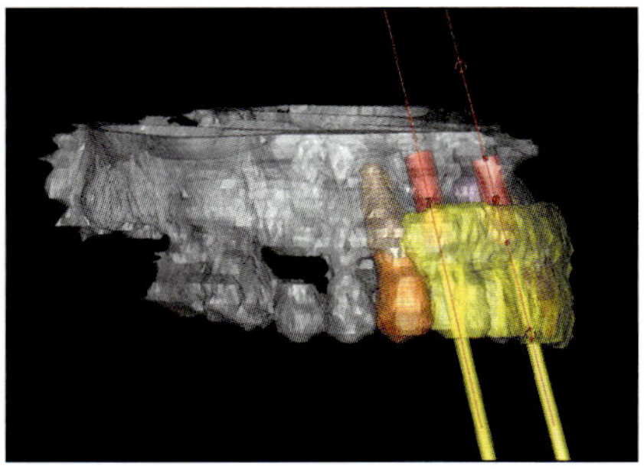

Right lateral view.

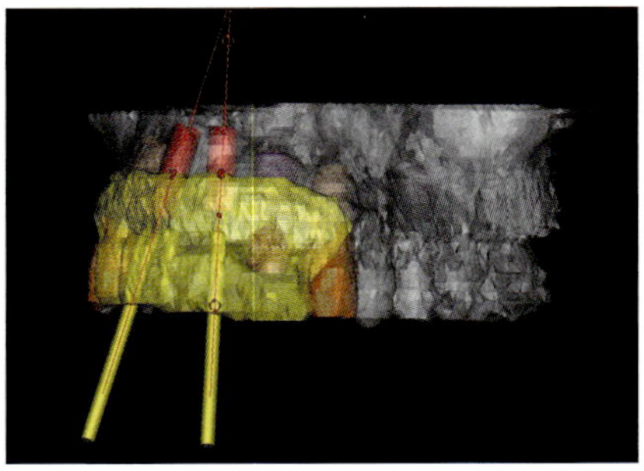

Left lateral view.

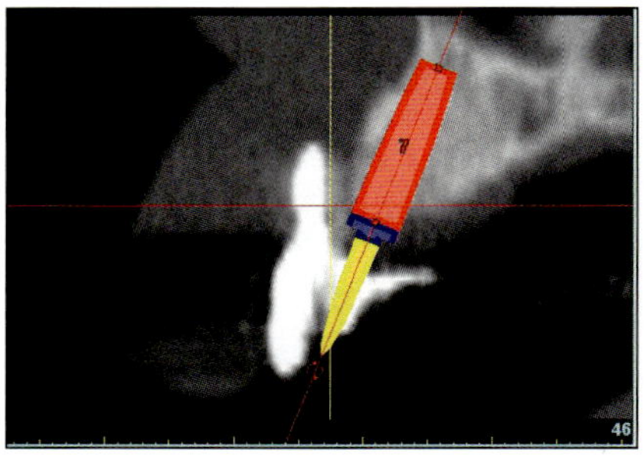

Cross-sectional view of the right lateral incisor post–site development.

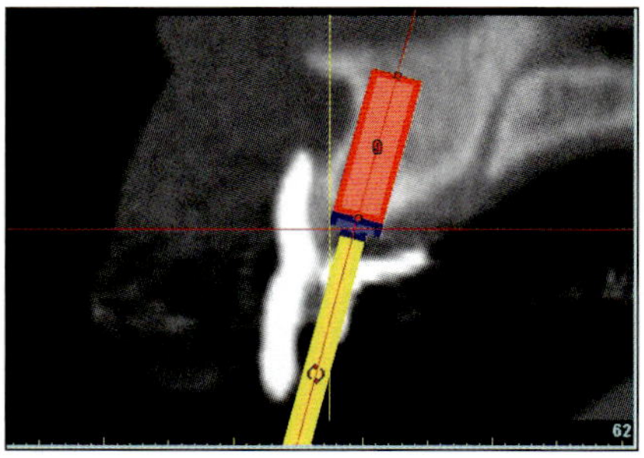

Cross-sectional view of the left central incisor.

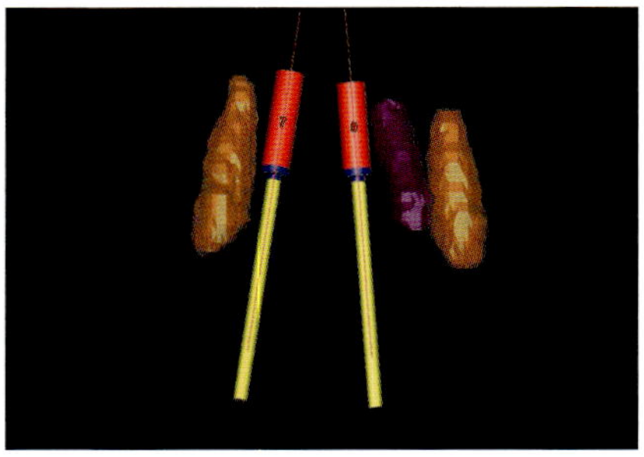

Mask of maxilla and mask of the scanning appliance removed. Natural canines and previous implant at the left lateral incisor site visualized.

PHASE V Medical Modeling

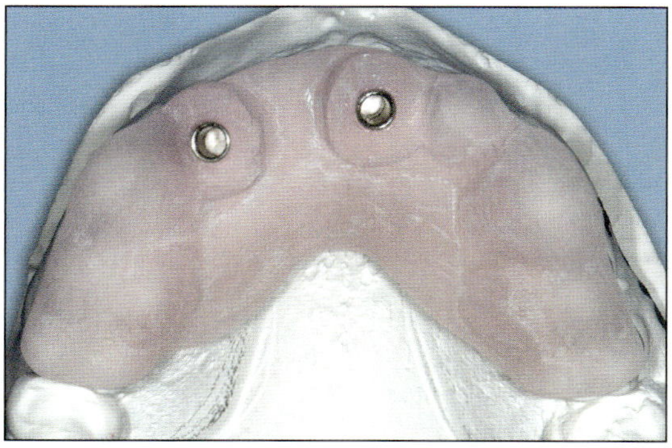

The 2-mm tooth-supported SurgiGuide on an accurate stone cast.

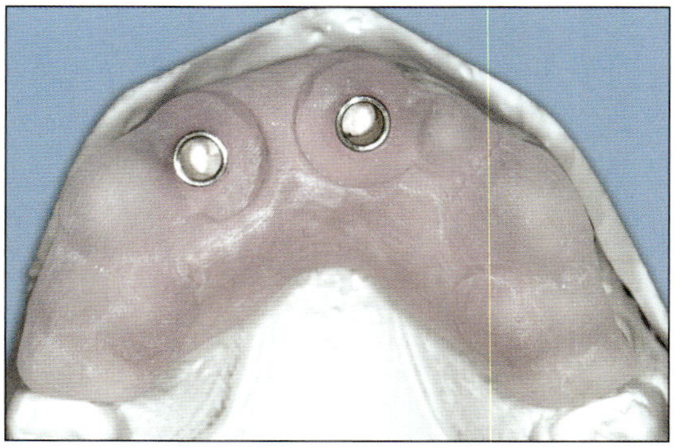

The 3-mm tooth-supported SurgiGuide on an accurate stone cast.

PHASE VI

Surgery

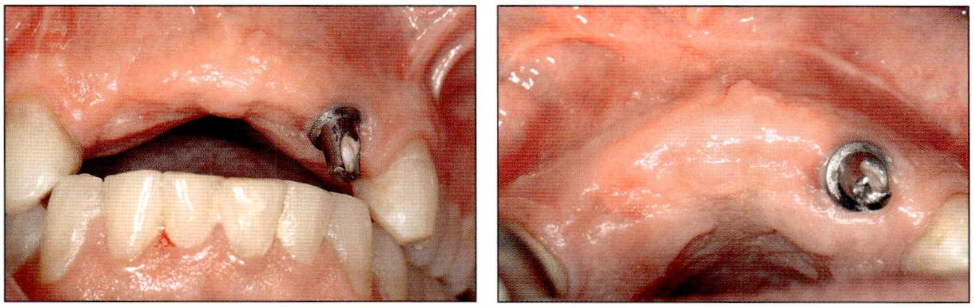

Views of the right lateral incisor site after site preservation/reconstruction.

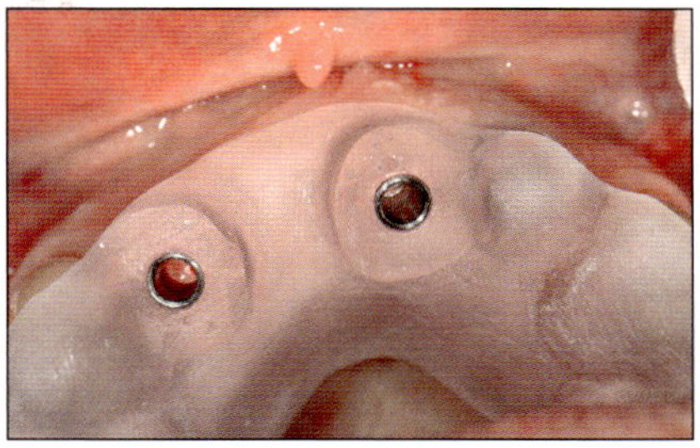

2-mm SurgiGuide in place.

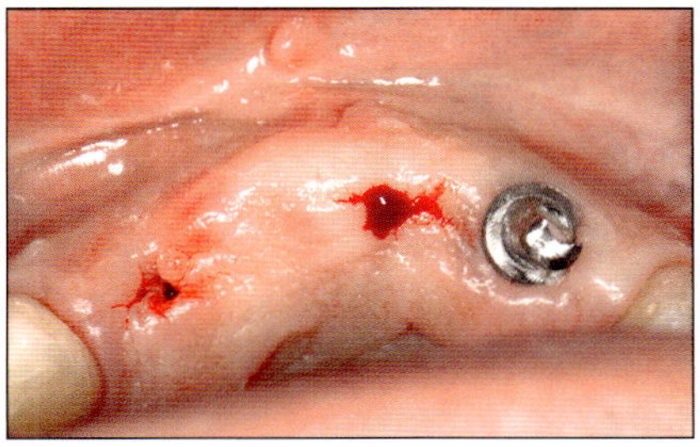

Minimally invasive approach. Punch access to the right lateral incisor and left central incisor sites.

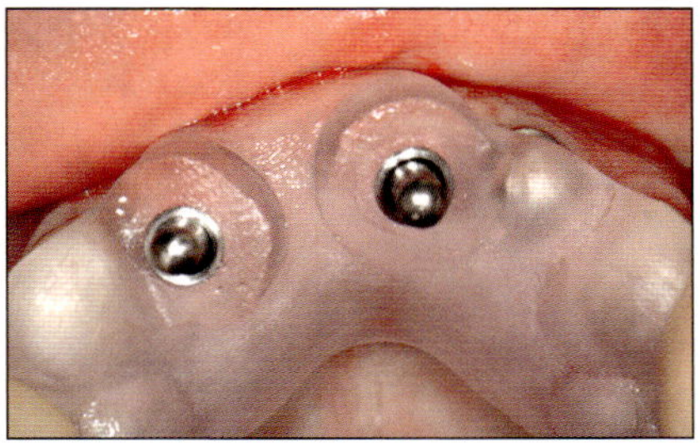

3-mm SurgiGuide with direction indicators in place.

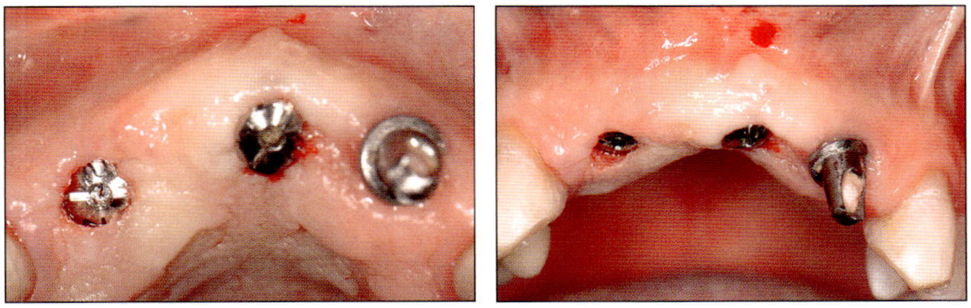

Implants placed at the right lateral incisor and left central incisor sites and healing abutments seated.

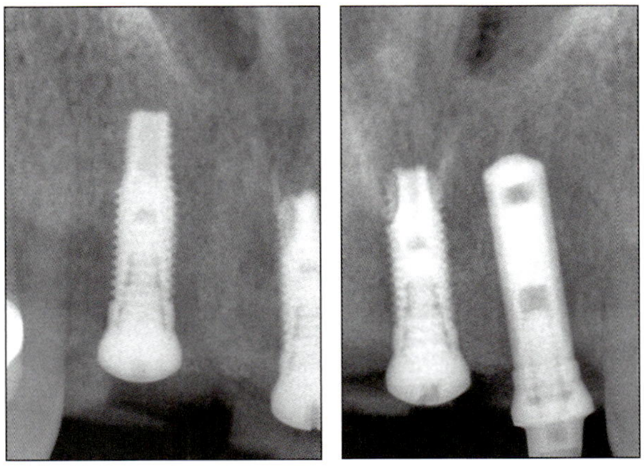

Radiographs of the right lateral incisor and the left central incisor sites after implant placement.

PHASE VII

Definitive Restoration and Supportive Maintenance

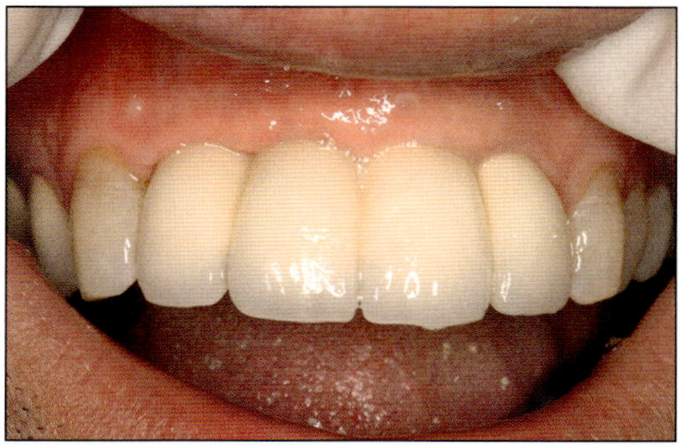

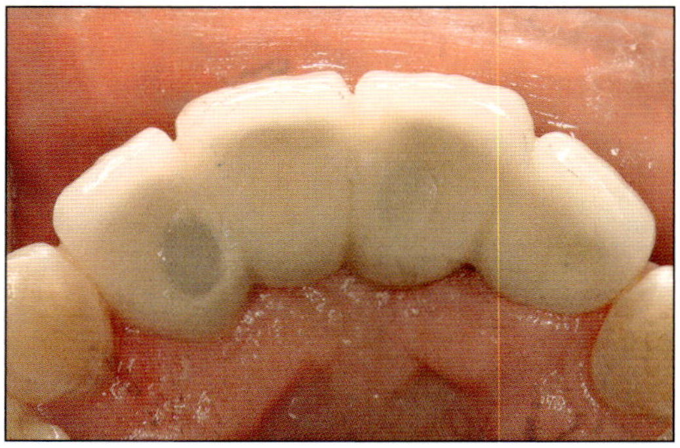

Definitive implant-supported fixed prosthesis from the right lateral incisor to the left lateral incisor. (Restoration by Dr Ken Milin, Winnetka, IL.)

Case 12 Mandibular Anterior Advanced Nonrestorable Caries

A 78-year-old woman presented with the chief complaint of fractured and nonrestorable decayed teeth resulting from xerostomia secondary to Sjogren syndrome. Her medical history was complex. The patient's needs and concerns were to have a stable-fitting, fixed, implant-supported prosthesis that would replace the hopeless mandibular anterior teeth and look similar to her natural dentition.

Diagnoses

- Nonrestorable dentition in the anterior mandible extending from the left canine to the right lateral incisor
- Horizontal crown fracture of the left canine
- Tooth–arch size discrepancy in mandible
- Xerostomia secondary to Sjögren syndrome
- Generalized moderate chronic periodontitis
- Wear and compensatory eruption from the left canine to the right lateral incisor
- Malocclusion (Angle Class I)

Case type: 2

- Gingival asymmetry with mucogingival deficiency at the right central incisor
- No bone loss at planned implant sites

Diagnostic inquiries

Clinical

- Tooth–arch size discrepancy and impact on final prosthesis design
- Anatomic considerations

Radiographic

- Bone quality
- Bone availability in the anterior mandible

Physical

- Ability to withstand elective dental surgery

Critical actions

- Diagnostic waxup after socket grafting to manage tooth–arch size discrepancy
- CT scan–based treatment planning
- Preoperative prosthetic outcome determination: Fixed implant-supported prosthesis

PHASE I Initial Diagnostics

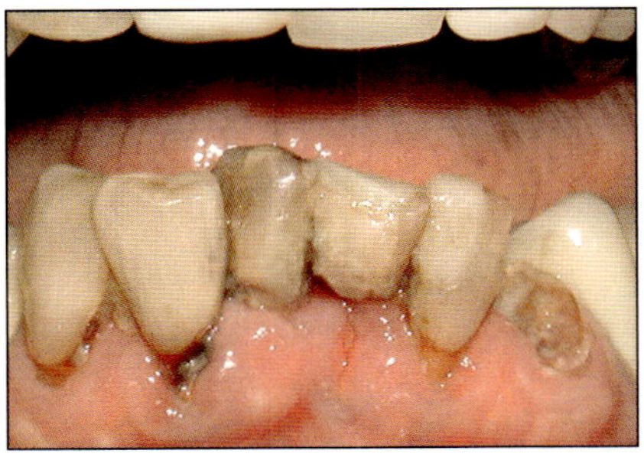

Preoperative view of the nonrestorable dentition extending from the mandibular left canine to the right lateral incisor.

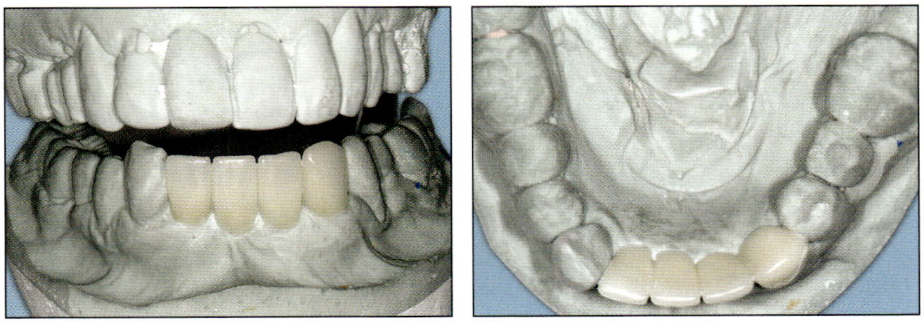

Diagnostic waxup performed after extraction and socket grafting. Tooth–arch size discrepancy managed with three incisors in the final plan.

PHASE II Scanning Appliance Fabrication

Second-generation scanning appliance used based on the diagnostic waxup.

PHASE III CT Scan and SimPlant Conversion

CT scans are taken, and the resulting DICOM files are processed into the SimPlant format. Masks of specific anatomic structures are created.

PHASE IV Eight-Step Treatment-Planning Process

CT scan of the mandible post–socket grafting. Masks of the mandible, natural mandibular left first premolar and right canine, proposed implants, nerves, and the scanning appliance are incorporated.

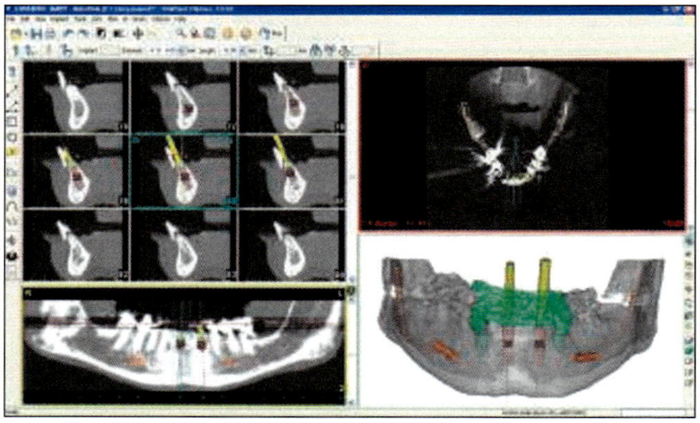

CT plan overview.

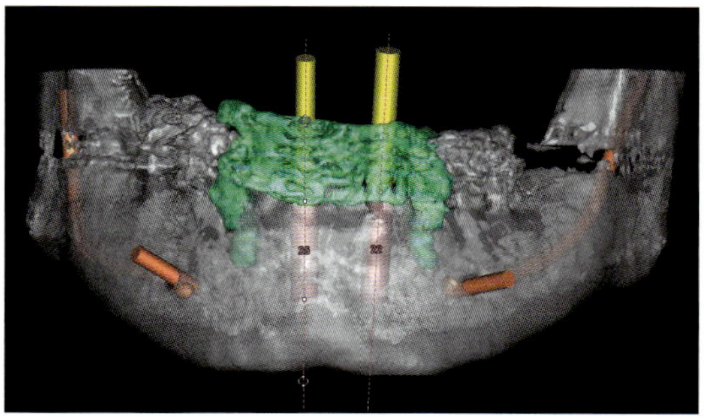

3D facial view. Transparency tool used.

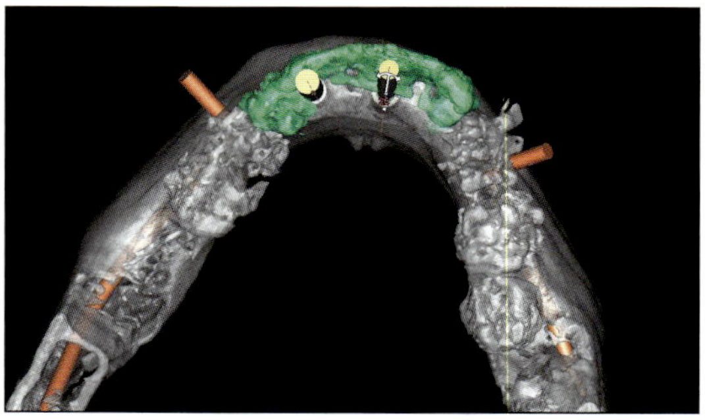

Occlusal view.

PHASE IV

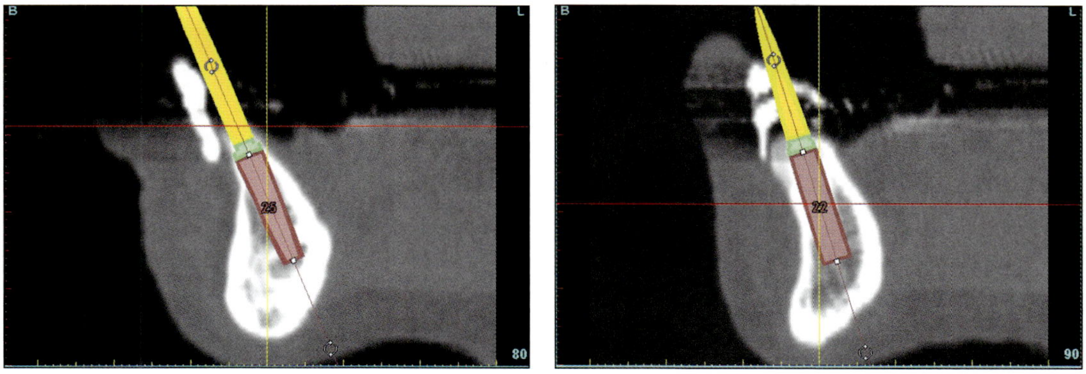

Cross-sectional views of implants at the sites of the left first premolar and right central incisor.

PHASE V Medical Modeling

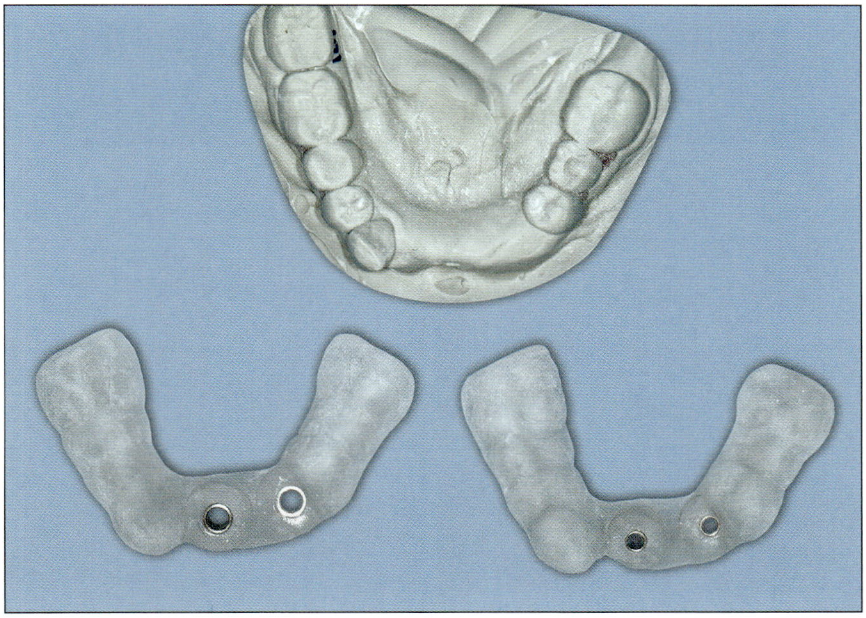

Tooth-supported SAFE SurgiGuide selected for surgery: 3-mm guide *(left)*, 2-mm guide *(right)*, accurate stone cast *(top)*.

PHASE VI

Surgery

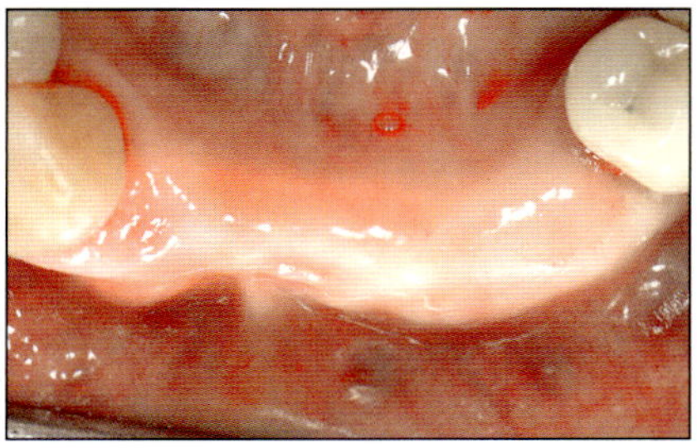

Occlusal view 6 months post–socket grafting and reconstruction.

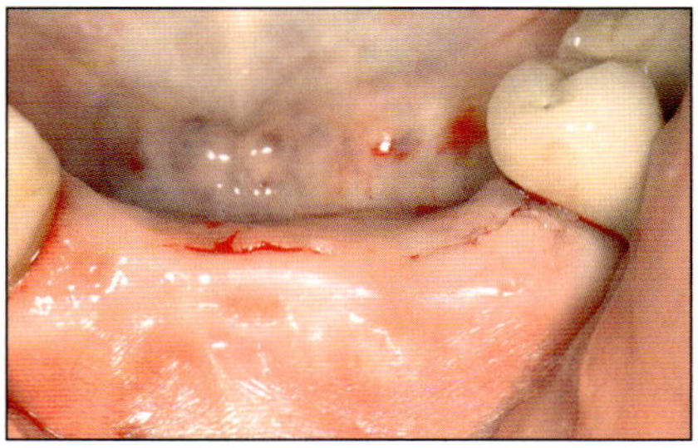

Minute incisions made to access bone of the anterior mandible.

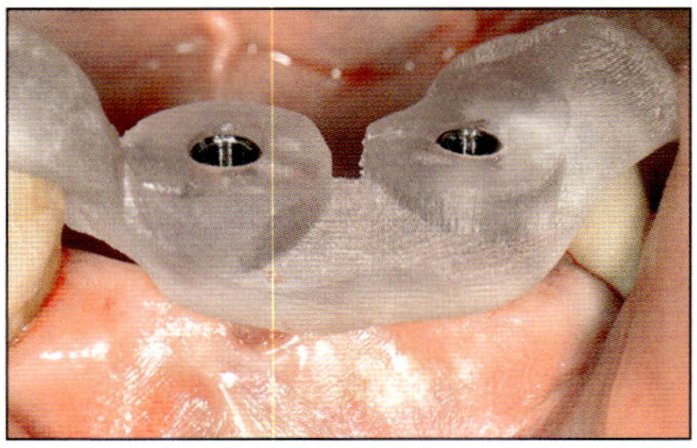

SurgiGuide (2 mm) in place.

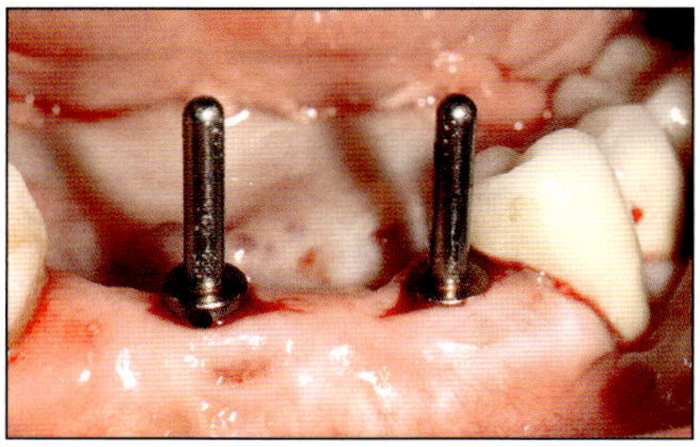

Implant direction indicators in place to maintain attached gingiva facial to implant positioning.

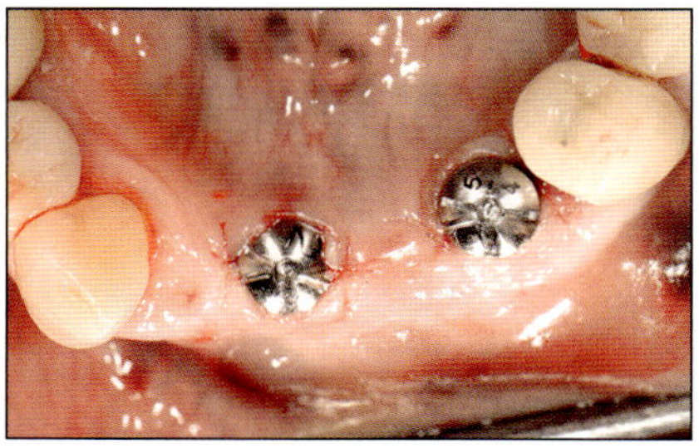

Implants placed at the 3-mm level in the sites of the mandibular left canine and right central incisor.

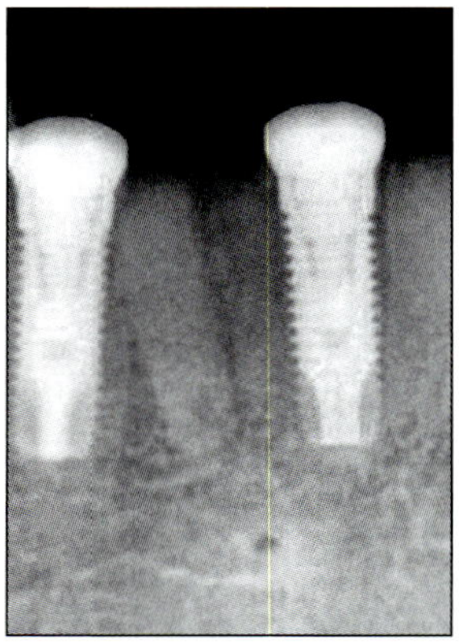

Immediate postoperative radiograph.

PHASE VII

Definitive Restoration and Supportive Maintenance

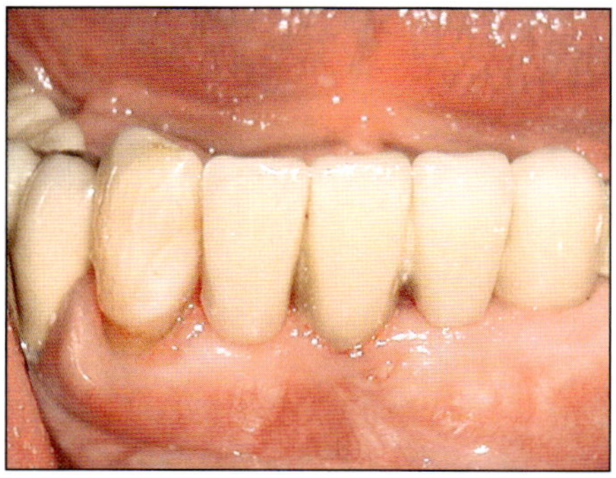

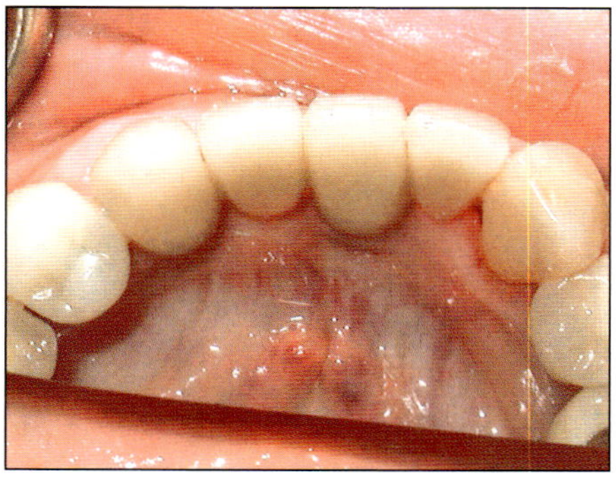

Final implant-supported fixed prosthesis. (Restoration by Dr Kevin Krug, Lombard, IL.)

Case 13 Generalized Aggressive Periodontitis

A 58-year-old woman presented with the chief complaint of generalized aggressive and progressive periodontitis. Her medical history was unremarkable. The patient had been struggling with maintaining her natural dentition for several years and was interested in alternative options for her ailing dentition. She had been comprehensively treated for periodontitis but demonstrated progressively mobile dentition with multiple endodontic pathologies and continued attachment loss. The patient's needs and concerns were to have a stable-fitting and fixed implant-supported prosthesis that would replace her compromised mandibular dentition.

Diagnoses

- Advanced disuse atrophy of the edentulous mandible
- Advanced residual ridge resorption
- History of generalized aggressive periodontitis

Case type: 5

- Significant horizontal and vertical bone loss

Diagnostic inquiries

Clinical

- Accurate denture
- Accurate ScannoGuide
- Final prosthetic outcome

Radiographic

- Position of mental foramen and nerves
- Extent and pattern of bone resorption
- Bone quality

Physical

- None

Critical actions

- Accurate mandibular denture and ScannoGuide fabricated
- Collaboratively based 3D CT scan treatment planning
- Preoperative prosthetic outcome determination: Fixed implant-supported prosthesis

PHASE I Initial Diagnostics

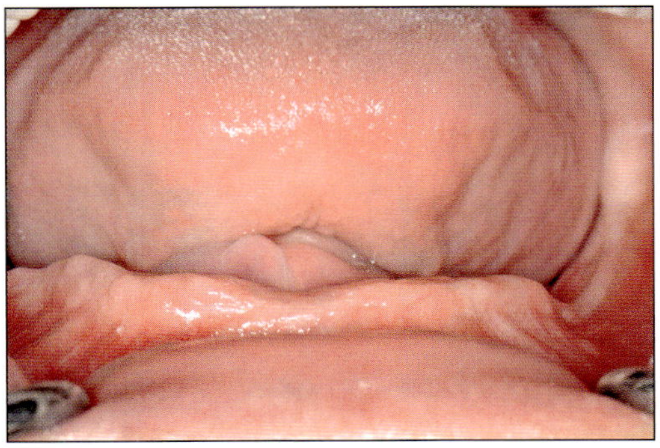

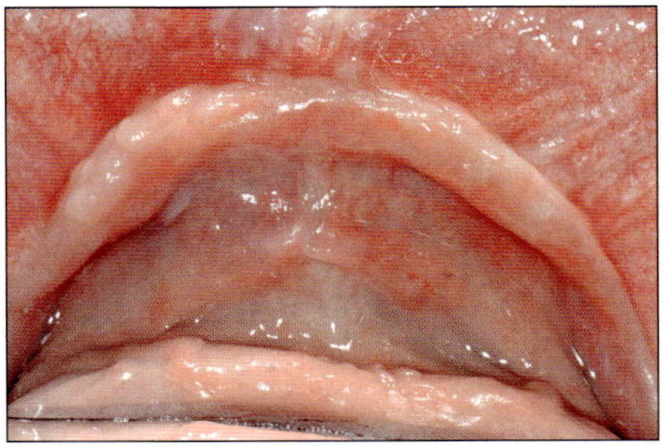

Pretreatment views: complete edentulism.

PHASE II Scanning Appliance Fabrication

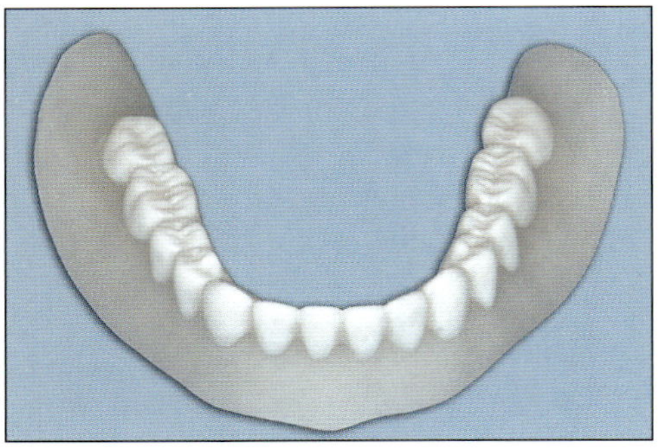

Third-generation ScannoGuide was fabricated to meet occlusal-prosthetic outcome requirements.

PHASE III CT Scan and SimPlant Conversion

CT scans are taken, and the resulting DICOM files are processed into the SimPlant format. Masks of specific anatomic structures are created.

PHASE IV Eight-Step Treatment-Planning Process

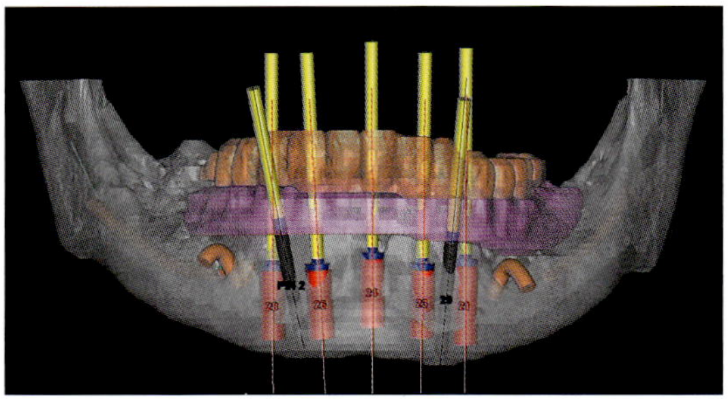

3D CT scan treatment planning.

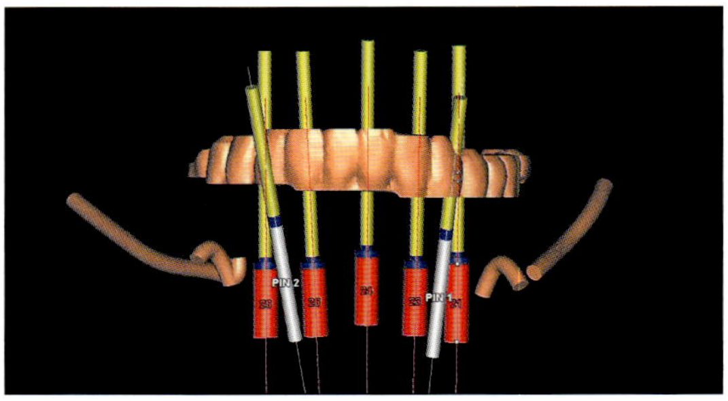

Masks of the mandible and denture base removed.

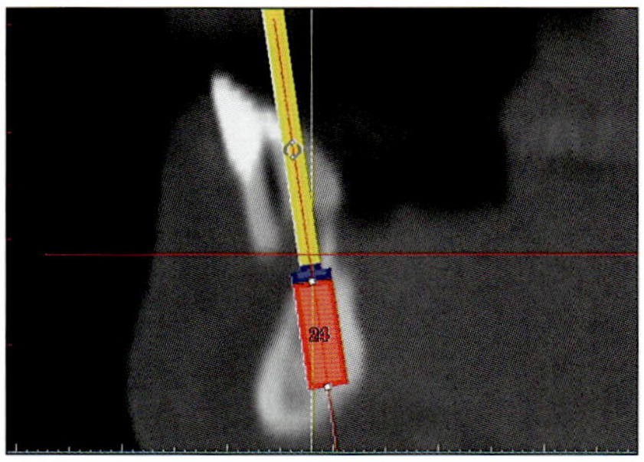

Cross section of implant. ScannoGuide is fully seated, revealing the density gradient differential between the denture base and the teeth.

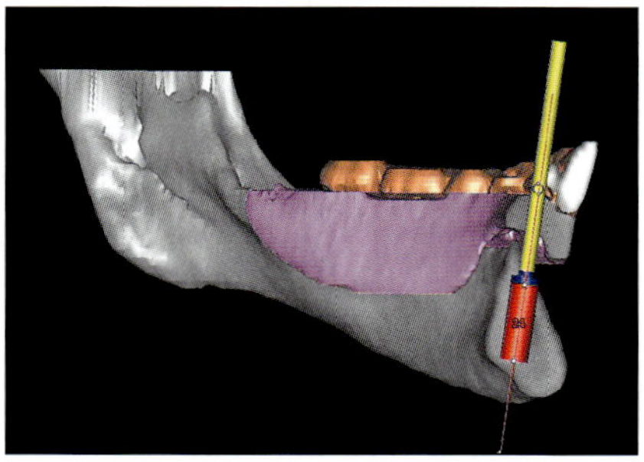

Clip art used to superimpose a cross section of the 2D image on the 3D image.

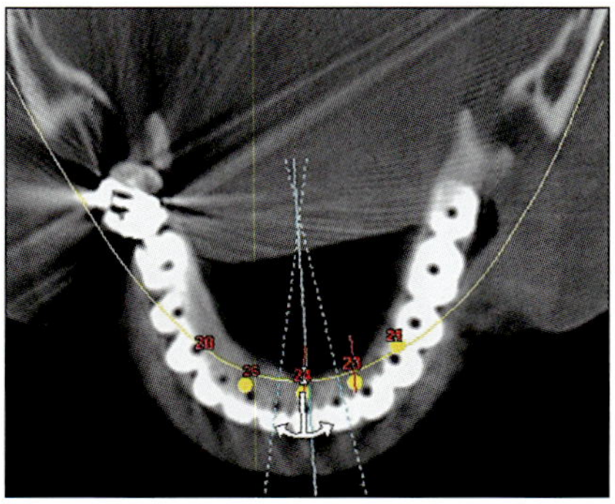

Axial view of implant emergence through planned tooth positions.

PHASE V Medical Modeling

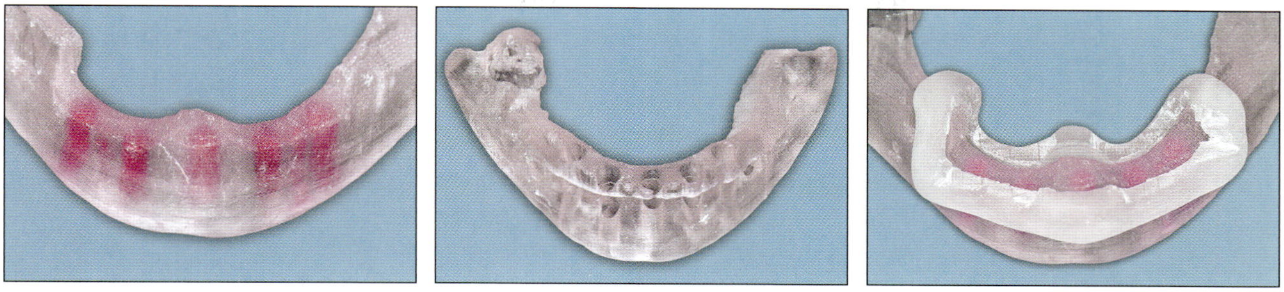

Stereolithographic bone medical model post–bone reduction showing planned implant sites highlighted with red dye *(left)*; osteotomy sites created for surgical dress rehearsal *(center)*; and bone reduction guide in place on medical cast *(right)*.

Bone-supported SAFE SurgiGuide. Note the variation in tube heights, which allows one drill length to be used for osteotomy site preparation.

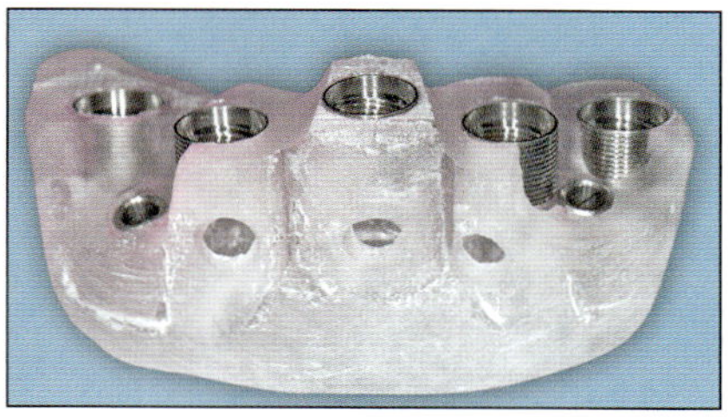

PHASE VI Surgery

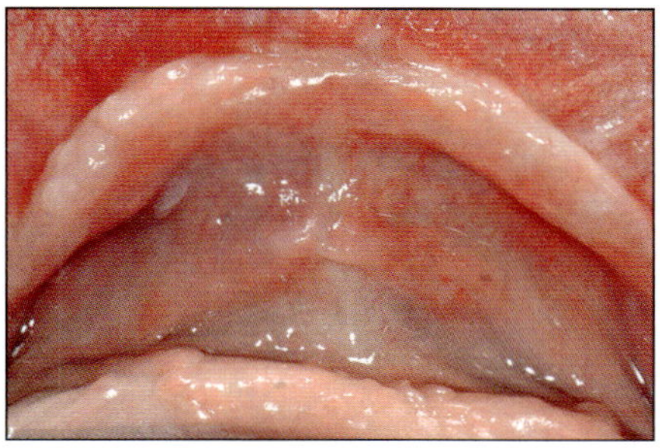

Initial preoperative view.

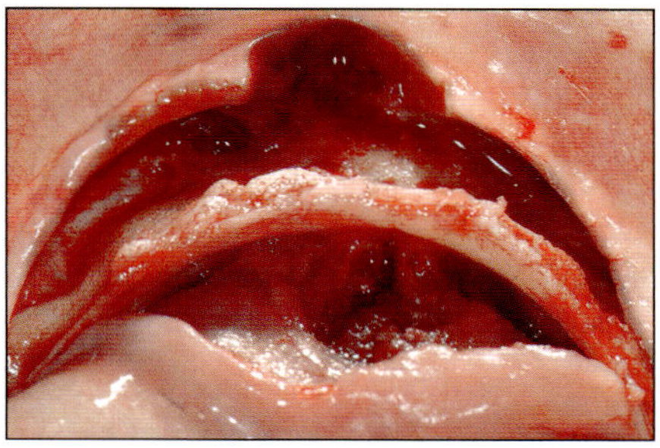

Flap reflection, revealing anatomy of the site.

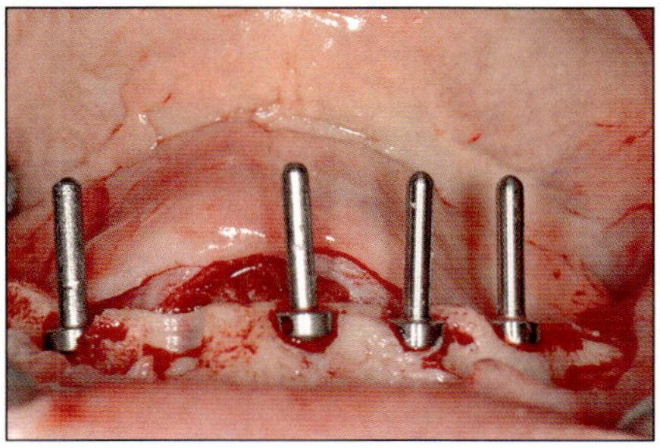

Precision osteoplasty performed via bone reduction guide.

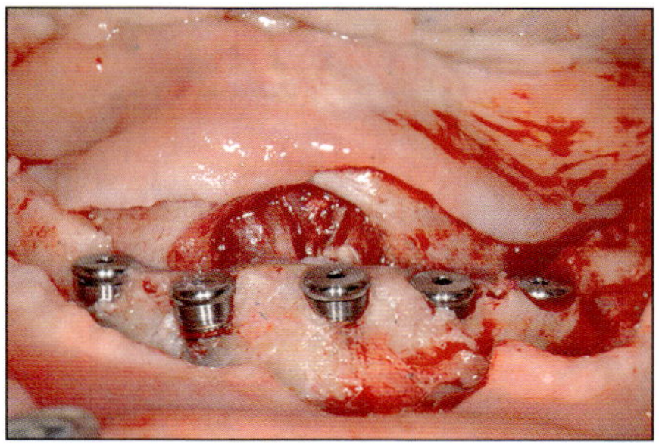

Osteotomy site preparation performed.

PHASE VI

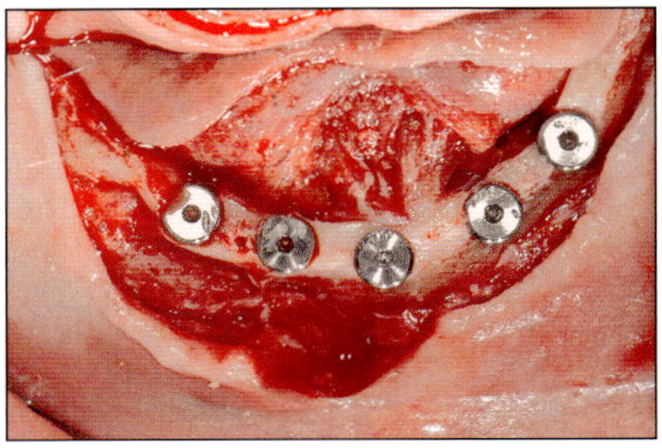

Implants placed via bone-supported SAFE SurgiGuide.

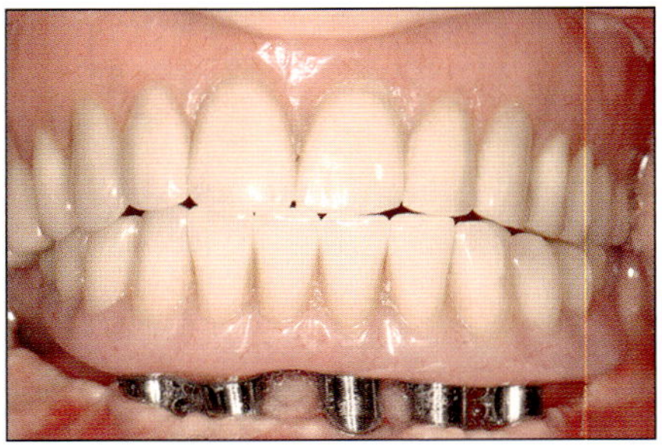

Immediate-load prosthesis finalized.

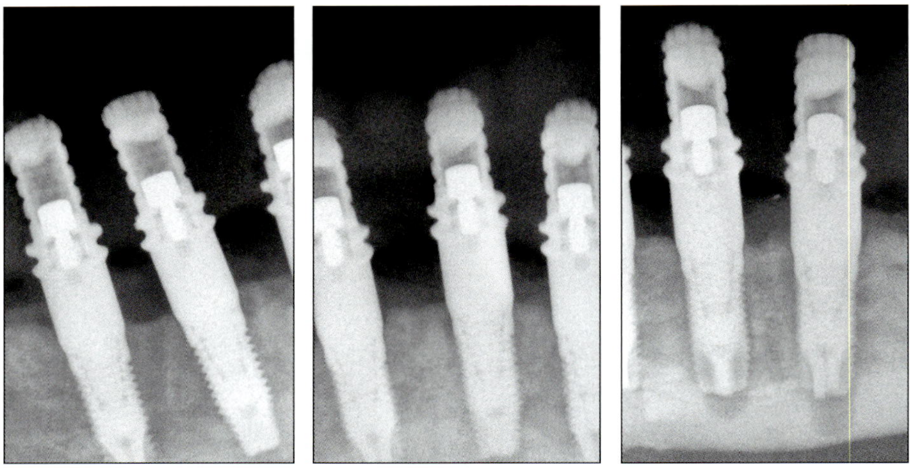

Immediate postoperative radiographs of the implants.

PHASE VII Definitive Restoration and Supportive Maintenance

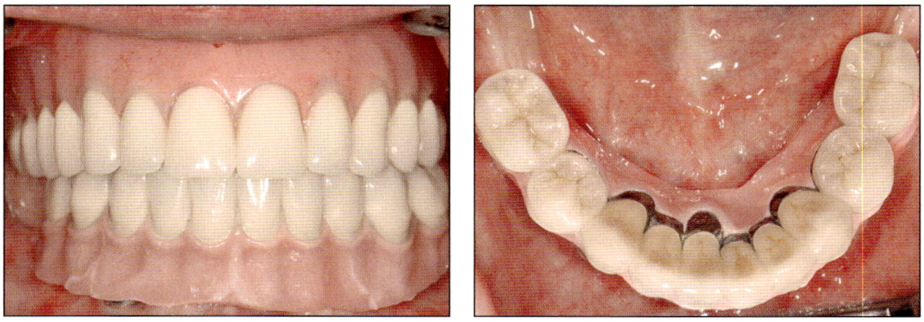

Definitive implant-supported fixed prosthesis. (Restoration by Dr John Petrie, Chicago, IL; laboratory technician: David Guelde, CDT, Clarkston, MI.)

Case 14 Fractured/Nonrestorable Mandibular First Molar

A 63-year-old man presented with the chief complaint of a nonrestorable mandibular left first molar. His medical history was unremarkable. The patient's needs and concerns were to have a stable-fitting, fixed, implant-supported prosthesis that would be maintainable long-term.

Diagnoses

- Horizontal fracture/nonrestorable mandibular left first molar
- Class I skeletal relationship
- Angle Class III molar tendency
- Periapical pathosis of the mandibular right first molar

Case type: 1

- Optimal final tooth position acceptable
- Acceptable gingival symmetry, volume, and color
- No horizontal or vertical bone loss

Diagnostic inquiries

Clinical

- Attachment loss associated with fracture?
- Adjacent or maxillomandibular teeth malposed?

Radiographic

- Extent of periapical pathosis
- Position of nerve
- Lingual bone anatomy (concavity?)

Physical

- None

Critical actions

- Ensure that the current molar tooth position is acceptable prosthetically to allow its use for the planned implant position
- Preoperative prosthetic outcome determination: Fixed implant-supported prosthesis

PHASE I Initial Diagnostics

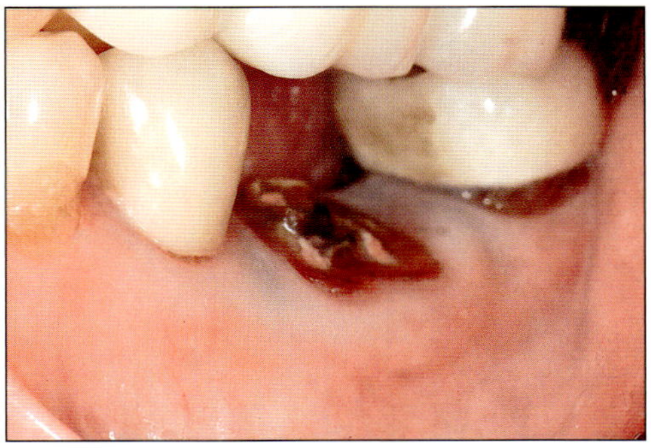

Pretreatment view of the mandibular left first molar.

PHASE II Scanning Appliance Fabrication

No scanning appliance was utilized.

PHASE III CT Scan and SimPlant Conversion

CT scans are taken, and the resulting DICOM files are processed into the SimPlant format. Masks of specific anatomic structures are created.

PHASE IV Eight-Step Treatment-Planning Process

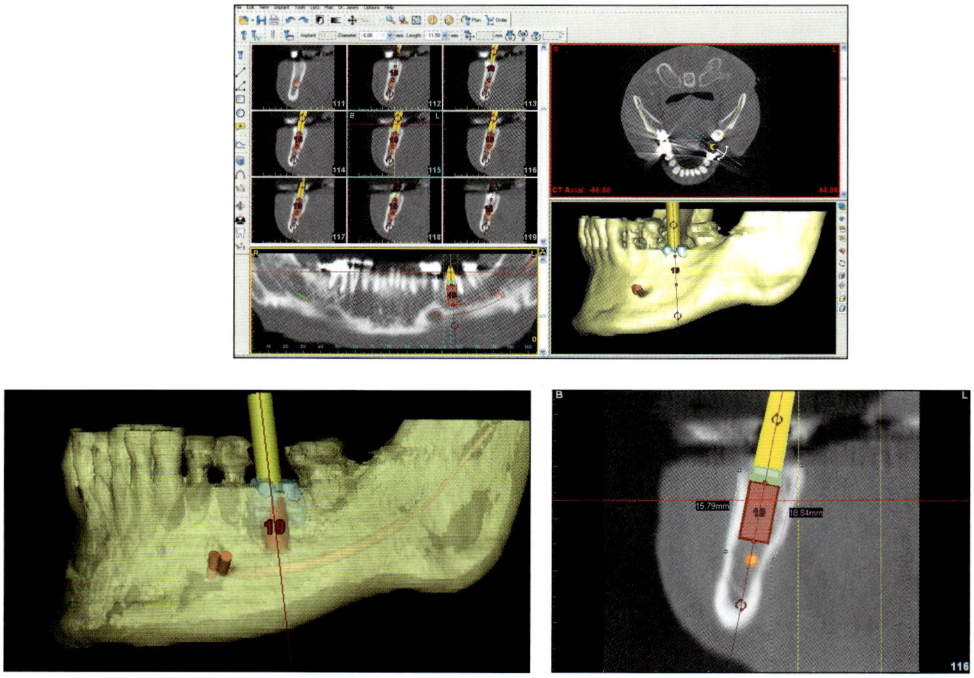

Cross-sectional view of planned implant position. Preoperative planning (ie, assessment of bone availability, anatomy, and position of nerve) analyzed three dimensionally.

PHASE V Medical Modeling

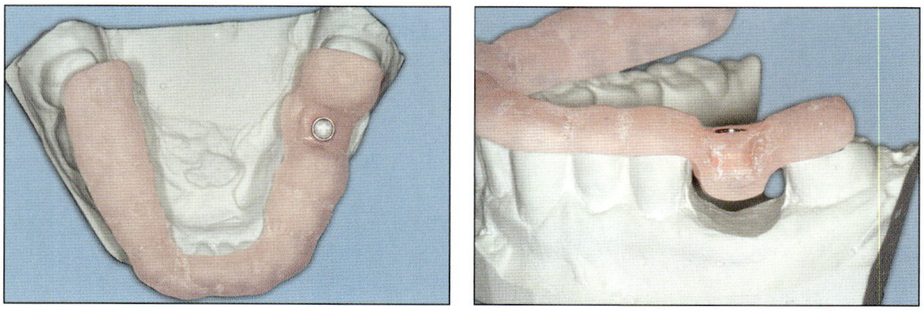

Tooth-supported SurgiGuide selected for surgery.

PHASE VI

Surgery

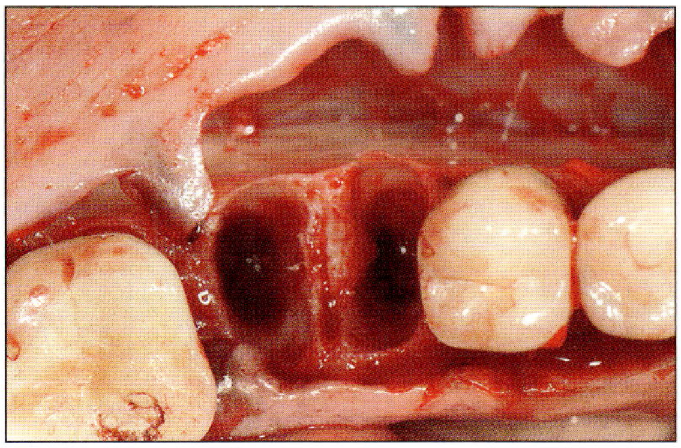

Atraumatic extraction.

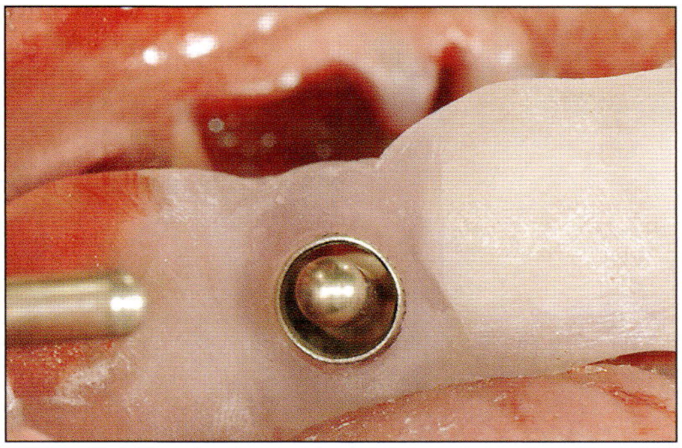

Tooth-supported SurgiGuide in place for precise osteotomy site preparation.

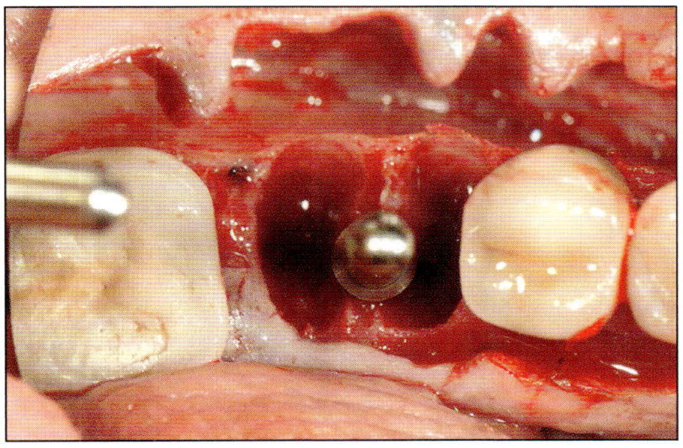

Precise osteotomy site preparation in furcation bone.

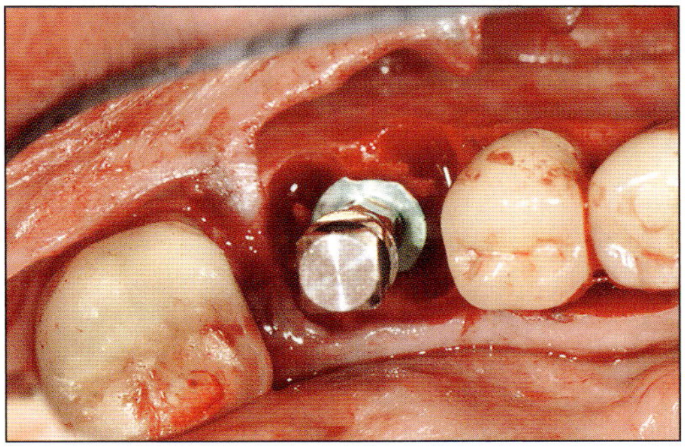

Immediate implant placement in furcation bone.

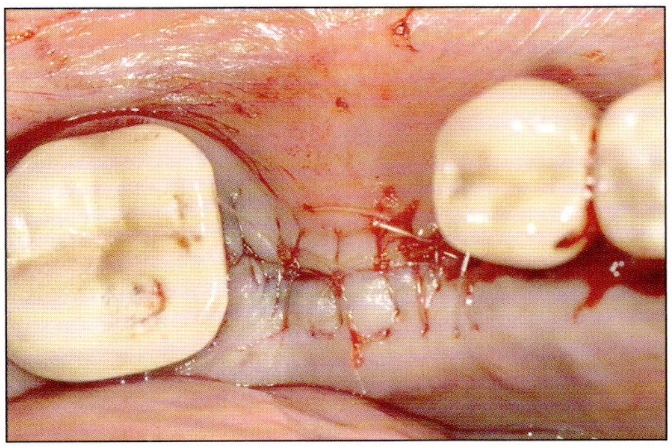

Primary closure following bone grafting.

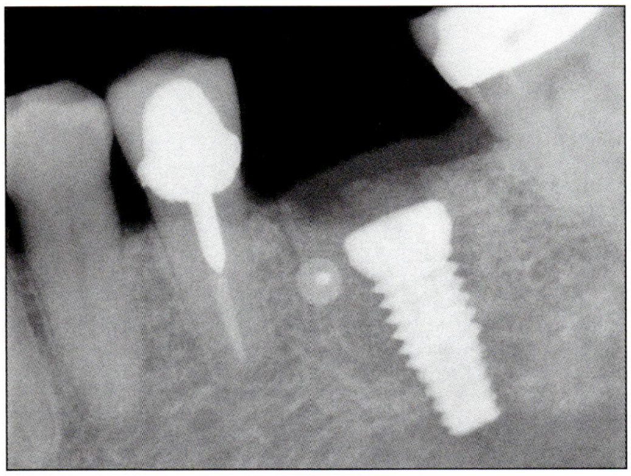

Direct postoperative radiograph demonstrating optimal positioning.

PHASE VI

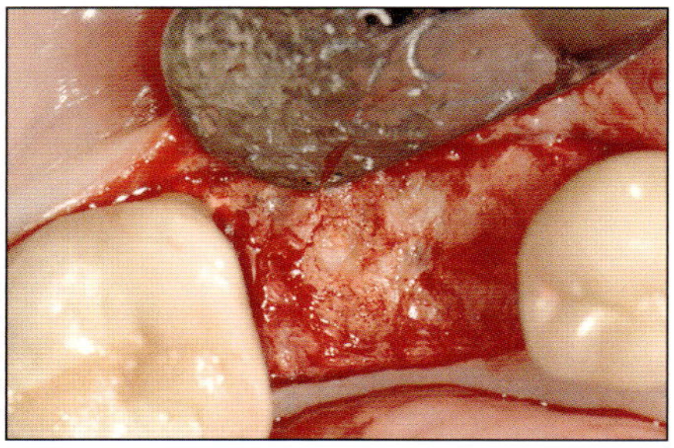

Uncovering procedure, stage 2 surgery. Bone healing is observed.

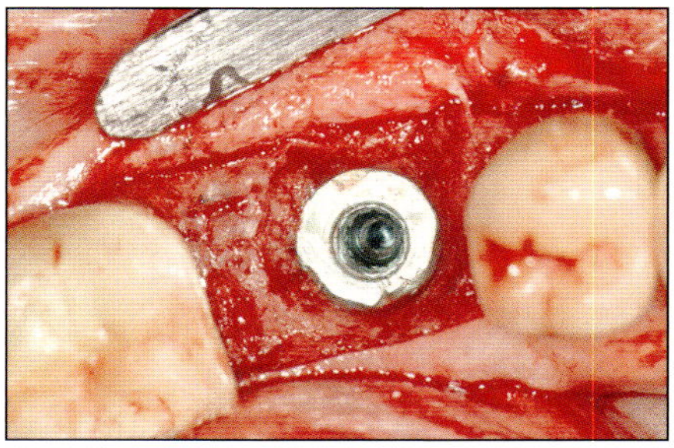

Exposure of implant.

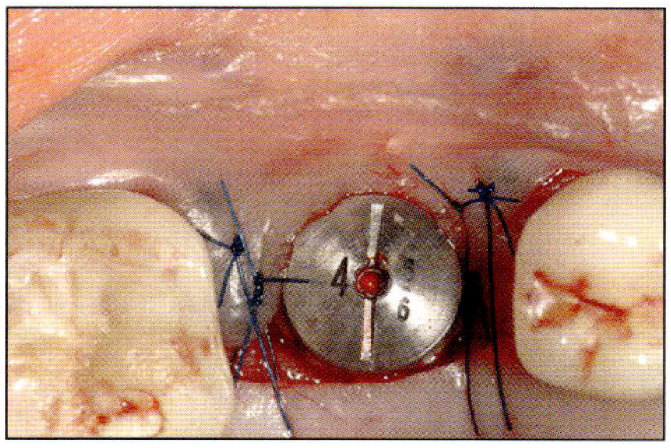

Placement of healing abutment and suturing.

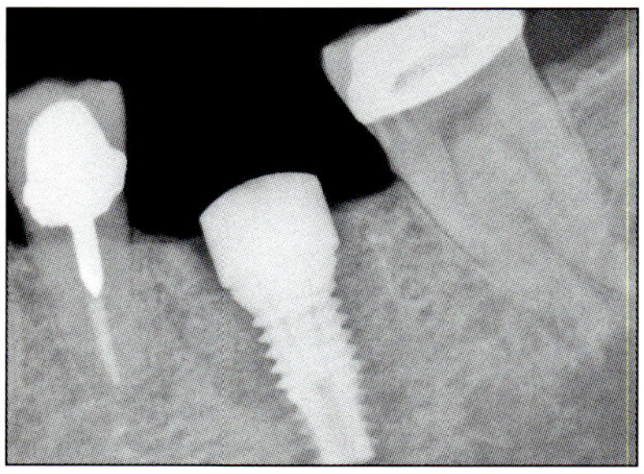

Radiograph taken at stage 2 surgery.

PHASE VII Definitive Restoration and Supportive Maintenance

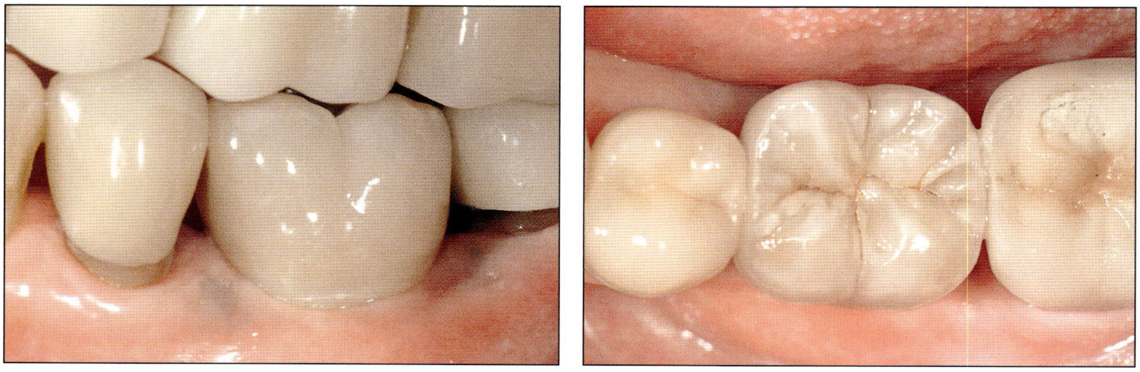

Definitive implant-supported fixed partial prosthesis at the site of the mandibular left first molar.

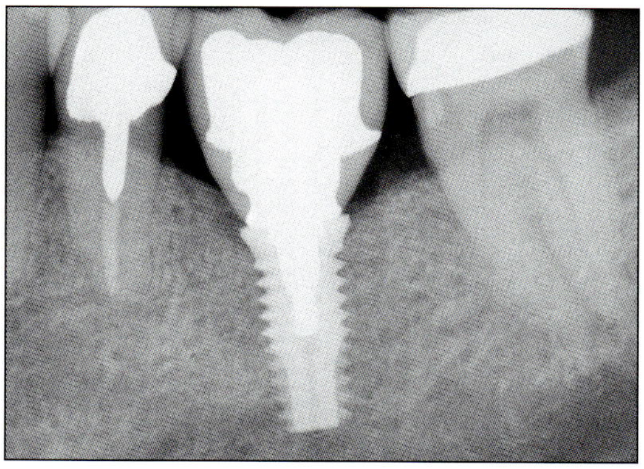

Final radiograph of implant and prosthesis. (Restoration by Dr Michael Morgan, Hinsdale, IL; laboratory technician: David Guelde, CDT, Clarkston,MI.)

9

SAFE SYSTEM AND IMMEDIATE SMILE

Philippe B. Tardieu, DDS
Veerle Pattijn, MSc Eng, PhD

Having achieved confidence and proficiency with using computer-guided implant placement, clinicians may want to take it to the next level by trying advanced options such as SAFE System and Immediate Smile. Both of these systems were invented by the author (PT) to improve accuracy and efficiency of implant treatment. This chapter explains the components of each system, describes a case example to illustrate their clinical application, and provides the rationale behind their development.

SAFE System

The SAFE (secure, accurate, flexible, ergonomic) System was developed for use in combination with surgical guides to provide more accurate guidance of drilling as well as implant placement. Under the standard protocol, a series of surgical templates and drills with increasing diameters are used to prepare the implant site. Each step requires the removal of one template and the placement of the next, which carries an inherent risk of misalignment. The SAFE System allows the use of only one surgical template and two specially designed drills. In addition, it provides a physical stop for both drilling and implant placement, which reduces the risk of drilling or placing the implant too deep. The SAFE System includes a surgical tray, guiding cylinders, a trephine, pilot and final drills, implant holders, and a storage box for the components.

SAFE System components

SAFE Surgical Tray

The SAFE Surgical Tray (Fig 9-1) is designed to represent the 16 tooth positions in a jaw, allowing the clinician to place the surgical components at the appropriate tooth positions before surgery to help eliminate errors during the surgical procedures. Titanium implant containers are also available to accommodate the change from a brand-specific fixture mount to the SAFE fixture mount. Once assembled, the SAFE Tray can be placed in the surgical box for sterilization of all components simultaneously.

Guiding and drilling cylinders

A *guiding cylinder* (Fig 9-2) is used to stabilize the drilling cylinder and guide implant placement. This titanium-alloy cylinder is glued inside the surgical guide and has three grooves on its internal surface that serve to stabilize the drilling cylinder. It measures 4 mm in height and has a 4.2-mm internal diameter and a 5.2-mm external diameter to allow implants to be placed as close as 2 mm apart.

The *drilling cylinder* (Fig 9-3) is a surgical stainless steel tube 5 mm in height that is placed inside the guiding cylinder to direct the drills during implant site preparation. The same drilling cylinder is used to guide each of the drills used to prepare the implant sites. Once the drilling procedures are completed, the drilling cylinder is removed, and the implants are placed using the guiding cylinder.

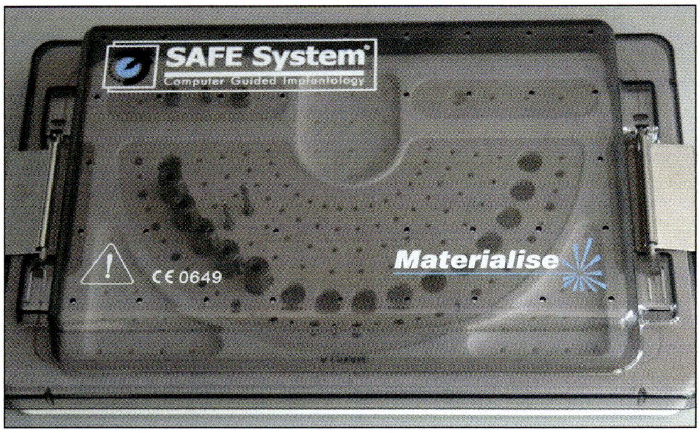

Fig 9-1 SAFE Surgical Tray and storage box.

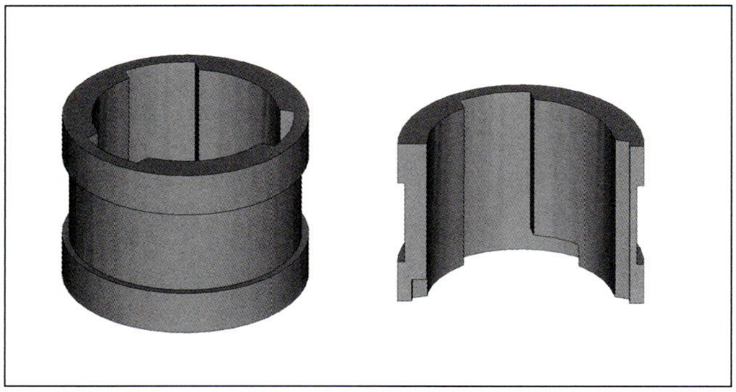

Fig 9-2 *(left)* Guiding cylinder. *(right)* Cross section of the guiding cylinder showing the grooves that stabilize the drilling cylinder.

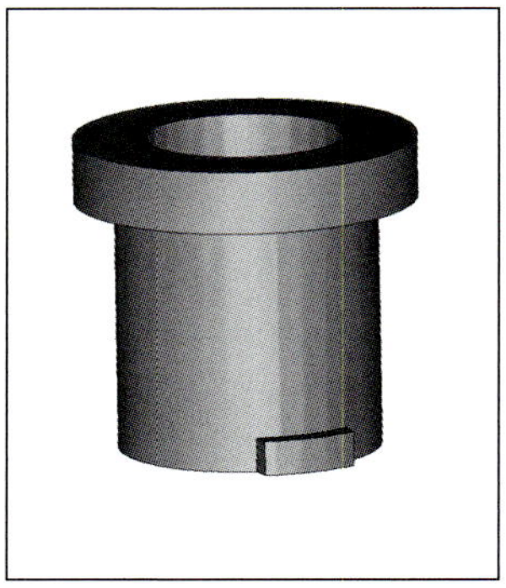

Fig 9-3 Drilling cylinder.

Trephine

The *trephine* (Fig 9-4) is designed to be placed over the pilot drill and fits inside the guiding cylinder. It is used to remove the soft tissue in a transmucosal procedure and to center the initial penetration of the pilot drill into the bone during flap elevation procedures.

Drills

The SAFE System requires only two drills to prepare an implant site: a staged (pilot) drill and a calibrating (final) drill. The thread, gouge drawing, and surface processing of these drills are optimized to increase their cutting capacity and prevent overheating during site preparation; however, irrigation with cool saline solution is still necessary. The stepped design of the drills allows each to be guided through the same drilling cylinder and the same surgical guide.

The diameter of the *pilot drill* (Fig 9-5) is 2 mm at the most apical 4 mm of its length, then increases to 2.7 mm. The *final drill* (Fig 9-6) is 3.15 mm in diameter and has a relief on its surface to prevent overheating due to friction.

Drills are available in seven different lengths, ranging from 10 to 25 mm. The most commonly used drills are those with lengths of 13, 15, and 18 mm. Each drill features a physical stop, which, in combination with the vertical position of the cylinders in the guide, controls the depth of the drilling.

Implant holders

With the SAFE System, the implant is directed to its planned position without the need for visual control, thanks to the use of a dedicated *implant holder* (Fig 9-7) that passes through the guiding cylinder. This implant holder has a flange at its proximal end that serves as a physical depth control stop. Currently, seven lengths of implant holders are available, ranging from 4 to 15 mm. The most commonly used are those with lengths of 6, 7, and 9 mm.

The SAFE System enables the placement of all implant brands with a standard platform of 4.1 mm, a 2.7-mm external hex, and a diameter ranging from 3.25 to 4.1 mm.

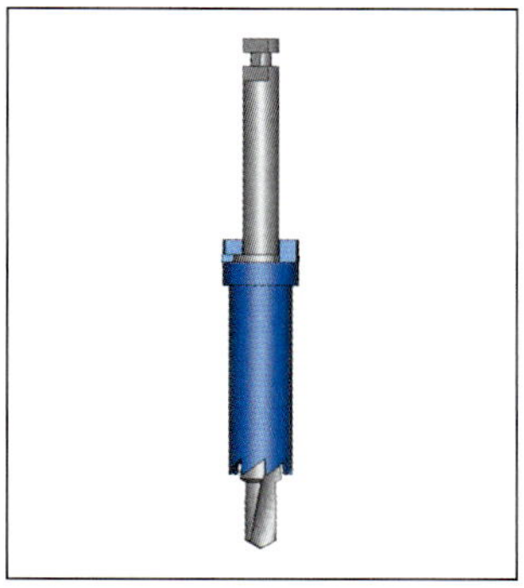

Fig 9-4 Trephine *(blue)* mounted on the pilot drill.

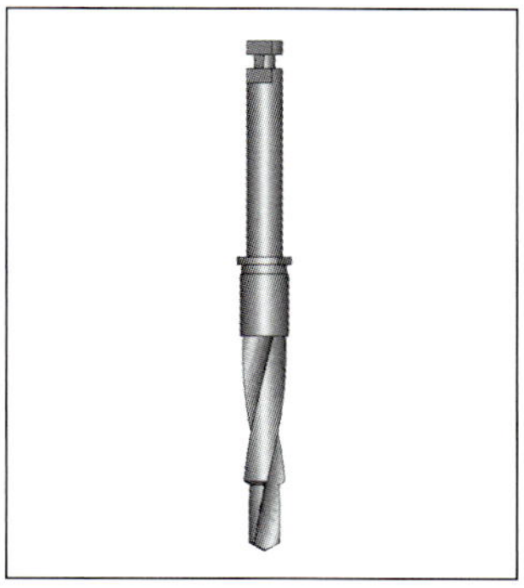

Fig 9-5 SAFE pilot drill.

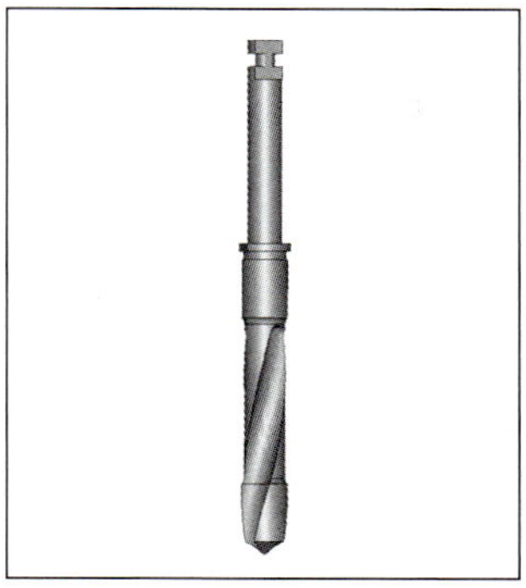

Fig 9-6 SAFE final drill.

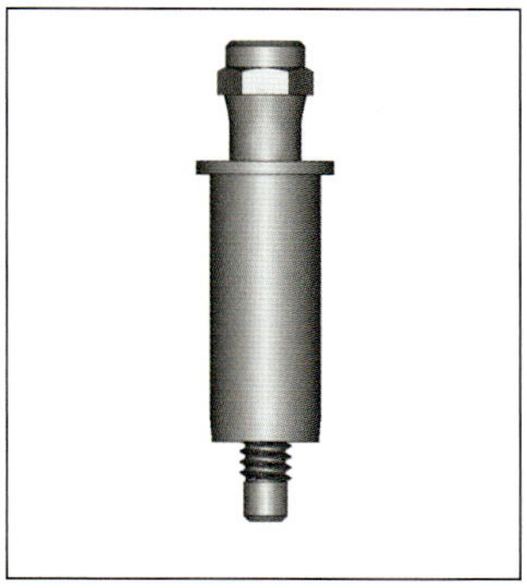

Fig 9-7 SAFE implant holder.

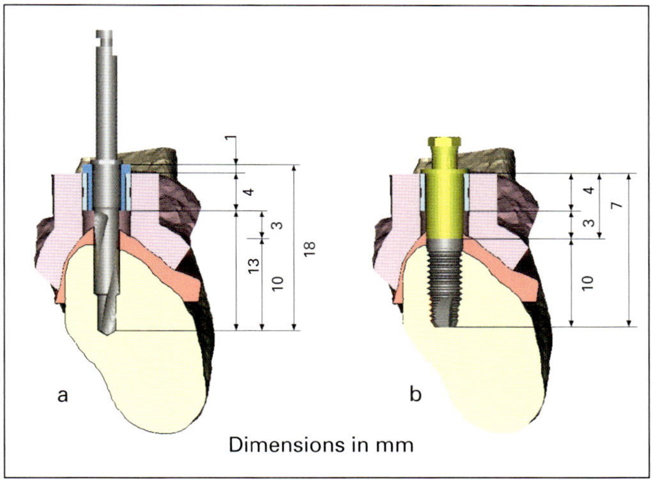

Fig 9-8 Cross section of bone and mucosa with mucosa-supported SurgiGuide and SAFE System components in place. *(a)* The guiding cylinder *(light blue)* is 4 mm in height and is mounted with its top surface level with the surface of the surgical guide *(light pink)*. The drilling cylinder *(dark blue)* is 1 mm longer than and placed inside the guiding cylinder. The pilot drill is used through the drilling cylinder and inserted until its flange contacts the top of the drilling cylinder. The length of the cutting portion of the drill (13 mm) is the sum of the length of the implant (10 mm) and the regulator (3 mm). The full length of the drill, from apex to flange, is the sum of the cutting portion and the drilling cylinder. *(b)* The implant holder *(yellow)* is used for placing the implant through the guiding cylinder *(light blue)*. The length of the implant holder (7 mm) is the sum of the height of the guiding cylinder (4 mm) and the regulator (3 mm).

Development of SAFE System

Height control and the regulator

Initially, the SAFE System guiding cylinders were placed directly on top of the bone because only bone-supported drill guides were in use. This approach assumed that the bottom of the guiding cylinder coincided with the top of the implant, and that the top of the implant was placed at the top of the crest of the bone. However, this would only work if the crest of the bone were perfectly even. Unfortunately, this happens very rarely, and errors in depth of implant placement were common.

In 2001, mucosa-supported SurgiGuide drill guides were introduced. With mucosa-supported guides, the bottom of the guiding cylinder could be placed on the surface of the soft tissue instead of bone. Initially the approach was to measure the thickness of the soft tissue and to plan the placement of the guiding cylinder based on that height. However, soft tissue thickness varies over the surface, and it was not clear which measurement should be taken into account: the highest, the lowest, or the average value. Moreover, the computer tools used to measure the soft tissue thickness were very accurate (up to 0.01 mm), but the drills and implant holders could not be used with this degree of precision. Finally, when measuring the soft tissue thickness on computed tomography (CT) images, measurements were made from the top of the bone to the top of the soft tissue. On 2D reconstructions, it is very difficult to precisely define the bone and soft tissue surfaces. It was clear that the position of the guiding cylinder could not be properly defined to accurately control depth during implant placement, even with mucosa-supported guides.

Two fixed reference points were needed. The first reference point could be easily identified as the bottom of the guiding cylinder. However, the second reference point could not be the surface of the soft tissue nor the surface of the crest of bone. The author determined that the second fixed reference point should be the top of the implant since it was easy to determine. He coined the term *regulator* to refer to the distance between the top of the implant and the bottom of the guiding cylinder (expressed as an integer in millimeters). The regulator determines the length of the drills and the implant holder (Fig 9-8). The length of the cutting portion of the drill is calculated by

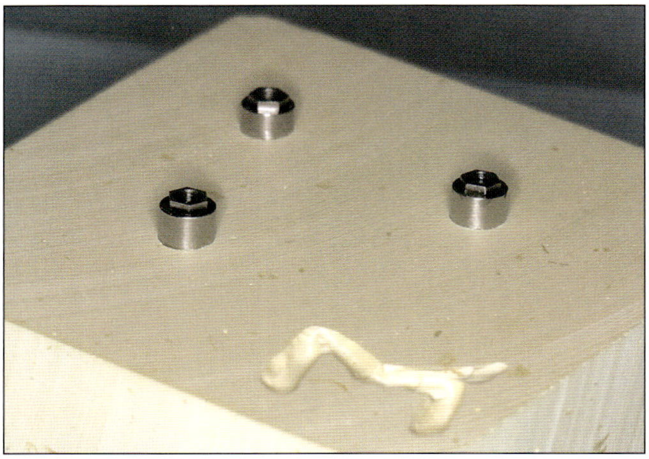

Fig 9-9 Master model with implant analogues.

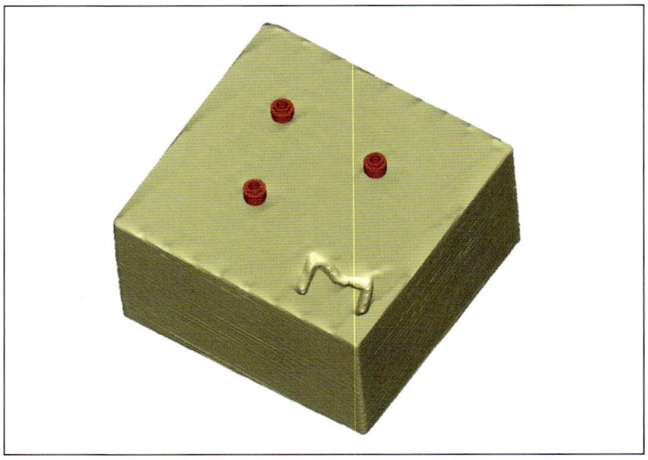

Fig 9-10 Superimposition of analogues on 3D image of the master model.

adding the implant length and the regulator, while the length of the drill from flange to apex is the sum of the cutting portion of the drill and the height of the drilling cylinder (5 mm). The length of the implant holder is determined as the sum of the regulator and the height of the guiding cylinder (4 mm). When the flange of the SAFE System implant holder reaches the top of the guiding cylinder, then the top of the implant is placed at exactly the right height. This measure is fully independent of the relationship between implant and surrounding bone or soft tissue.

The regulator distance can be adjusted to allow the same drill to be used regardless of the implant length, but should be limited to allow drills and implant holders to be easily manipulated in the mouth of the patient. However, it must be remembered that the regulator should be larger than the soft tissue thickness to avoid interference between the bottom of the guiding cylinder and the soft tissue. Today, all values are calculated by Materialise Dental; the surgeon receives a guide that indicates the measurements for the regulator, drill, and implant holder needed for each implant in the treatment plan.

Establishing the accuracy of the SAFE System

The precision of computer-guided implant placement is often measured by superimposing preoperative CT images showing planned implant placement on postoperative CT images of the placed implants to find the deviation between the plan and the result. However, this deviation could result from errors occurring in any number of steps during the whole process (eg, scanning, production of the guide, or positioning of the guide); it does not necessarily provide information about the accuracy of the guiding system itself.

The author therefore set out to measure the deviation resulting from the guiding system itself, ie, the SAFE system, using a unique test. A master model was made out of polyurethane plaster (Polyurock, Metalor), which does not expand while hardening. Three holes were made in the master model in a triangular pattern using a 4-mm-diameter trephine. A General Electric LightSpeed 16 scanner was used to take a CT scan, using the same parameters as for a jaw examination. A conversion was done from the DICOM file to the SimPlant format. After scanning, three analogues with an external hex were placed in the holes (Fig 9-9). An optical image of the master model with

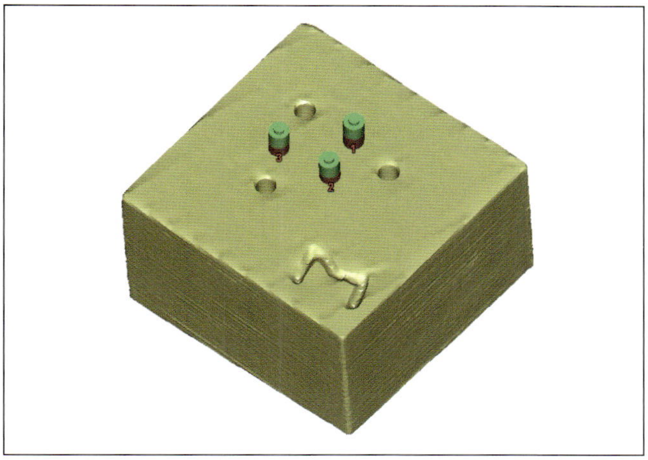

Fig 9-11 Planning of implants performed in SimPlant.

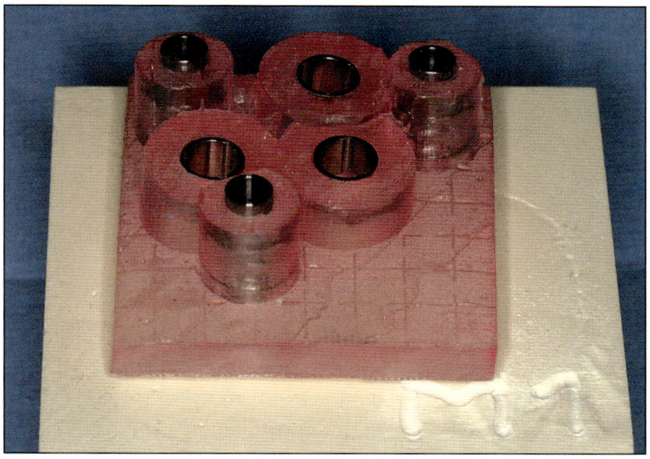

Fig 9-12 Screw-retained SurgiGuide with SAFE System in place on the model.

analogues was taken with a D-200 Dental 3D Scanner (3Shape) and superimposed on the CT image. This method was used to create a 3D model of the master cast with analogues (Fig 9-10) while reducing the possibility of error due to metal-scattered images.

Three hex pickup impression copings were placed on top of the implant analogues on the master model and connected using polyurethane plaster to make a transfer model, from which duplicate models were made.

Three implants were planned by the surgeon using the CT data (Fig 9-11), and three SurgiGuides were ordered from Materialise Dental. The stabilization of the SurgiGuide was accomplished on the three implant analogues using screw-retained nonhex temporary cylinders included in the stereolithographic surgical guide (Fig 9-12). This step allowed for stabilization of the guide, ruling out the possibility that error could be caused by malpositioning of the guide. The normal SAFE System sequence was used to place three implants per model using a SurgiGuide and SAFE System components. One surgeon placed the implants in three different models, using a unique SurgiGuide for each model.

After the guided implant placement, a CT scan was taken of each model. The SimPlant planning was superimposed onto these CT images by registration of the implant analogues supporting the guide. Four deviation parameters between the planned and placed implants were defined and calculated: global, lateral, depth, and angle (Fig 9-13).

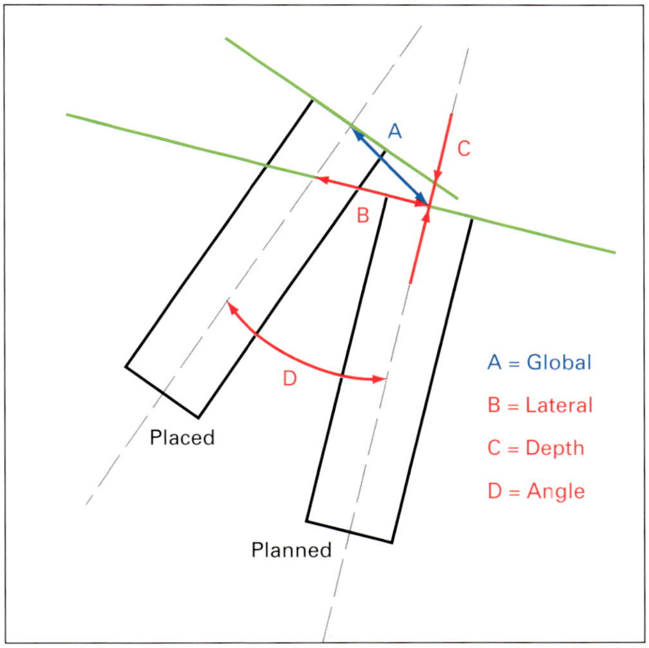

Fig 9-13 The *global parameter* (A) is defined as the distance between the coronal centers of the planned and placed implants. To determine the *lateral deviation* (B), a plane through the occlusal center and perpendicular to the longitudinal axis of the planned implant is defined. The lateral deviation is calculated as the distance between the occlusal center of the planned implant and the intersection of this plane and the longitudinal axis of the placed implant. For the *depth deviation* (C), a plane through the occlusal center and perpendicular to the longitudinal axis of the placed implant is defined. The depth deviation is the distance between the coronal center of the planned implant and the intersection of this plane and the longitudinal axis of the planned implant. The *angle parameter* (D) defines the 3D angle between the longitudinal axes of the implants.

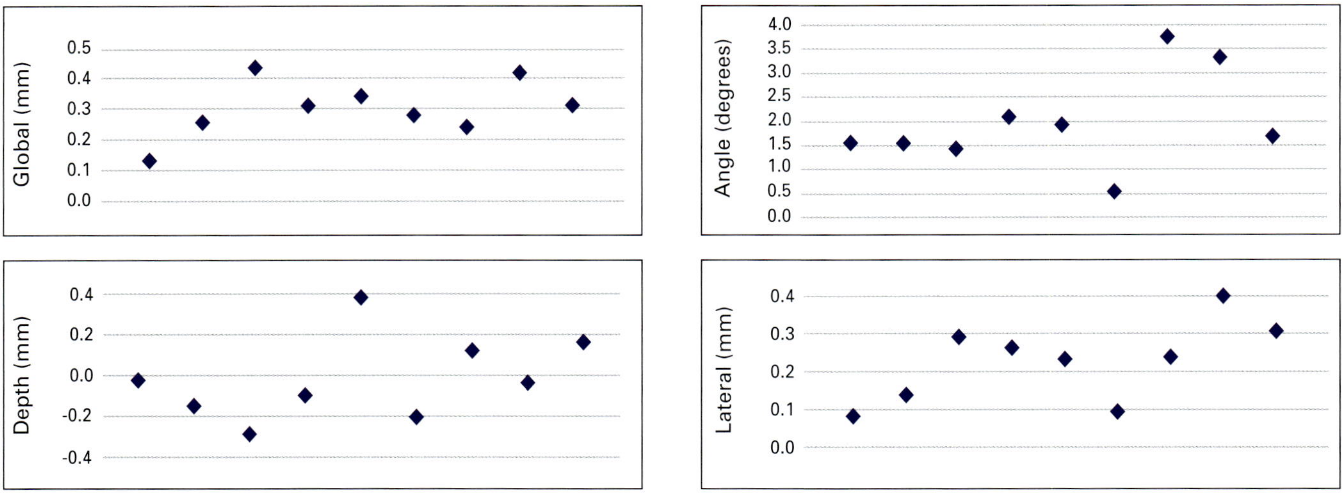

Fig 9-14 Deviations measured between planned implants and implants placed with a SurgiGuide and SAFE System. Note that the values for depth can be either positive or negative; a positive value indicates that the implant is placed less deep than planned, whereas a negative value indicates that the implant is placed deeper than planned.

Table 9-1 Deviation between planned implants and placed implants

Parameters	Mean (SD)
Global (mm)	0.30 (0.09)
Angle (degrees)	2.00 (1.00)
Depth (mm)*	0.17 (0.10)
Lateral (mm)	0.23 (0.11)

*Given as an absolute value.

Figure 9-14 presents the deviations measured between planned implants and implants placed using a SurgiGuide and the SAFE System. The mean value and standard deviation of each parameter are presented in Table 9-1. Statistical analysis showed that there is no significant difference between the three guides, indicating that the reproducibility of the manufacturing process for the guides is very good. This test, while limited in scope, indicated that the SAFE System itself will produce only a small margin of error when comparing the placement of implants with the planning.

SAFE System case example

This case example illustrates the surgical steps for implant placement to replace six missing maxillary anterior teeth (Fig 9-15a) using a tooth- and mucosa-supported surgical guide and the SAFE System.

First, a scanning appliance (ScannoGuide) is fabricated by your lab (Fig 9-15b). The patient then is sent to a center to have a CT scan taken, and the DICOM file obtained is converted into a SimPlant file to plan the implant placement (Fig 9-15c). A SurgiGuide supported by mucosa and the neighboring teeth is ordered. The guide is equipped with titanium guiding cylinders in which drilling cylinders will be placed (Fig 9-15d). The depth control for drilling and implant placement is provided in the design of the stereolithographic guide, and Materialise Dental sends the surgeon indications of which drills and implant holders to use for each implant to be placed (Fig 9-15e). All components needed for the surgery are placed at the appropriate tooth positions in the surgical tray before the procedures begin (Fig 9-15f).

A trephine is slipped over a pilot drill to remove the soft tissue and to mark the bone (Fig 9-15g). Drilling cylinders are placed inside the guiding cylinders. Drilling is performed until the pilot drill is blocked by the physical depth control stop (Fig 9-15h). This procedure is repeated using the final drill (Fig 9-15i).

The drilling cylinders are removed from the stereolithographic guide. The implants are placed using the implant

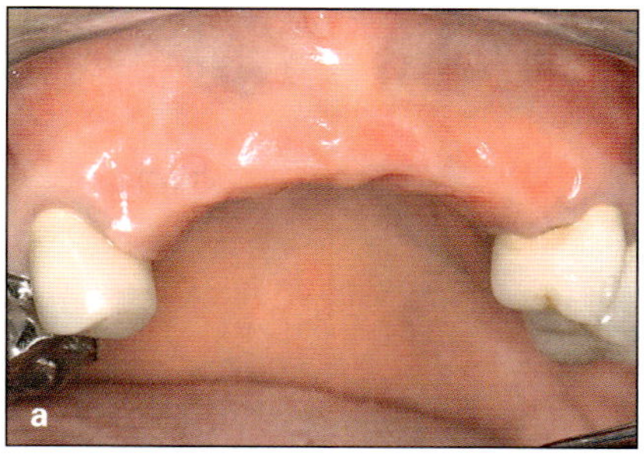

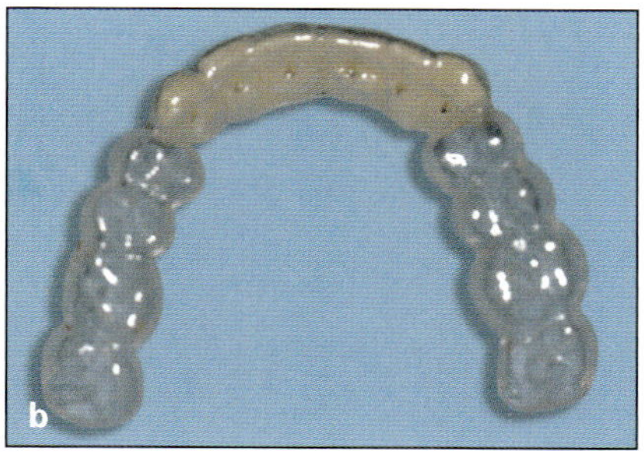

Fig 9-15a *(near right)* Clinical view of the patient before treatment.

Fig 9-15b *(far right)* ScannoGuide for visualization of the six missing teeth in CT images.

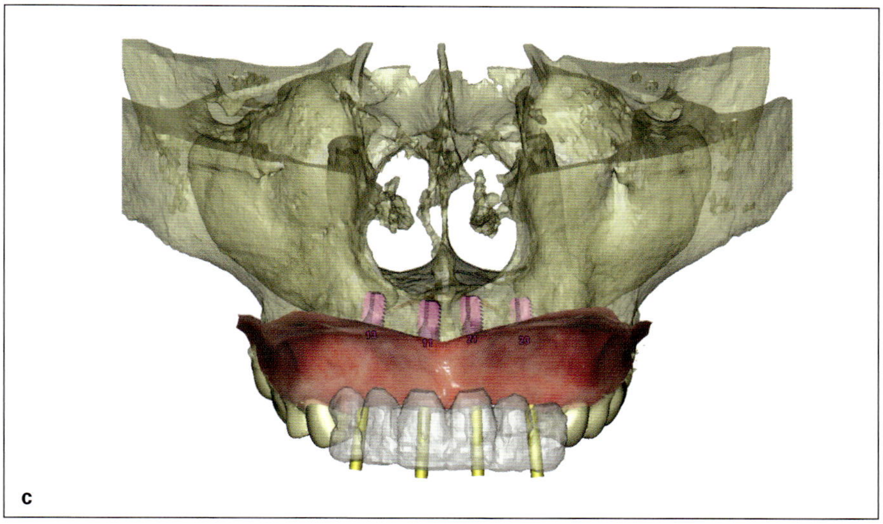

Fig 9-15c SimPlant 3D model of the bone, ScannoGuide, soft tissue, and planned implant placement.

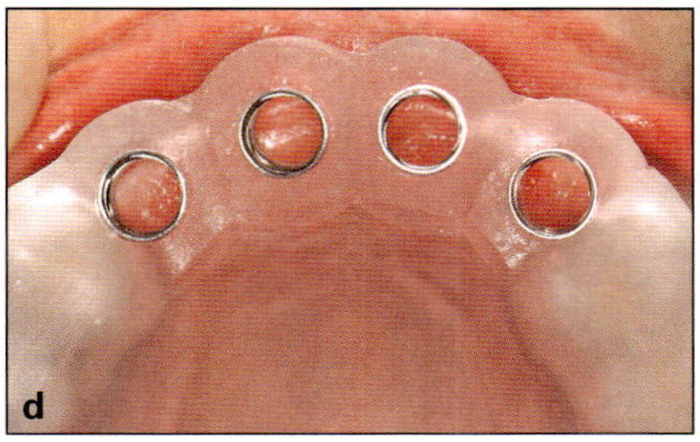

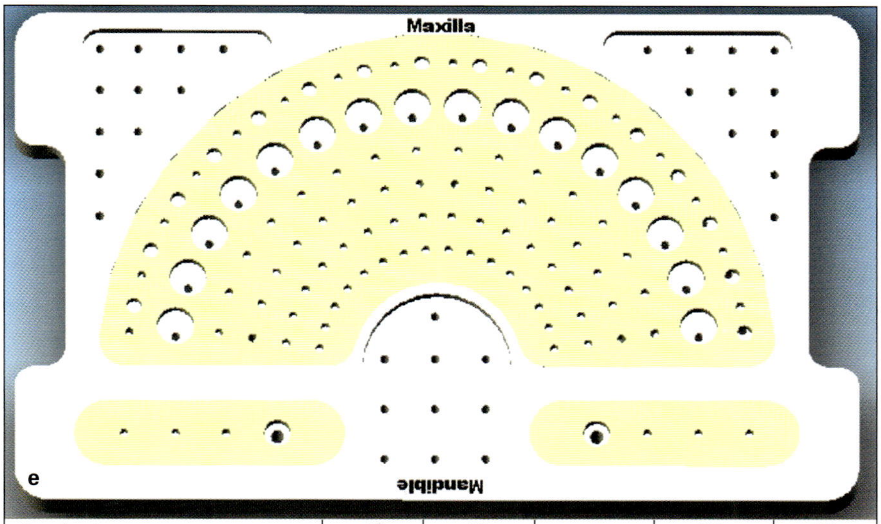

Implant	13	11		21	23
Planned implant length (mm)	13				
Planned implant diameter (mm)	4.10				
Placement of SAFE SurgiGuide with internal tubes screwed in					
Drill needed (L=mm)	**Drilling**: 18				
Removal of internal tubes – Implant placement					
Implant holders (H=mm)	**Implant placement:** 9				

Fig 9-15d Tooth- and mucosa-supported SurgiGuide in place.

Fig 9-15e Form provided by Materialise Dental containing information about which components to use in the surgery.

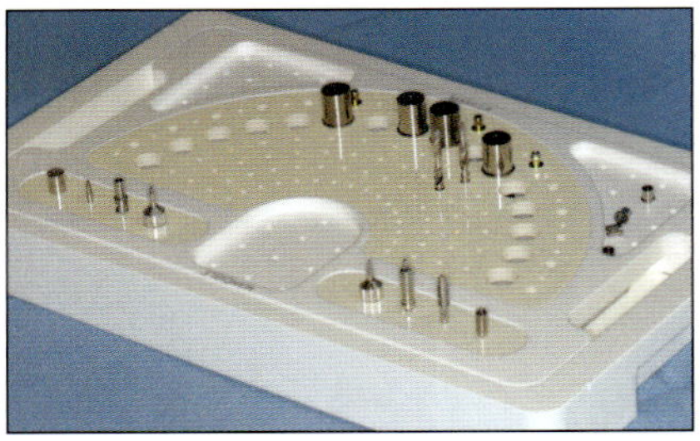

Fig 9-15f SAFE Surgical Tray with the components arranged for surgery.

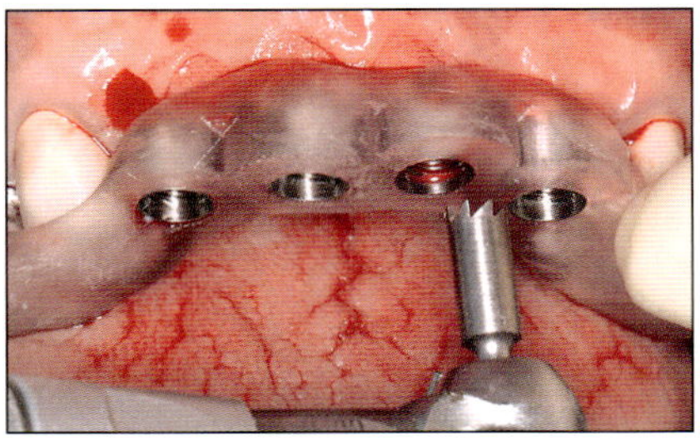

Fig 9-15g Use of the trephine through the guiding cylinders prior to drilling.

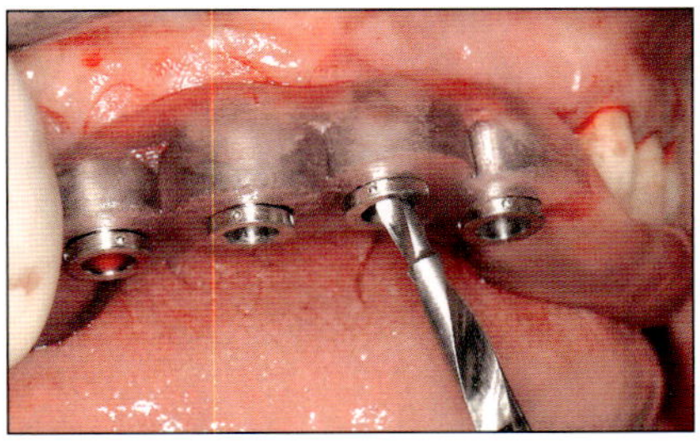

Fig 9-15h The pilot drill is used through the drilling cylinders to make the initial osteotomies.

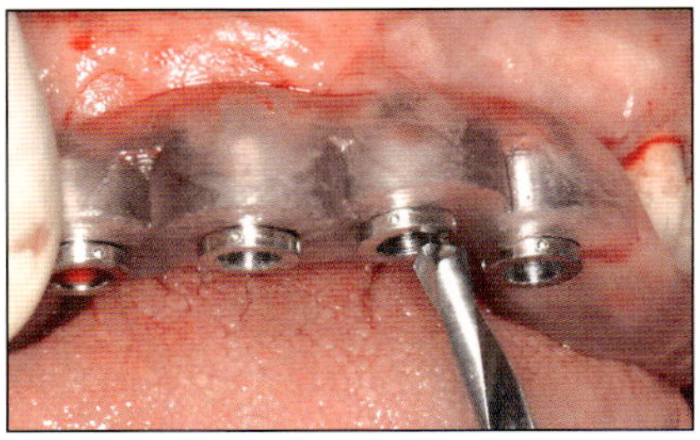

Fig 9-15i The final drill is used through the drilling cylinders to complete the osteotomies.

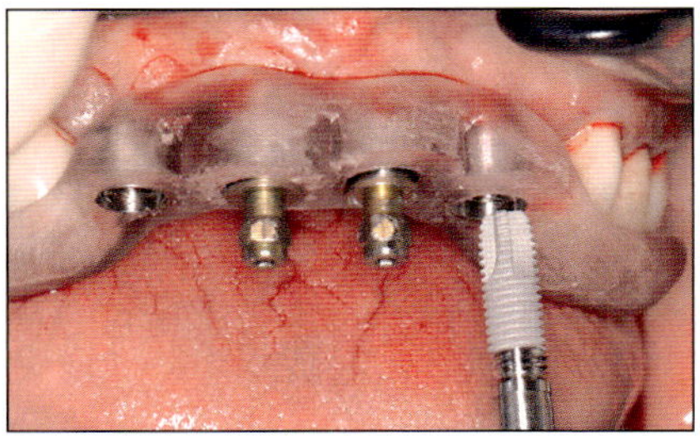

Fig 9-15j The implants are placed using implant holders.

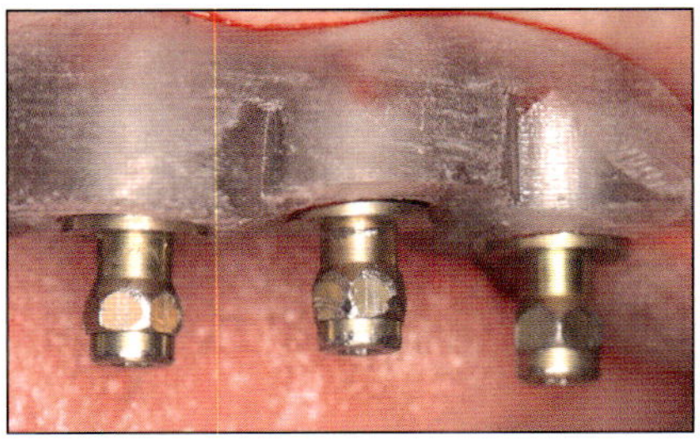

Fig 9-15k The implant holders are tightened until they contact the flange of the guiding cylinders to ensure the implants are in the correct final position.

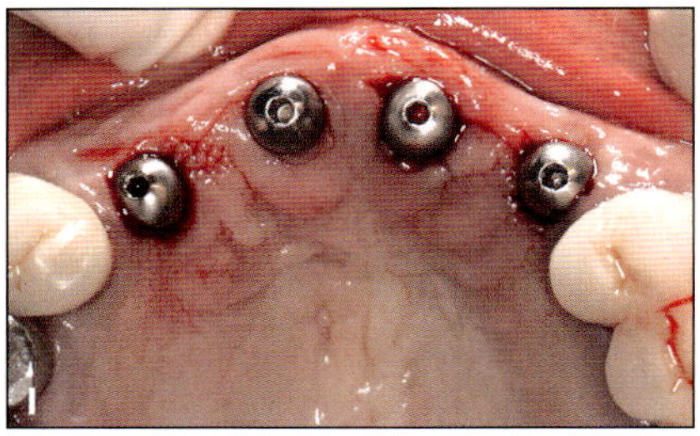

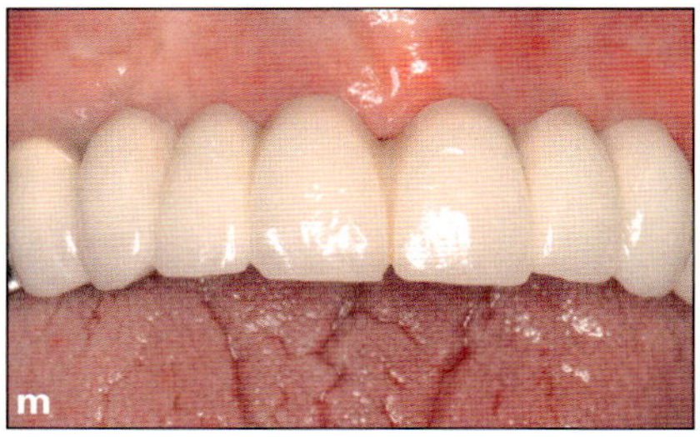

Fig 9-15l The healing abutments are positioned on the implants.

Fig 9-15m Clinical view 2 months after surgery with definitive prosthesis in place.

holders and the guiding cylinders (Fig 9-15j). Once all implants are in position, the implant holders are tightened until the flange contacts the cylinder using 50-N/cm torque (Fig 9-15k). Healing abutments are placed over the implants (Fig 9-15l). Figure 9-15m shows the clinical result with the prosthesis in place 2 months after surgery.

Summary

The SAFE System provides drilling and implant placement guidance in position, angulation, and depth with only one surgical template and two drills. Moreover, the surgical tray allows the easy transfer of the implant planning to the surgery. The currently available system has been designed for standard external hex implants. However, several implant manufacturers with internal retention implants have already adapted their components to make them compatible with internal connections. In addition, SAFE System leads the way to minimally invasive surgery, trans-sinus implant placement (by allowing avoidance of the lateral sinus windows and accurate access to the back wall of the sinus), and the Immediate Smile procedure, which is discussed in the next section.

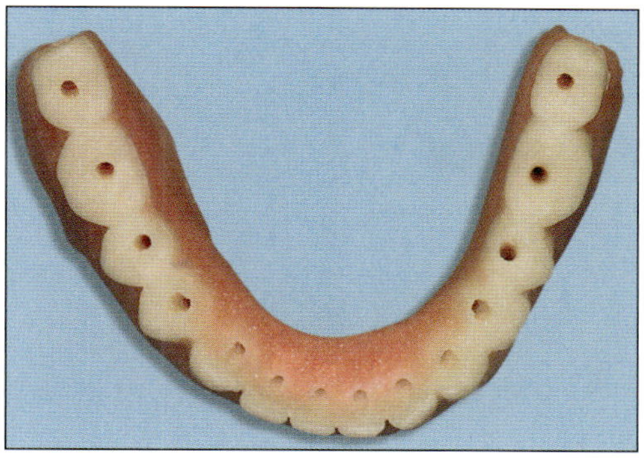

Fig 9-16a *(above)* Radiopaque scanning appliance.

Fig 9-16b *(right)* SimPlant project showing the CT scan images with implant planning and a 3D model of the bone, planned implants, and scanning appliance.

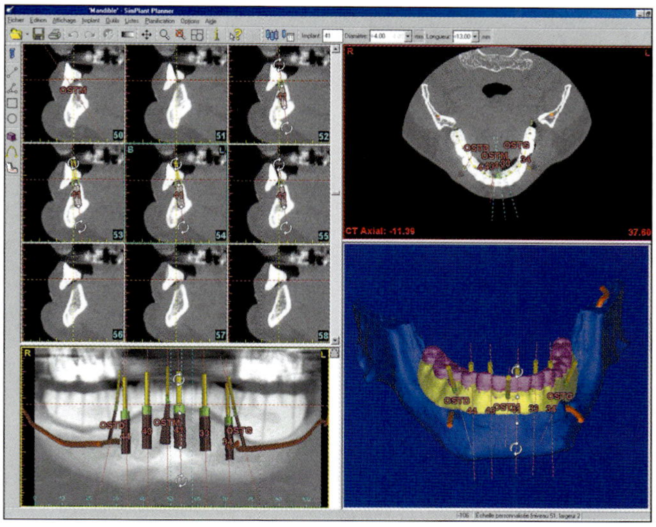

Immediate Smile

The Immediate Smile procedure allows clinicians to use SimPlant technology to place a provisional screw-retained restoration in the same appointment as implant placement. This is a safe and accurate way to increase patient satisfaction by reducing the time and cost associated with implant placement and restoration, while also limiting pain and, when working through the mucosa, the need for flaps and sutures. Moreover, the supracrestal vasculature is respected, and the underlying bone is kept intact.

Despite all of these advantages, the clinician should take the following five points into consideration before undertaking the procedure:

1. The clinician must fully understand the mechanics involved in immediately loaded implants. The success of immediate loading is primarily based on the full and immediate stabilization of implants inside the bone. This is related to several factors, such as size and number of implants, relative position of implants to each other, bone quality, implant surface texture, occlusion and related forces, and tongue pressure.
2. Precision in implant placement is crucial and can only be achieved with guidance systems such as the SurgiGuide SAFE System.
3. Relative vertical deviations of the implants must be minimized so that a restoration fabricated before surgery can be placed at the time of implant placement with good passive fit.
4. To allow fabrication of the restoration before surgery, the implant positions as planned on the CT images should be transferred accurately to a model for the dental technician. By using stereolithography, a digital cast with prepared sites for the implants as planned can be produced. For fully edentulous patients, even the soft tissue can be simulated in the digital cast, and the scan template can be used to transfer the occlusion.
5. The provisional prosthesis must be fabricated to allow final adjustments at placement since implant positioning will never be completely identical to the planning.

Immediate Smile procedure

The Immediate Smile procedure is described and illustrated in this section using a clinical case example of a patient with a fully edentulous mandible.

Implant planning

The starting point for fabrication of the provisional prosthesis is high-precision computer planning that communicates the ideal positions of the implants in the patient's jaw according to the planned prosthesis. The first step is to have the dental lab manufacture a radiopaque scanning appliance in accordance with the diagnostic tooth setup (Fig 9-16a). This template is worn by the patient during the CT scan, allowing the predetermined prosthetic setup as well as the mucosal situation to be visualized in the images. A SimPlant project containing the CT scan information and 3D models of the bone volume, mucosa, and planned prosthesis is created, and implant placement is planned using the SimPlant software, taking into account both biomechanical and esthetic considerations (Fig 9-16b).

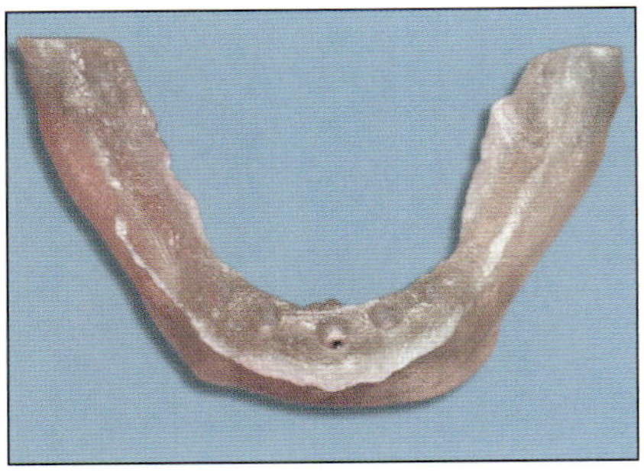

Fig 9-16c Digital cast provided by Materialise Dental.

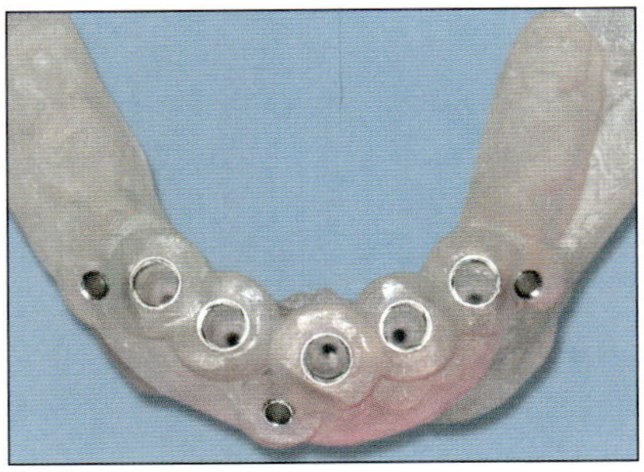

Fig 9-16d Mucosa-supported SurgiGuide with SAFE System components positioned on the digital cast.

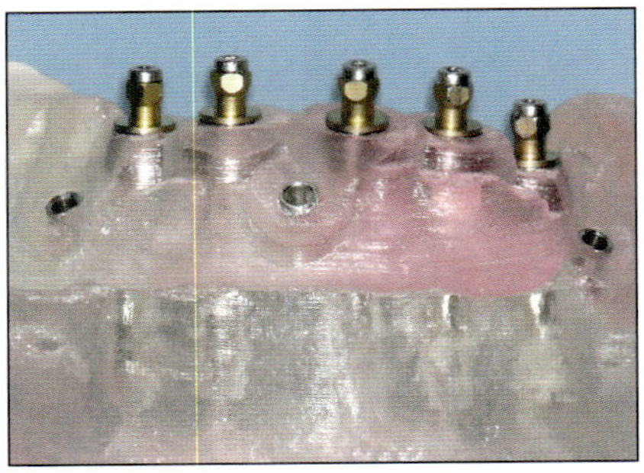

Fig 9-16e Placement of the implant analogues using the SAFE implant holders and according to the SimPlant plan.

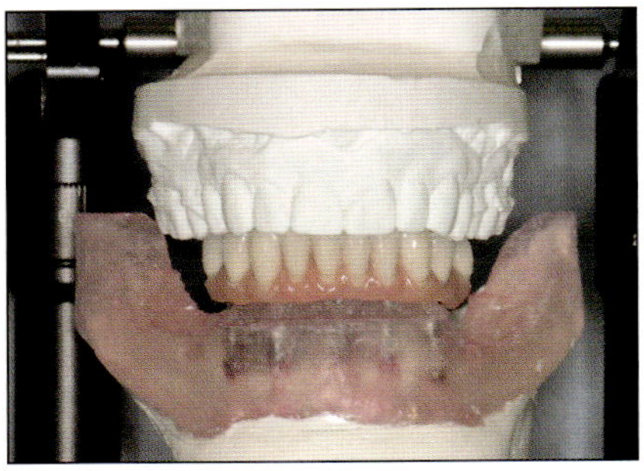

Fig 9-16f The model, scanning appliance, and a cast of the opposing arch are mounted on the articulator in order to transfer the occlusion.

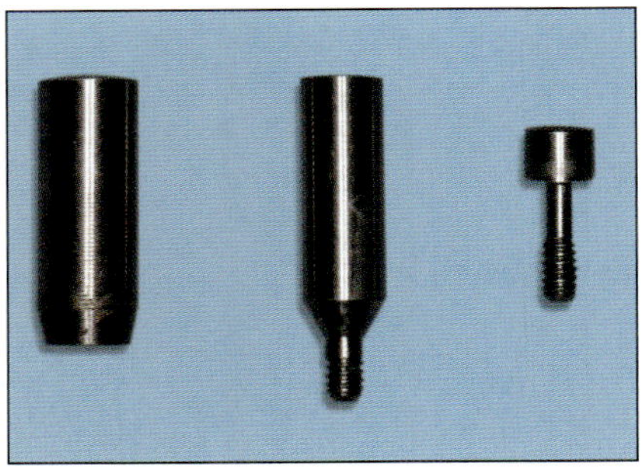

Fig 9-16g Immediate Smile components: *(left)* cylinder, *(center)* centering screw, *(right)* retention screw.

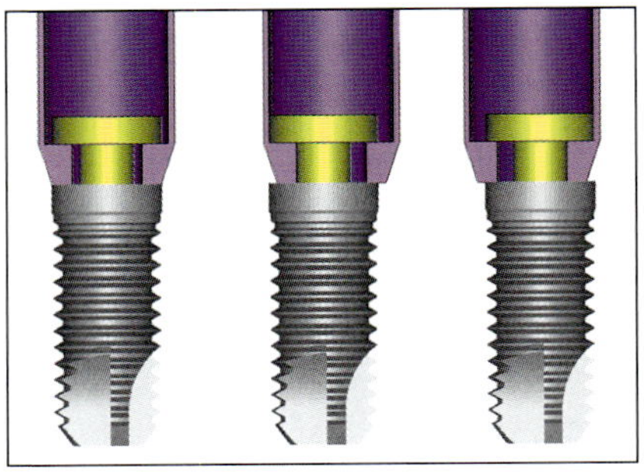

Fig 9-16h Once the cylinder is mounted on top of the flat implant, it can be adjusted to allow a lateral deviation of up to 0.5 mm, then is fixed with the retention screw.

Presurgical laboratory phase

Based on the computer implant planning, Materialise Dental delivers a digital cast (Fig 9-16c) and a SAFE System–compatible SurgiGuide (Fig 9-16d). The digital cast is a stereolithographic model of the patient's jaw containing prepared sites in the same position and orientation as the implant sites planned on the CT images.

The SurgiGuide and SAFE System implant holders are used to place the implant analogues at the correct position, orientation, and depth inside the model (Fig 9-16e), and the analogues are glued in place. The scanning appliance is placed on the implant analogues, and the model is mounted on the articulator together with a cast of the opposite arch to check the occlusion (Fig 9-16f).

The analogues, like the implants to be used in the Immediate Smile procedure, have an internal connection and a flat surface, which allows the use of specially designed Immediate Smile components (cylinder, centering screw, and retention screw) that provide compensation for inevitable small lateral deviations (Figs 9-16g and 9-16h). Once the occlusion has been checked and the scanning appliance removed, the cylinders are placed on the flat surfaces of the implant analogues and centered using the centering screws (Fig 9-16i). A provisional acrylic prosthesis is fabricated in the conventional way using the model, analogues, and cylinders (Fig 9-16j). A metal or carbon framework can be incorporated in the provisional prosthesis for increased strength in the maxilla.

Fig 9-16i *(near right)* The cylinders are centered on top of the implant analogues using centering screws.

Fig 9-16j *(far right)* Occlusal view of the provisional prosthesis.

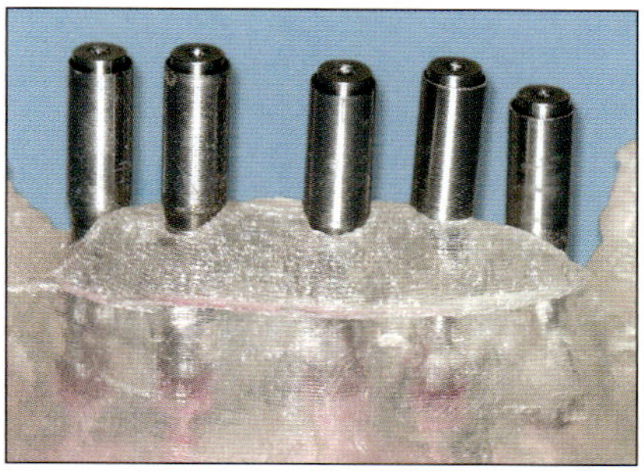

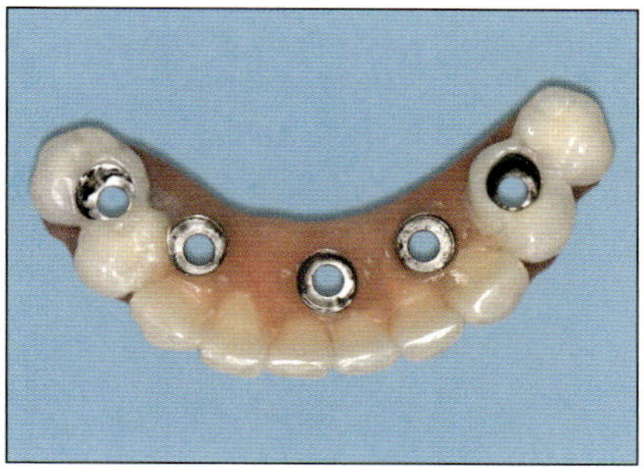

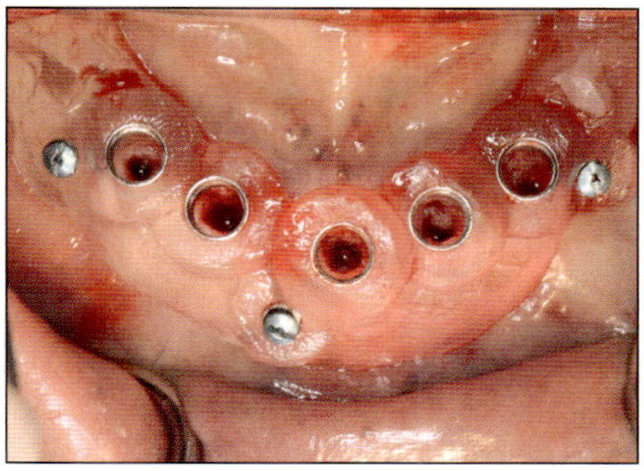

Fig 9-16k SurgiGuide fixed with three osteosynthesis screws in the patient's mouth. The SAFE trephine has been used to remove the soft tissue and center the pilot drill in the bone.

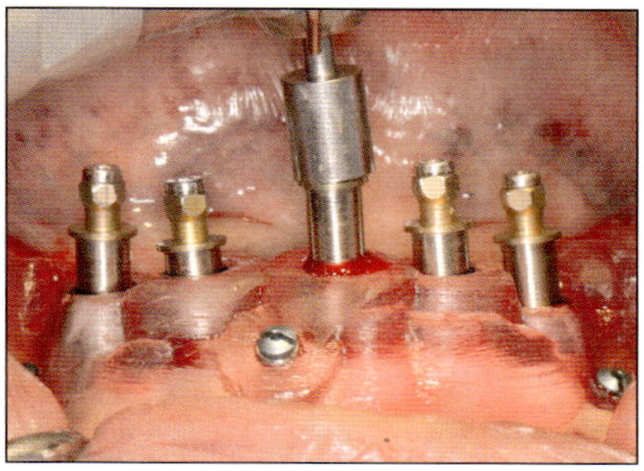

Fig 9-16l Implant placement using the SurgiGuide and SAFE implant holders.

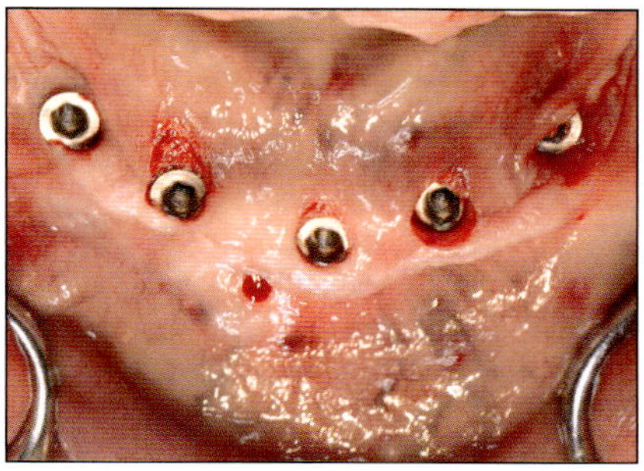

Fig 9-16m Occlusal view of implants directly after placement.

Fig 9-16n *(near right)* Occlusal view of the provisional restoration secured to the implants using the Immediate Smile components. Note that the retention screws are not centered in the cylinders, which indicates that the lateral tolerance was needed and allowed for passive fit of the prosthesis.

Fig 9-16o *(far right)* Occlusion of provisional prosthesis with opposing arch.

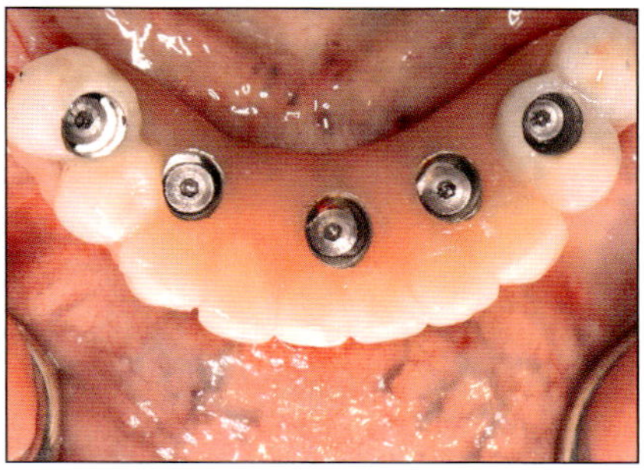

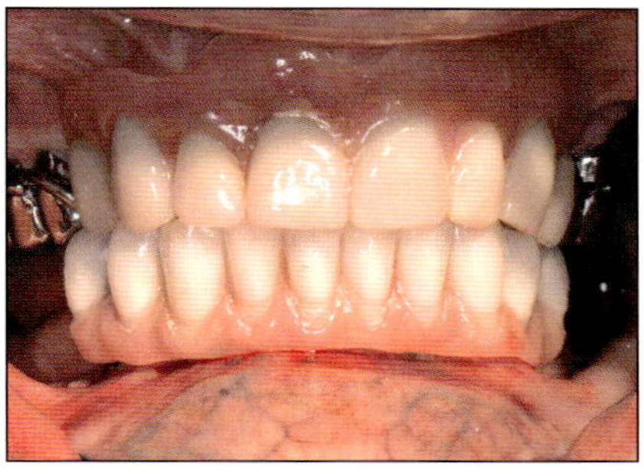

Surgery and placement of provisional prosthesis

The SurgiGuide is placed using an occlusal template and secured by several osteosynthesis screws (Fig 9-16k). For this case, a flapless approach was chosen; therefore, the SAFE trephine is used to remove the soft tissue, gain direct access to the bone, and center the pilot drill in the bone. The SAFE pilot and final drills are used to prepare the implant sites. The drilling cylinders are removed, and, because of the high density of the bone, bone tapping is performed through the guiding cylinders. Implants are placed using the SAFE implant holders to control their position and depth (Fig 9-16l), and the SurgiGuide is removed (Fig 9-16m).

The provisional prosthesis is placed using the Immediate Smile cylinders and retention screws, with which any required lateral adaptation of the prosthesis is performed (Fig 9-16n). Once a good passive fit is obtained, the retention screws are tightened. The occlusion is checked and any required small adjustments are made (Fig 9-16o). The use of an acrylic provisional restoration allows modification at this stage if one or more of the implants deviates from the planned position more than the tolerance incorporated in the Immediate Smile components. In such circumstances, the cylinder corresponding to the deviated implant is removed from the provisional, and the cylindrical site is enlarged in the area of the deviation. The prosthesis is placed back on the implants, the cylinder is secured to the implant using the retention screw, and additional acrylic is used to fill the void left by the adjustment.

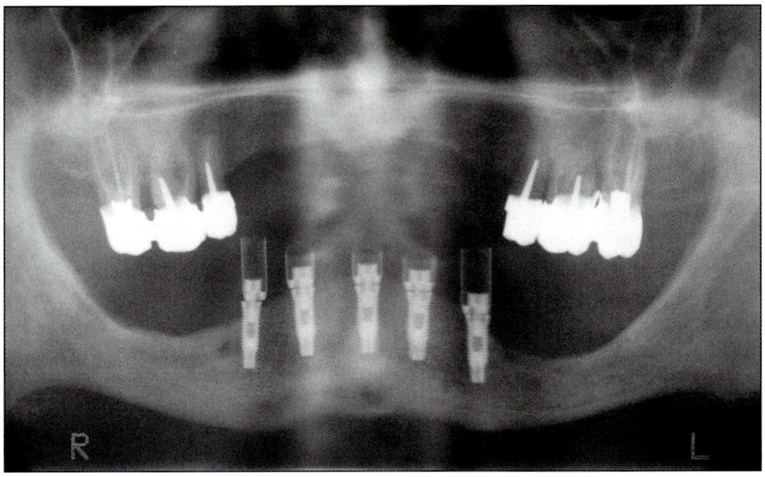

Fig 9-16p Postoperative panoramic radiograph showing the lateral deviation of the Immediate Smile components on the implants.

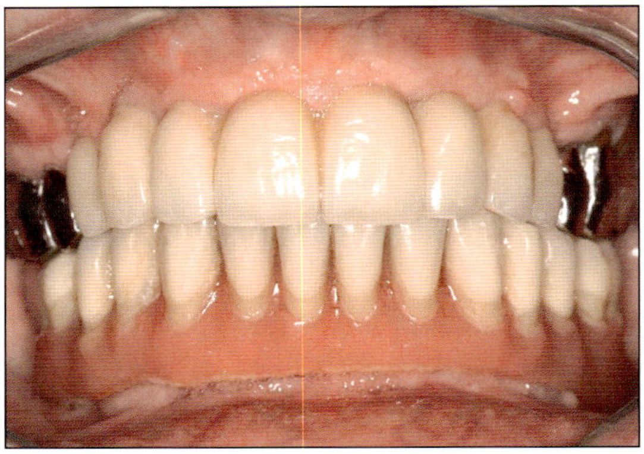

Fig 9-16q The definitive restoration in the patient's mouth after 2 years of function.

Finally, a panoramic radiograph is taken to check the positioning of the Immediate Smile components on the implants (Fig 9-16p).

Definitive restoration

A few weeks after surgery, a definitive restoration with a metal framework is fabricated. Figure 9-16q shows the final restoration in the patient's mouth after 2 years of function.

Summary

Partial as well as full cases can be treated using the Immediate Smile procedure. As long as the number of implants in the procedure is limited to five or fewer, the above-described protocol results in sufficiently precise implant placement to obviate the need for adaptation of the provisional prosthesis beyond adjustment of the cylinders. If more than five implants are required, there are likely to be more deviations at the time of implant placement; however, because further adaptation of the provisional acrylic prosthesis is possible (as described above), such cases still may be treated successfully in one appointment.

Development of Immediate Smile protocol

The test described in this section, which was based on an actual patient CT treatment plan (Fig 9-17), was carried out during the development of the Immediate Smile protocol. It was designed to evaluate the accuracy of the Immediate Smile procedure and components and to determine the more preferable of two possible procedures for creating the model jaws used to construct the provisional prosthesis. The first method (T1) was to create a stereolithographic model without prepared implant sites in the laboratory (Fig 9-18a). The model would be sent to the clinician, who would place the SurgiGuide on the model, drill the holes, and place fake implants using the SAFE implant holders (Fig 9-18b). The second method (T2) was that described in the previous case example, ie, the implant sites were created in the lab based on the planned implant placement (Fig 9-19a). The digital cast was sent to the clinician, who placed and glued implant analogues in the prepared sites using the SurgiGuide and SAFE implant holders (Fig 9-19b).

In both cases, Immediate Smile cylinders and centering screws were placed on the fake implants/implant analogues (Fig 9-20a), and a resin block was created on the cylinders, representing the provisional prosthesis (Figs 9-20b and 9-20c). For both methods, the same SurgiGuide

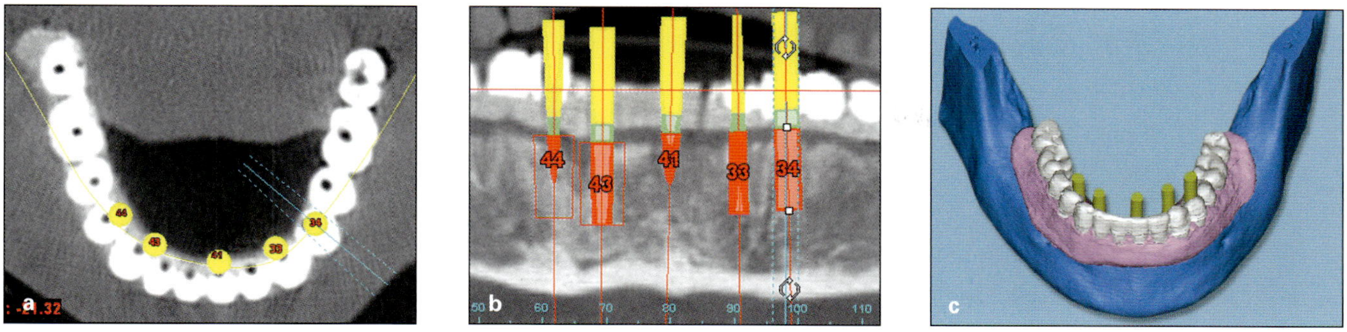

Fig 9-17 SimPlant planning used for Immediate Smile developmental testing. *(a)* Axial view showing scanning appliance and planned implant placement. *(b)* Panoramic reconstruction showing planned implants. *(c)* 3D image of bone, teeth, denture base, and implants.

Fig 9-18 T1 technique. *(a, clockwise from top left)* Laboratory model without prepared implant sites, mouth model, and SurgiGuide. *(b)* Laboratory model following drilling and placement of fake implants.

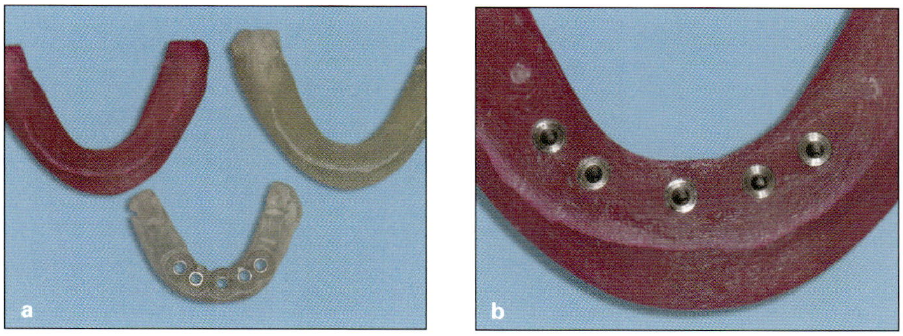

Fig 9-19 T2 technique. *(a, clockwise from top left)* Laboratory model with prepared implant sites, mouth model, and SurgiGuide. *(b)* Laboratory model following placement of implant analogues.

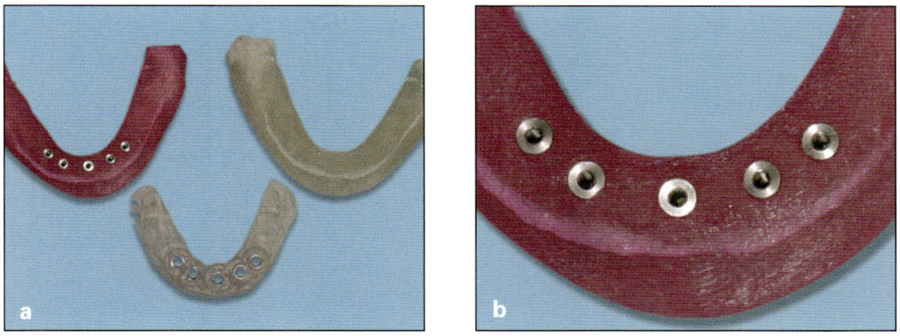

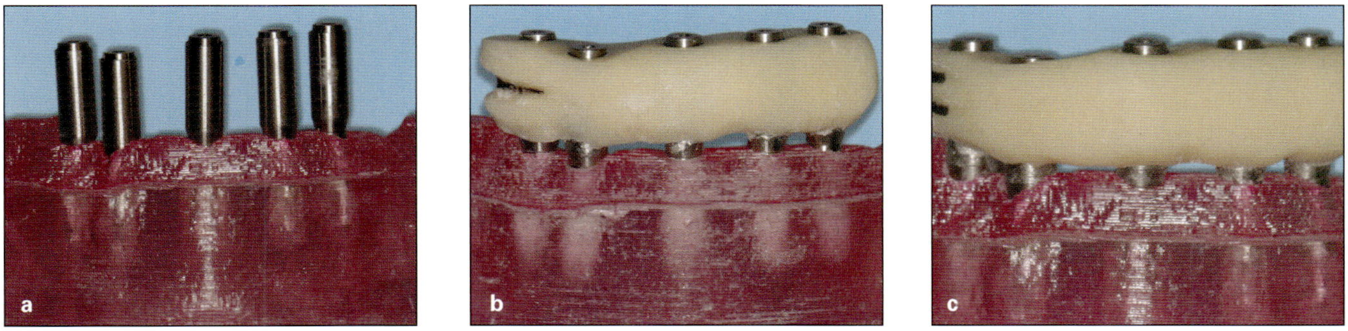

Fig 9-20 Fabrication of the resin block, representing the provisional prosthesis. *(a)* Immediate Smile cylinders in place on a laboratory model. Resin block in place on the T1 *(b)* and T2 *(c)* laboratory models.

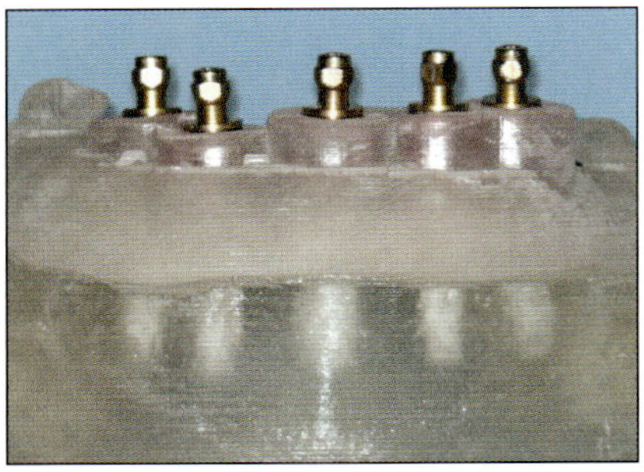

Fig 9-21 Placement of implants in a mouth model using the same SurgiGuide used for the placement of implants in the laboratory model.

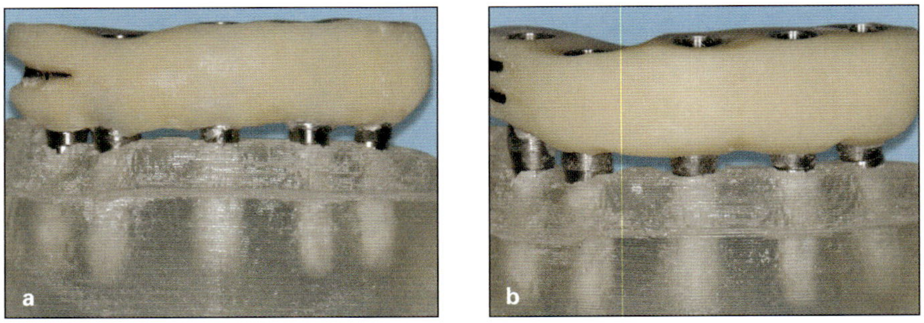

Fig 9-22 Frontal view of resin block in place on the T1 *(a)* and T2 *(b)* mouth models, showing good vertical adaptation.

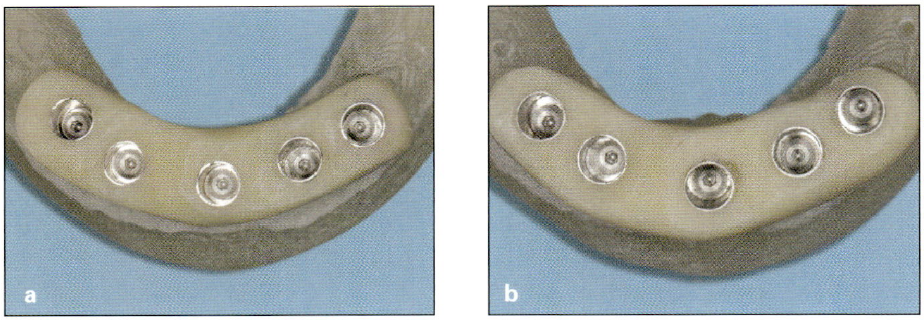

Fig 9-23 Occlusal view of resin block in place on the T1 *(a)* and T2 *(b)* mouth models, illustrating the horizontal deviation of the screw and cylinder assembly.

used for the placement of implants in the laboratory model was used to prepare and place implants on another model, which represented the patient's mouth (Fig 9-21). The prefabricated Immediate Smile prosthesis was then placed in position to compare adaptation and accuracy for each procedure (Figs 9-22 and 9-23). Both resin blocks could be manually secured onto the implants with an acceptable fit. However, the author experienced a less passive fit with the T1 model compared with the T2 model.

CT scans of all four models were obtained to determine the precise position of the implants. The analysis used the same four deviation parameters used in the SAFE System test (see Fig 9-13) and included the following comparisons:

1. Original CT plan versus actual CT scan of placed implants on all models (Table 9-2). For all four models, all implants were placed to a shallower depth than planned. This means that the depth difference between planned and placed implants is in the same direction for each implant. To perform a statistical analysis, the models were split in two groups. The first group contains the models for which a SurgiGuide was used to drill the implant holes, whereas the second group contains only the model with prepared holes. The difference between the two groups is statistically significant only for the deviation parameters *global* ($P < .0005$) and *depth* ($P < .05$).
2. Implant analogues placed in T2 laboratory model versus implants placed in models using SurgiGuide for drilling the implant holes (both T1 models and T2 mouth model) (Table 9-3). The average values for the deviation parameters *global*, *depth*, and *lateral* are lower than those reported for the comparison between the implants in models using SurgiGuide and the planned implants (see Table 9-2); moreover, these differences are statistically significant ($P < .005$).
3. Implants placed in the corresponding laboratory and mouth models (T1 laboratory versus T1 mouth, T2 laboratory versus T2 mouth) (Table 9-4). The deviation parameters *angle* and *depth* are significantly different ($P < .05$). The average depth value is lower for the T1 procedure than for the T2 procedure. But for the T2 procedure all depth variations are in the same direction, which will result in a lower effective depth difference and therefore an absence of small gaps between the prosthesis and the implants.
4. The differences in the distances between the coronal centers of the implants in the T1 models versus in the T2 models (Table 9-5). These values are less than 0.5 mm, the tolerance allowed by the Immediate Smile cylinders and screws.

Table 9-2 Deviation between placed and planned implants on all models

Parameters	Means (SD)				
	T1L	T1M	T2M	T1L, T1M, and T2M	T2L
Global (mm)	1.29 (0.11)	1.16 (0.18)	1.27 (0.06)	1.24 (0.13)	0.96 (0.19)
Angle (degrees)	1.45 (0.84)	1.72 (0.75)	3.07 (2.18)	2.08 (1.50)	1.64 (0.54)
Depth* (mm)	0.82 (0.27)	0.94 (0.18)	1.03 (0.24)	0.93 (0.23)	0.69 (0.24)
Lateral (mm)	0.93 (0.30)	0.67 (0.10)	0.67 (0.27)	0.76 (0.26)	0.60 (0.26)

*Given as an absolute value.
L = laboratory model; M = mouth model.

Table 9-3 Deviation between implant analogues placed in T2 model versus implants placed in SurgiGuide models

Parameters	Mean (SD)
Global (mm)	0.69 (0.28)
Angle (degrees)	2.39 (1.42)
Depth (mm)*	0.46 (0.28)
Lateral (mm)	0.46 (0.22)

*Given as an absolute value.

Table 9-4 Deviation between implants placed in corresponding laboratory and mouth models

Parameters	Mean (SD)	
	T1 models	T2 models
Global (mm)	0.71 (0.25)	0.76 (0.41)
Angle (degrees)	1.10 (0.38)	3.05 (1.81)
Depth (mm)*	0.19 (0.09)	0.62 (0.34)
Lateral (mm)	0.67 (0.28)	0.43 (0.27)

*Given as an absolute value.

Table 9-5 Difference in the distances between the coronal centers of the implants in the T1 and T2 models

Implants	T1 models (mm)	T2 models (mm)
1–2	0.1673	0.2001
2–3	0.0265	0.4005
3–4	0.1976	0.0331
4–5	0.3105	0.4690

The following conclusions can be drawn from this study:

1. Using a SurgiGuide to prepare the implant holes in the stereolithographic model for the lab procedure (T1) is less accurate than using implant analogues in previously prepared sites (T2).
2. Either procedure results in deviations that are within the lateral tolerance of Immediate Smile components, hence allowing placement of the provisional prosthesis.
3. The implant-to-implant depth variation is limited and ensures a good fit of the prefabricated provisional prosthesis in both cases. The T1 technique results in smaller depth deviation than the T2 technique; however, the direction of the depth deviation using the T2 technique is consistent for all implants placed, limiting the overall depth error.
4. The implant-to-implant deviation is limited and allows prosthesis placement.
5. The lateral deviation allowed by Immediate Smile components, together with the inherent elasticity of the bone and the acrylic provisional prosthesis, seems to be sufficient to compensate for any lateral and vertical discrepancies.

Both studied techniques are accurate enough to allow for a successful Immediate Smile procedure; however, having the sites prepared in the laboratory simplifies the process and is therefore now the standard procedure.

10

ADVANCED CASE PLANNING WITH SIMPLANT

Scott D. Ganz, DMD

During the past 20 years, software applications for diagnosis and treatment planning have evolved with the concomitant acceptance of computed tomography (CT) and cone beam CT (CBCT) technology. CBCT is widely used to understand and appreciate patient anatomy, while prepackaged software can serve as an excellent aid in the evaluation of potential implant receptor sites or assessment for bone grafting procedures. However, it is the synergy between CBCT data and advanced interactive planning software such as SimPlant (Materialise) that fully empowers clinicians with the tools to achieve true restoratively driven implant dentistry through proper planning. This chapter presents the state of the art in diagnosis, treatment planning, and CT-derived surgical guidance. Two cases are presented—one involving the restoration of a single missing maxillary lateral incisor and the other restoration of a completely edentulous maxilla—to illustrate concepts and interactive software tools that can be used effectively to plan almost any case involving multiple implants for partial or fully edentulous presentations. Additionally, the use of this technology affords clinicians a powerful means of communicating with all members of the implant team and an effective marketing tool as well.

Case 1: Congenitally Missing Maxillary Lateral Incisor

A 33-year-old woman presented with a congenitally missing maxillary right lateral incisor. Her medical history was unremarkable. At the clinical examination, she exhibited limited interarch space. Also, the site of the missing incisor lacked a papilla and exhibited obvious facial concavity (Fig 10-1a). The patient had been wearing a space-maintaining appliance for approximately 1 year, and the orthodontist had done well in maintaining the space. The patient had already seen several clinicians to assess the options available for replacing the missing tooth. Periapical radiographs revealed adequate mesiodistal distance at the crest of the ridge for implant placement. However, the apex of the right central incisor tooth was slightly convergent and appeared to be encroaching on the available space. Interestingly, the patient presented for consultation with a disk containing data from a CBCT scan previously obtained with an i-CAT machine (Imaging Sciences).

Planning phase

The CT scan data and its use within the proprietary software (i-CAT Vision) was helpful for visualizing the potential implant receptor site. However, to enhance the diagnostic information, the data was imported into an interactive treatment-planning software program that has advanced features (SimPlant).

For the missing lateral incisor site, it was important to consider the available bone volume, the bone quality, and the proximity of adjacent tooth roots. Cross-sectional views aid in determining the available bone volume and assessing the density of the bone (Fig 10-1b). To make the connection between the implant location and the desired tooth restoration, it is useful to have the patient wear a radiopaque scanning appliance at the time the scan is taken. Because the CBCT scan was taken before the patient

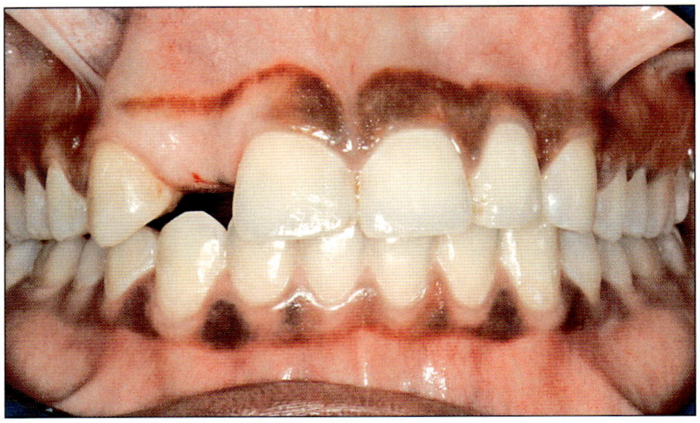

Fig 10-1a Retracted view of patient showing the missing maxillary right lateral incisor. Note the facial concavity, mesiodistal space, and zone of keratinized tissue at the site of the missing tooth.

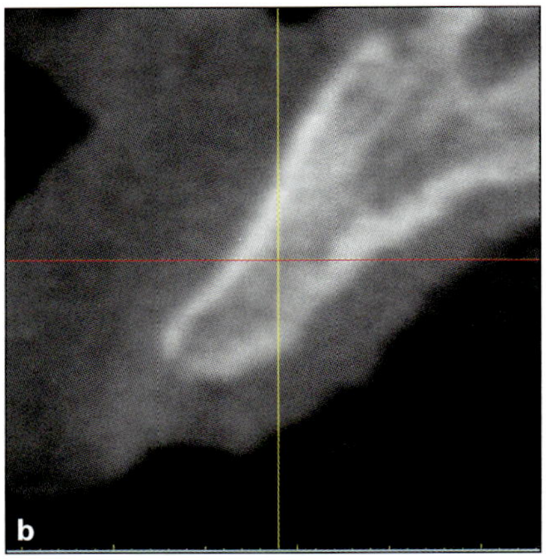

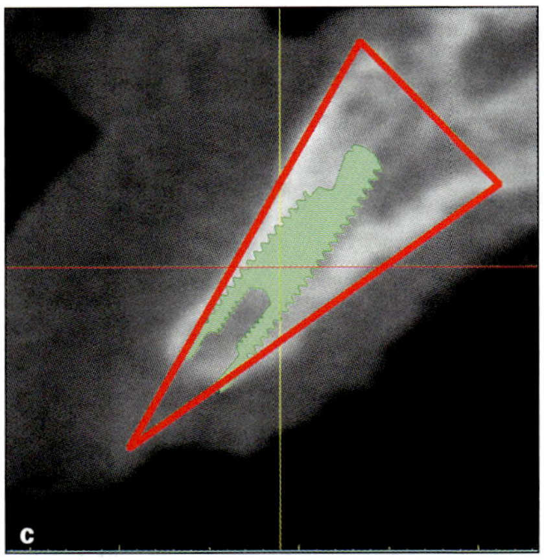

Fig 10-1b CBCT cross-sectional view after scan data was imported into SimPlant software.

Fig 10-1c Simulated realistic implant placed within the triangle of bone (TOB).

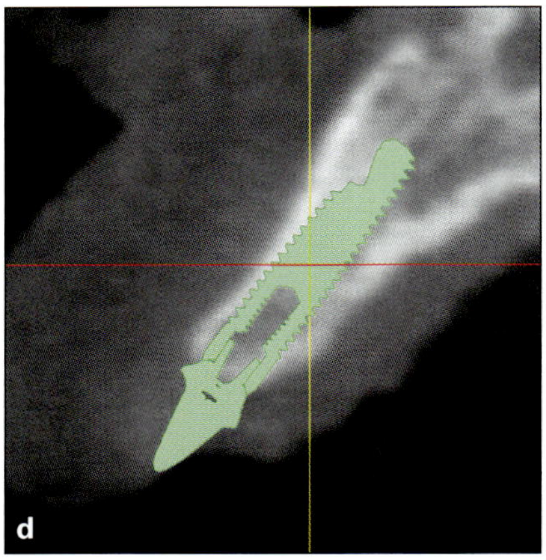

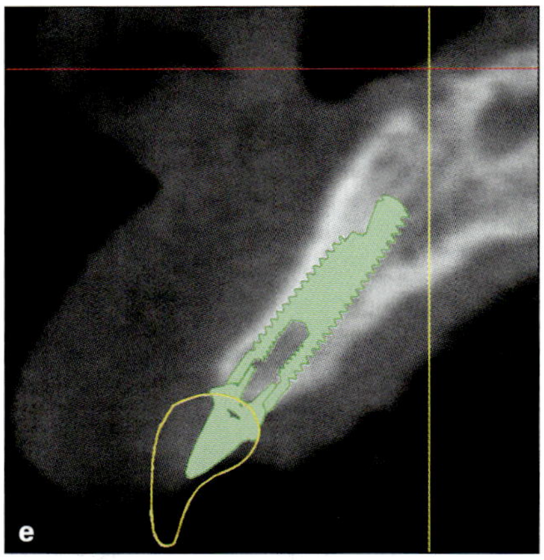

Fig 10-1d Cross-sectional slice of implant and attached realistic abutment.

Fig 10-1e Realistic implant, abutment, and virtual tooth.

presented for consultation, the connection between the implant and the restorative position could not be established with great accuracy, even with a simulated abutment projection. However, innovative new tools that can facilitate the process have recently been incorporated into the software.

In 1992, the author first postulated that the planning process can be facilitated through visualization of a zone that defines the available volume of bone for implant placement, known as the *triangle of bone* (TOB) (Fig 10-1c). By means of interactive planning tools, a realistic implant can be placed within the TOB to help ascertain implant length and width, and a realistic abutment can be placed within the schematic cross-sectional view. The clinician can select these from a library of virtual components (supplied by individual implant manufacturers) that includes most implants currently available, along with straight, angled, overdenture, and screw-receiving abutments (Fig 10-1d). Since the ultimate goal is the tooth to be replaced, the implant direction and the restorative components must project within the restorative envelope as defined by another innovative tool, known as the *virtual tooth* (Fig 10-1e).

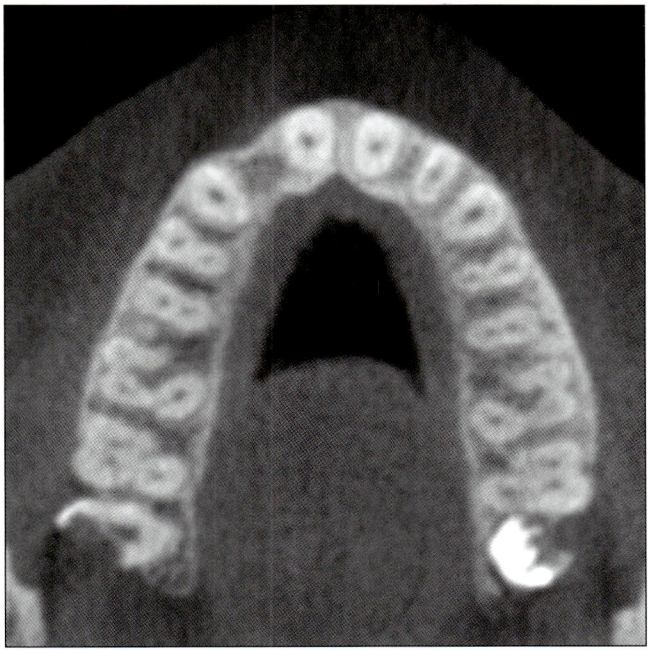

Fig 10-1f Axial view illustrating the so-called restorative dilemma associated with the surrounding maxillary root morphology.

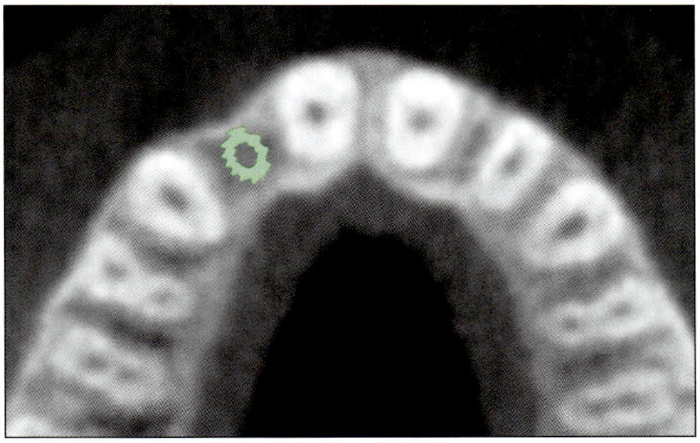

Fig 10-1g Implant placed to bisect the intertooth space within the existing alveolar bone.

The CT scan data from the i-CAT machine was then reconstructed within SimPlant to slice through the maxilla in the axial plane, allowing for a visual inspection of the surrounding anatomy and root morphology (Fig 10-1f). The morphologic characteristics of the individual tooth roots at the level of the alveolar crestal bone are clearly defined in the axial view. It is this view that demonstrates the restorative dilemma, ie, the difficulty of restoring natural tooth form on round implants (Fig 10-1g). The application of this imaging technology provides tools to develop new paradigms for implant-to-tooth spacing, implant-to-implant spacing, and proximity to other adjacent structures. The panoramic, cross-sectional, and axial images afford a process of assimilation for proper diagnosis and treatment planning. However, they still represent only two-dimensional (2D) reconstructions from the CT dataset.

Visualization of the patient's anatomy in true three-dimensional (3D) form was accomplished using the powerful, feature-rich software engine provided by SimPlant. The inspection of a virtual 3D model of the patient's maxilla can be exponentially enhanced with a variety of new interactive tools. Rotating the 3D maxilla reveals the surrounding bony topography, root eminences, and concavity in the area of the missing tooth (Fig 10-1h). The 3D model can be rotated in any position, allowing for ultimate inspection and appreciation of the site. The use of advanced masking or "segmentation" allows for the separation and colorization of specific anatomic structures, which intensifies diagnostic capabilities. The ability to create "selective transparency" is invaluable diagnostically because the outer bone can be made semi-transparent to reveal the underlying surrounding opaque tooth roots (Fig 10-1i).

As noted earlier, the goal is the tooth that is to be replaced; therefore, the development of the virtual tooth is an important evolutionary step toward virtual implant planning (Fig 10-1j). The virtual tooth can be scaled to fit the space and allow inspection of the contact areas, the distance to the alveolar crest, and the esthetics. Improved features of the SimPlant software have made it easier to remove the bone entirely in order to gain access to anatomy previously hidden from view (Fig 10-1k). Accurate placement of a virtual realistic tapered implant (Tapered Internal Implant, BioHorizons) from the manufacturer library was made possible by these advanced modalities. The coronal position of the implant, which was suspect in the original periapical radiograph (see Fig 10-1d), can be easily evaluated. The yellow abutment projection is helpful in identifying the overall spatial position of the implant as it points toward the envelope of the proposed tooth. Removing the bone entirely helps to finalize the position of the implant and abutment projection. The body and thread design of the implant are in full view.

In addition, and perhaps of most importance for this case, is the assessment of apical proximity to the adjacent tooth roots. Adding selective transparency allows for unparalleled appreciation of the implant, the abutment projection, and the virtual tooth in various views (Figs 10-1l

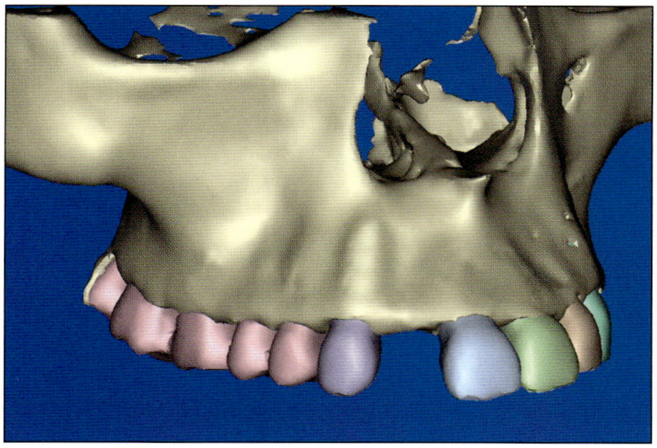

Fig 10-1h The 3D reconstruction is helpful in visualizing the patient's anatomy. The lateral 3D view shows the surrounding root eminences and amount of bone available for implant placement.

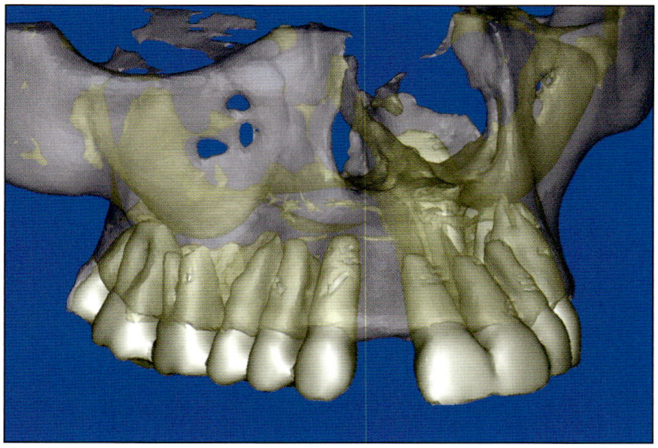

Fig 10-1i With the use of the selective transparency and segmentation tools, the adjacent roots can be separated from the surrounding structures and bone.

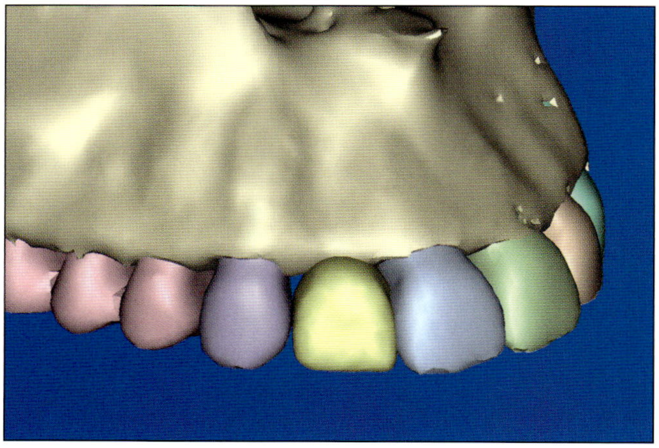

Fig 10-1j Virtual tooth replacing the missing lateral incisor.

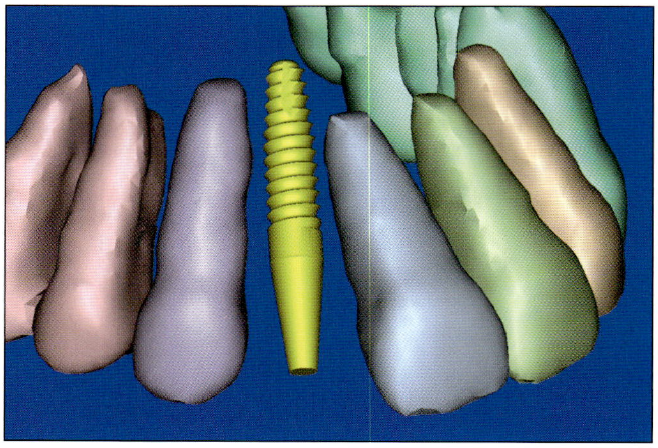

Fig 10-1k A tapered implant with an abutment projection (yellow) is used for the apical positioning.

and 10-1m). This method is especially useful in planning implants near natural teeth. The occlusal view affords additional examination of the relationship of the abutment and the virtual tooth to the adjacent teeth and greatly facilitates restoratively driven planning (Fig 10-1n).

The anti-rotational feature of the implant can be adjusted to be consistent with the desired abutment for a cement-retained restoration. This rotational position has been defined by the author as the *fifth dimension*, allowing the "flat" aspect of the internal hex to be oriented toward the facial (Fig 10-1n). The next step was to replace the generic abutment projection with a realistic abutment from the implant library. A precontoured straight abutment was evaluated for proper marginal positioning as dictated by the orientation of the flat aspect of the internal hex rotation toward the facial (Fig 10-1o). If the intraoral position of the implant places the hex in a different orientation, the margins of the abutment would not be in the proper position for completion of the restoration, in which case a custom abutment would be required.

Additional information can be obtained by slicing through the 3D model with the Virtual Tooth, a process in SimPlant called *clipping*. This highly diagnostic view provides information about the implant receptor site that was previously inaccessible (Fig 10-1p). While clinicians unfamiliar with standard CT images may find it difficult to interpret the information they provide, 3D images are easily understood. The labial/buccal and palatal/lingual cortical thickness surrounding the dense trabecular bone can be evaluated to ensure proper positioning of the implant within the TOB (Fig 10-1q). Note that the realistic abutment (for a cementable restoration) has been rotated to orient the lower premachined margin toward the facial and the higher margin toward the palate so that it fits within the envelope of the virtual tooth. The virtual implant library can aid clinicians in planning cases with a va-

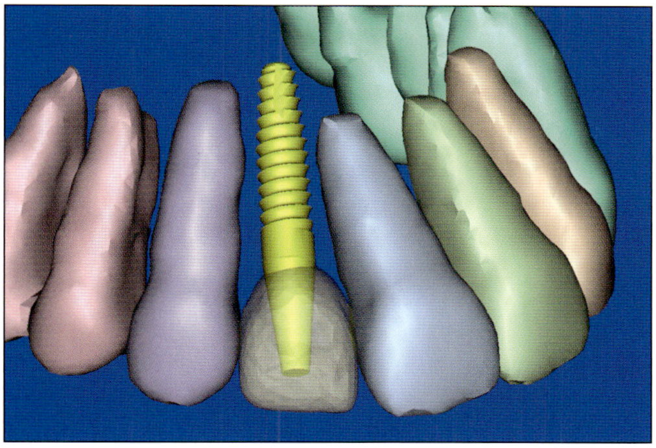

Fig 10-1l Selective transparency allows the simulated abutment to be seen through the virtual tooth.

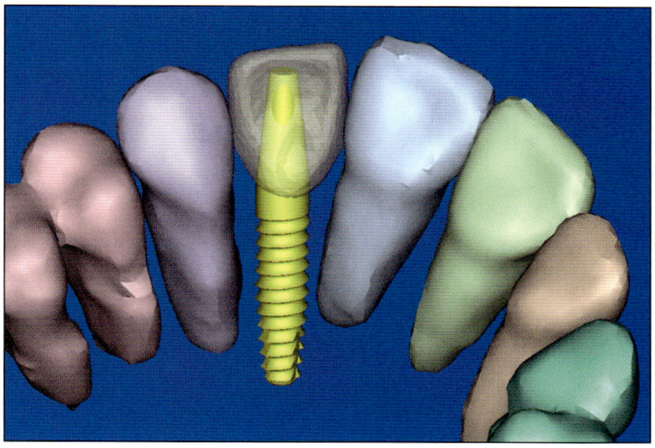

Fig 10-1m The lingual view allows further assessment of the implant placement.

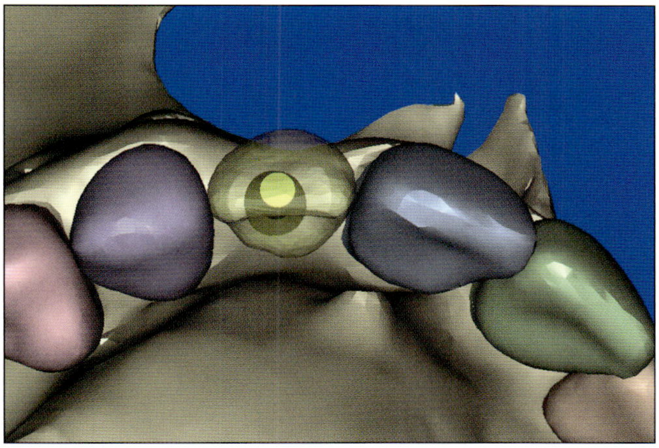

Fig 10-1n The occlusal view of the virtual tooth and abutment projection aids in positioning the implant within the restorative envelope.

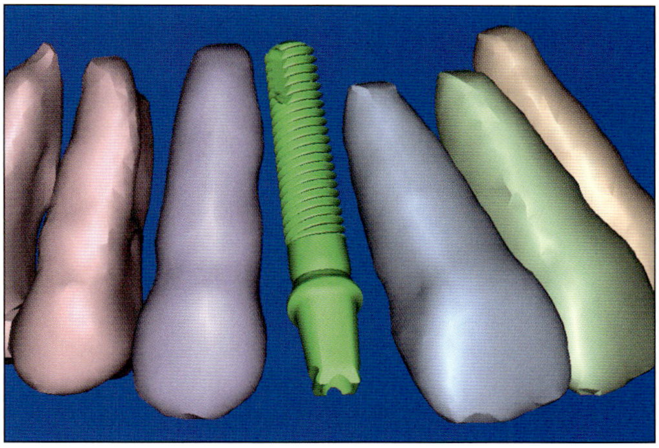

Fig 10-1o The realistic implant and precontoured abutment in proximity to the adjacent roots.

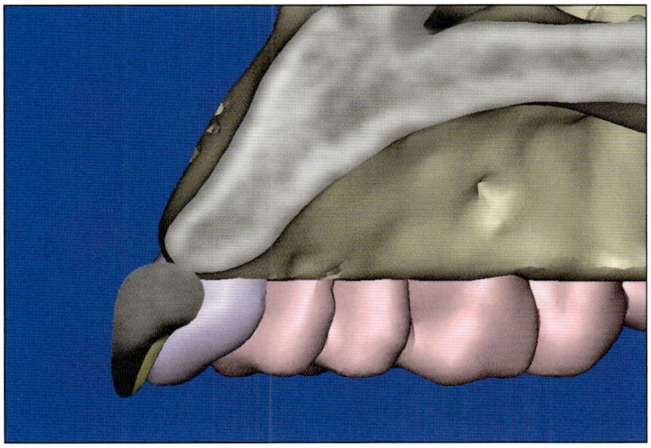

Fig 10-1p With the use of the clipping function, the 3D reconstruction slices through the maxilla and the virtual tooth.

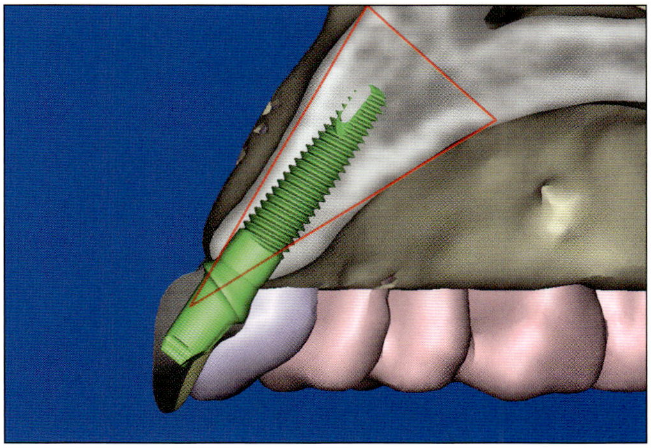

Fig 10-1q The realistic implant and precontoured abutment within the TOB.

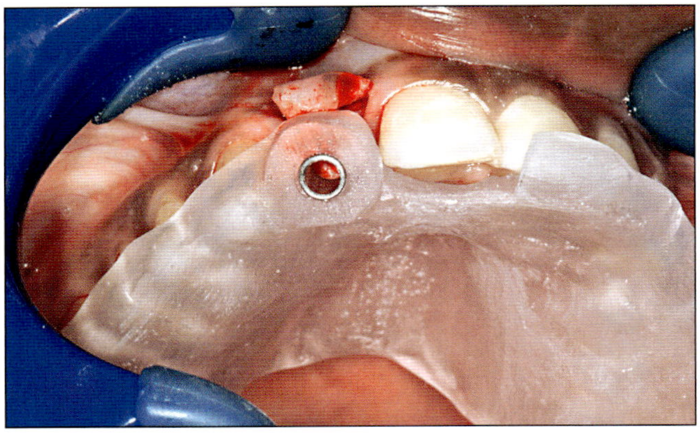

Fig 10-1r The tooth-supported guide seated intraorally, allowing for precision drill guidance.

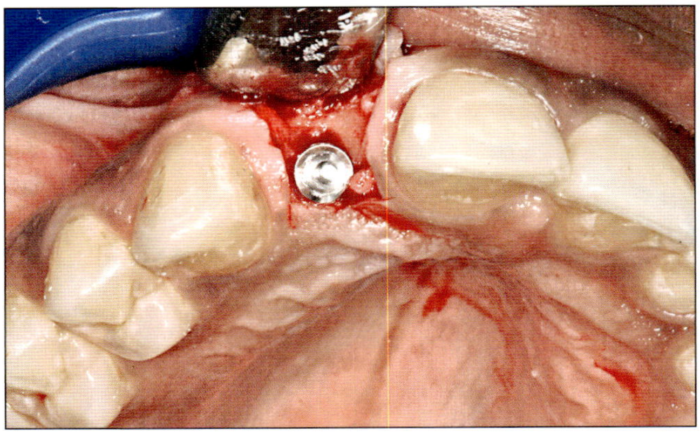

Fig 10-1s The implant has been placed into the bone with the flat aspect of the internal hex rotated toward the facial.

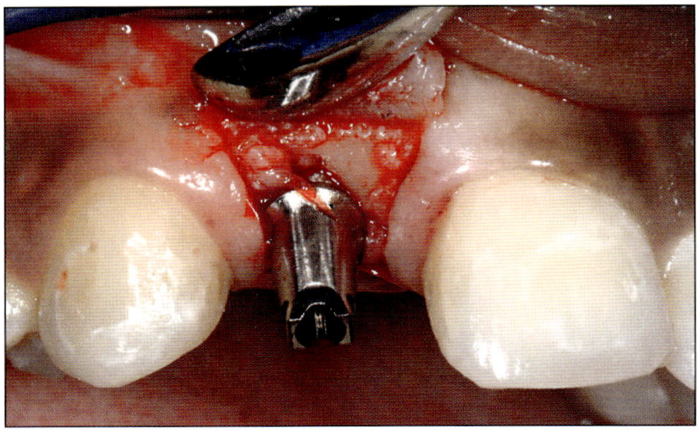

Fig 10-1t Seated intraorally, the precontoured abutment mimics the position in the virtual planning.

riety of implants and prosthetic components, giving new meaning to the concept of preoperative prosthetic planning. This assessment is representative of how these 3D tools can be used to define new paradigms for implant planning, serving as an excellent educational opportunity for all members of the implant team.

Surgical phase

Once the plan has been reviewed in all available views and the implant position established, this information can be shared with the patient and, if applicable, members of the implant team. The widespread use of computers and high-speed Internet access allow for quick and easy exchange of this important information, within the constraints of the Healthcare Information Portability and Accessibility Act (HIPAA). When this technology becomes incorporated into daily practice, its value goes well beyond its excellent diagnostic capability and empowers clinicians with a powerful communication and marketing tool. Moreover, the images can be easily incorporated into an impressive presentation that helps patients understand the treatment recommendation.

Because the apex of the maxillary right central incisor root was in close proximity to the implant, it was advisable to place the implant with the aid of a CT-derived surgical guide. Once the patient accepted the treatment plan, the data was sent via email for fabrication of the CT-derived surgical templates to link the virtual plan to the surgical procedure (SurgiGuide, Materialise). The surgical templates can be bone supported, tooth supported, or mucosa supported depending on the software application used. For this case, a tooth-supported guide was necessitated by the partially edentulous condition.

The tooth-supported guide was fabricated by means of a stereolithographic process. Surgical guidance is supplied by the 5-mm-tall stainless steel cylinder, which varies in diameter based on the drills to be used to create the osteotomy (Fig 10-1r). Three different templates were used for the classic SurgiGuides, corresponding to the three different manufacturer-specific drills used for sequential osteotomy preparation. After the elevation of a conservative mucoperiosteal flap to expose the underlying bone, the osteotomy was created with the use of sequential drills and guides. A 3.75-mm diameter × 13-mm length implant (Tapered Screw-Vent, Zimmer) was placed according to the CT plan (Fig 10-1s). The bone density and bone

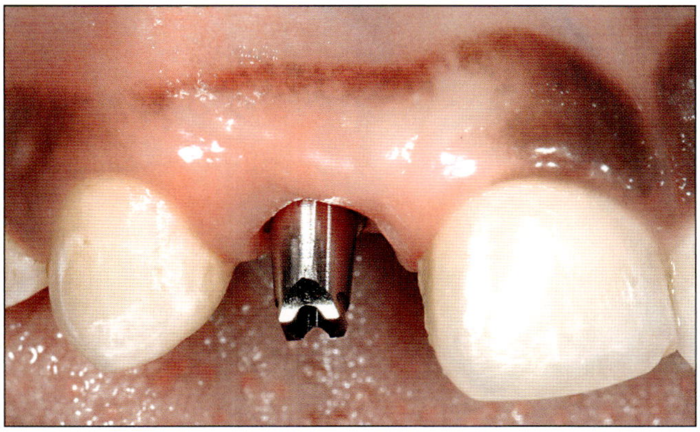

Fig 10-1u The soft tissue response was excellent after an adequate healing phase.

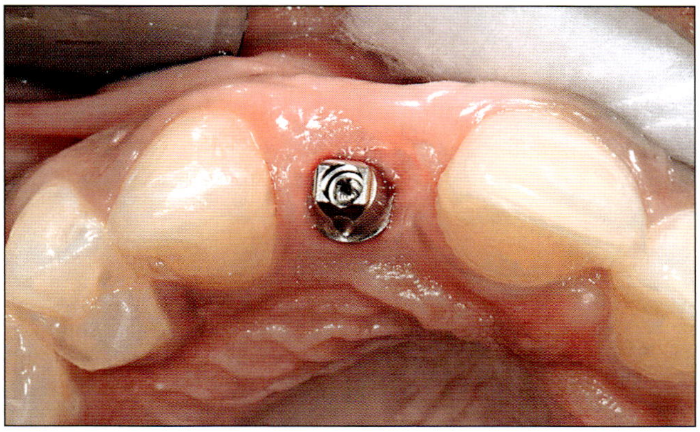

Fig 10-1v The facial-palatal width was well-maintained.

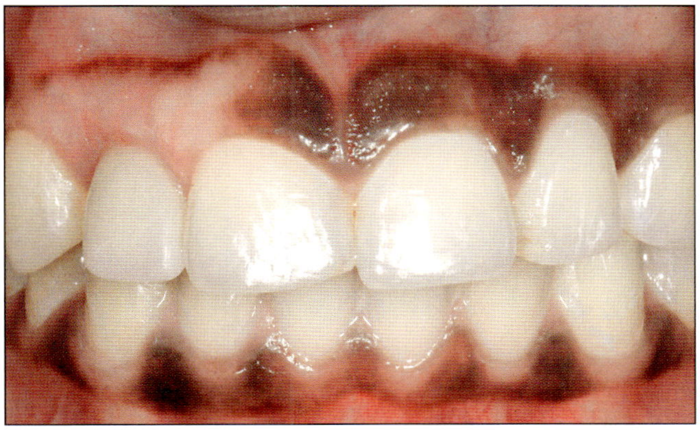

Fig 10-1w Retracted view of the completed metal-ceramic restoration.

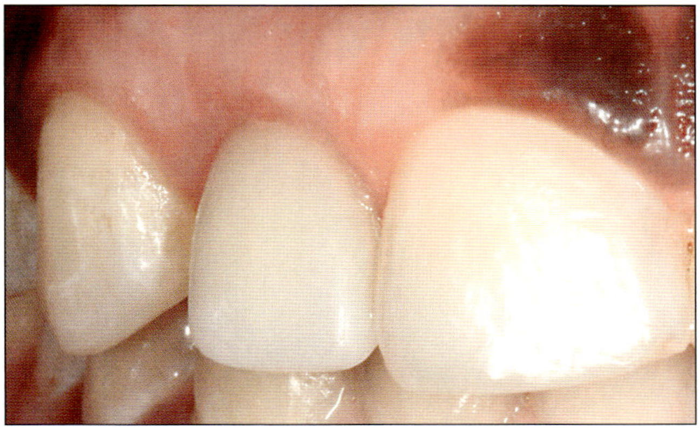

Fig 10-1x Close-up view demonstrating excellent adaptation of the interdental papillae.

topography had been previously assessed using the CT data. The excellent fixation properties of the implant, combined with the CT-derived plan, established that the implant could be immediately restored. Based on the use of the advanced planning features of the SimPlant software, the implant was rotated so that the flat aspect of the internal hex connection was oriented toward the facial. A precontoured stock abutment was ready at the time of surgery and then secured to the implant for immediate provisionalization (Fig 10-1t).

Our ability to assess the restorative requirements of the receptor site was greatly enhanced by the development of the Virtual Tooth feature and the use of realistic abutments that can be positioned within the envelope of the desired tooth position. The position of the actual abutment intraorally matched that of the virtual plan (see Fig 10-1o) and allowed adequate distance between the premachined margins of the abutment and the adjacent teeth, which is important for papilla preservation.

Restorative phase

After a sufficient healing period of approximately 2 months, the provisional restoration was removed, revealing mature soft tissue contours that were well-maintained interproximally (Fig 10-1u). Because of the excellent preoperative prosthetic planning, there was no need to remove the original stock precontoured abutment. A snap impression coping from the restorative kit provided by the manufacturer was used for an abutment-level impression, leaving the soft tissue interface undisturbed. The analogue was then sent to the laboratory for fabrication of a metal-ceramic restoration. The occlusal view revealed preservation of the facial aspect of the alveolar ridge and spatial placement of the implant (Fig 10-1v). The definitive porcelain-fused-to-metal restoration displayed a favorable emergence profile and excellent adaptation of the interdental papillae (Figs 10-1w and 10-1x). This predictable result was achieved through proper restoratively driven planning made possible by the technologic advances of the CBCT and the SimPlant software platform.

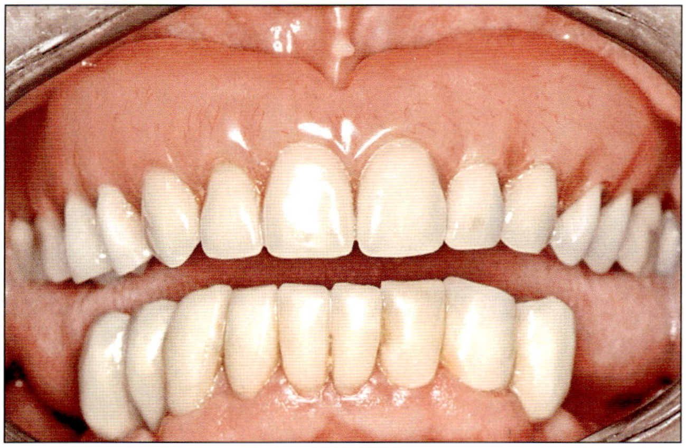

Fig 10-2a Preoperative maxillary complete denture.

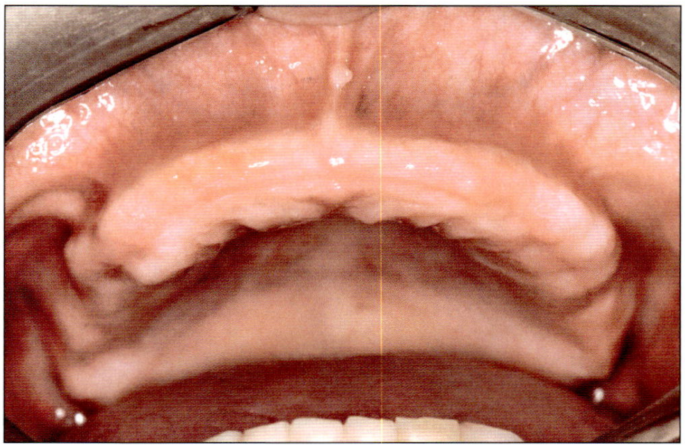

Fig 10-2b Preoperative retracted view of maxillary edentulous alveolar ridge.

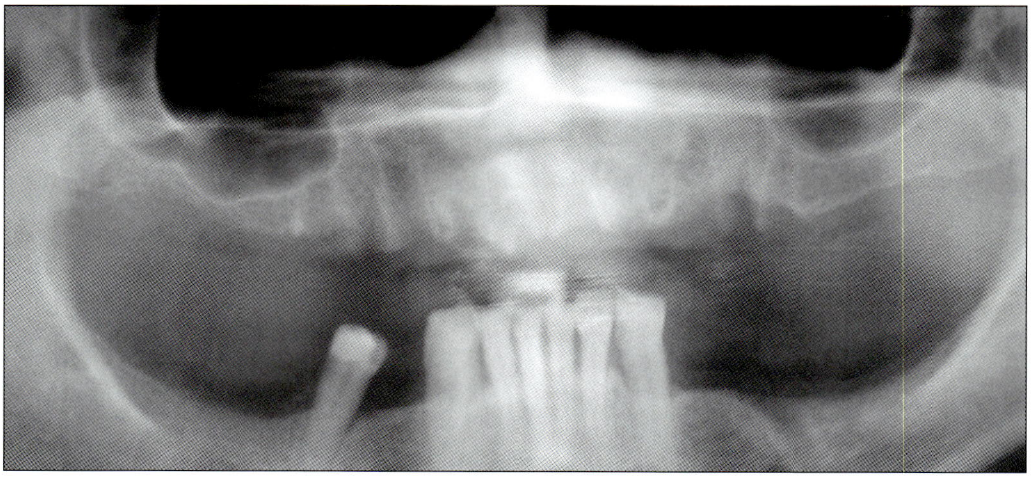

Fig 10-2c Preoperative panoramic radiograph, revealing poorly healed maxillary extraction sites.

Case 2: Immediate-Load Maxillary Fixed Restoration

A 55-year-old woman presented with a problematic maxillary complete denture that she had been wearing for approximately 4 years. The patient had heard that implants might be an option to help support a fixed restoration but was never offered this treatment alternative by her local dentist. She was very unhappy with her removable denture and wished to have a fixed restoration if possible. She was a nonsmoker in good general health and her medical history was unremarkable.

Clinical exam revealed a complete maxillary denture and periodontally compromised mandibular teeth (Fig 10-2a). The underlying maxillary alveolar ridge exhibited good demarcation between keratinized and nonkeratinized tissue with areas of convex and concave bone topography posteriorly (Fig 10-2b). The preoperative panoramic radiograph revealed outlines of previous extraction sites and an irregular bone pattern in the maxilla. The mandibular molars and premolars were missing with the exception of a single premolar remaining on the right side (Fig 10-2c). Following the clinical and preliminary radiographic evaluation, the patient was informed that she could be a candidate for maxillary implants. The final determination could only be confirmed via CT scan analysis of the residual bone. The patient agreed, and a scan was scheduled. Prior to the scan, a barium sulfate scanning appliance was fabricated from a duplicate of the patient's existing maxillary complete denture.

Planning phase

A complete arch restoration raises additional concerns in planning dental implants that were easily addressed with SimPlant. The CT scan revealed significant features of the

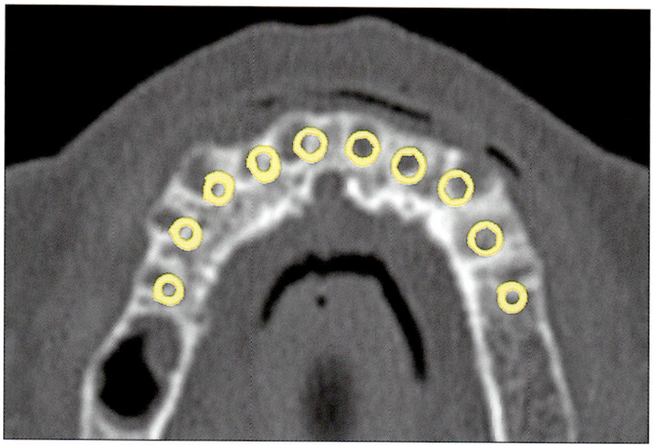

Fig 10-2d Axial view with simulated placement of 10 implants in the maxilla.

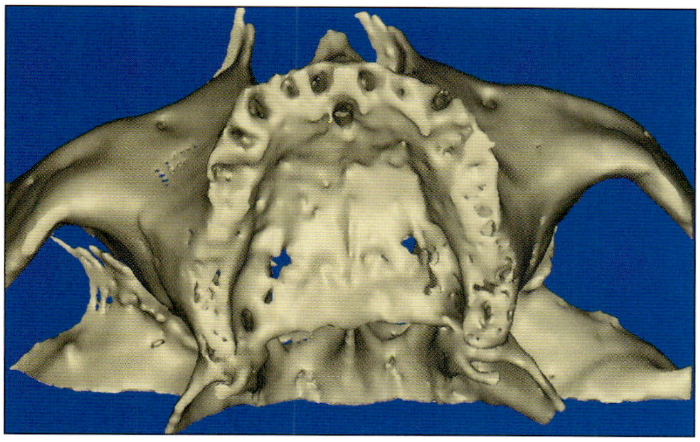

Fig 10-2e 3D reconstruction occlusal view of edentulous alveolar ridge.

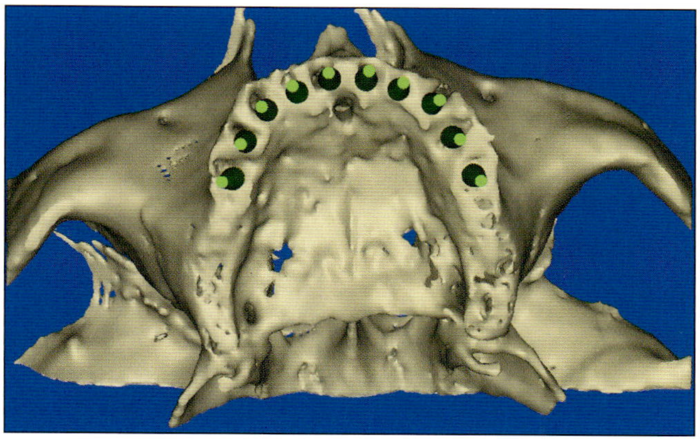

Fig 10-2f 3D reconstruction with simulated placement of 10 implants with abutment projections.

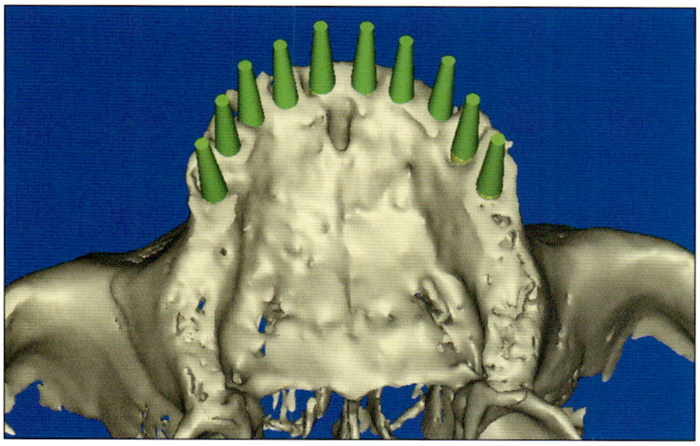

Fig 10-2g Rotation of the 3D view allows for inspection of the potential implant receptor sites.

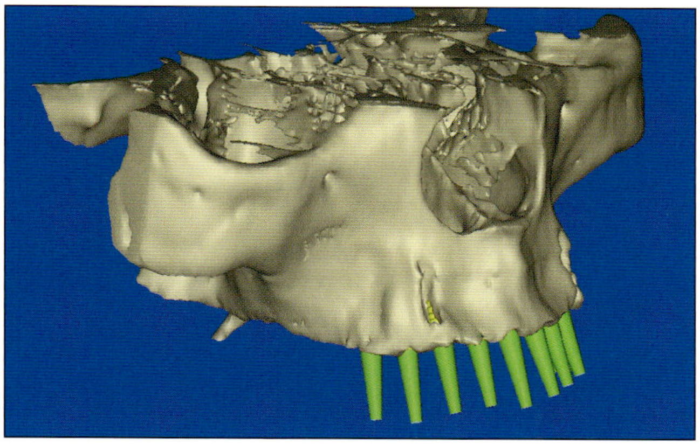

Fig 10-2h Lateral view of the 3D reconstruction with abutment projections. Note the fenestrations in the canine areas.

underlying alveolar ridge anatomy that could not have been visualized with conventional 2D radiography. After a careful examination using all available views within SimPlant, 10 potential implant receptor sites were identified (Fig 10-2d). The axial 3D reconstruction displayed residual unhealed socket sites with dehiscence of the facial cortical plate evident in the areas of the maxillary right and left canines, demonstrating irregular bone protuberances that were painful to the patient under the pressure of her existing denture. These irregularities are readily apparent in the 3D reconstruction (Fig 10-2e). The simulated implants were placed with abutment projections to aid in the planning process (Fig 10-2f). The advantages of being able to manipulate and rotate the 3D model for proper visualization are amplified when multiple implants are planned within the variations of the maxillary arch topography (Figs 10-2g and 10-2h).

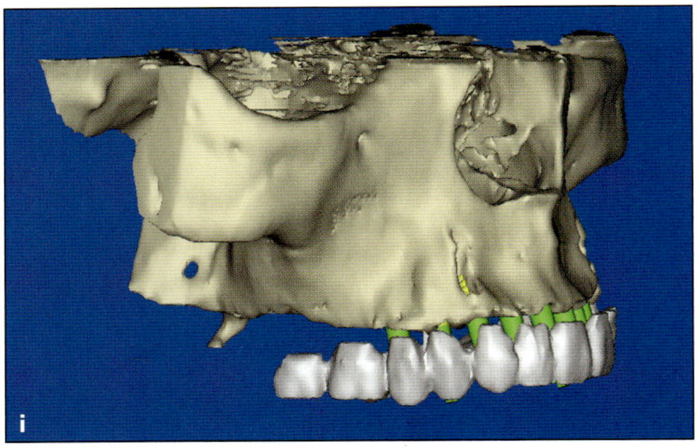

Fig 10-2i The lateral view reveals the full contoured radiopaque teeth, allowing for visualization of the restorative embrasures.

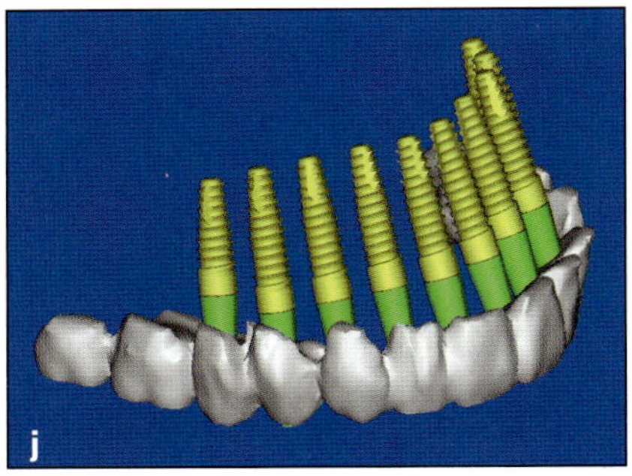

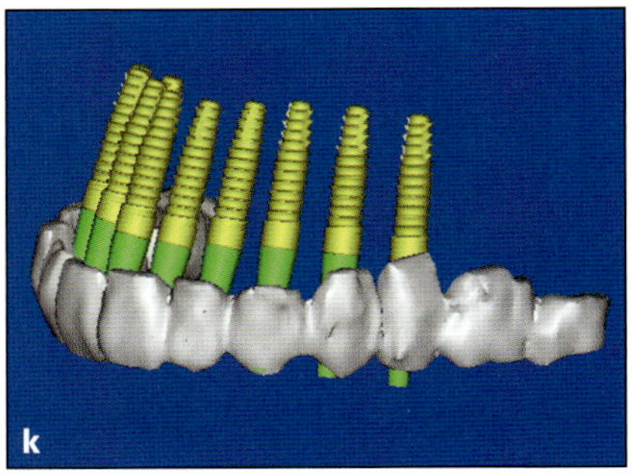

Figs 10-2j and 10-2k With the bone "removed," the realistic implants can be visualized within the envelope of the radiopaque scanning appliance.

As in Case 1, the implants were first placed in the 2D axial and cross-sectional plane views, then brought into the powerful interactive 3D model views for final placement. The importance of using a barium sulfate scanning appliance for this full arch reconstruction cannot be overemphasized. The ability to visualize the desired tooth position in relation to the underlying bone is an essential step in restoratively driven planning. Using the 3D software dialogue, it was easy to activate and deactivate various 3D volumes that were created during the planning process. The lateral view of the maxillary arch reveals the scanning appliance with sculpted teeth and embrasures (Fig 10-2i). Removing the bone entirely allowed for each individual implant (with an abutment projection) to be positioned properly within the body of the radiopaque tooth to avoid embrasures or undesirable faciolingual angulations (Figs 10-2j and 10-2k). The tooth-contoured radiopaque template allows the clinician to tweak the position of each implant for precision placement (Fig 10-2l). Each implant was placed according to the TOB concept to maximize surrounding bone volume and within the restorative envelope of the radiopaque template. This was confirmed in the 2D cross-sectional views of the implants with abutment projections simulated to assist with the ultimate trajectories of each implant (Figs 10-2m and 10-2n).

Because the canines are essential for long-term maintenance of the arch form, simulated implants were placed in these sites in spite of the obvious lack of adequate facial cortical bone. The ability to fixate these implants would depend on the implant type, thread design, management at time of surgery, and skill of the clinician. Additionally, the treatment plan must include grafting procedures to cover any exposed threads with appropriate bone graft and/or membrane for adequate regeneration. These techniques are beyond the scope of this chapter.

SimPlant as a diagnostic and planning tool has continued to evolve with the addition of important features that add new layers of sophistication. In 1994, the author introduced a unique concept that would allow a set of "virtual teeth" to be transposed over the CT scan images for better correlation between the bone and the desired tooth position. From this basic concept and through many years of development (combined with the improved graphics capabilities of today's high-powered, lower-cost computers), a Virtual Tooth tool became available in SimPlant Version 10. Although this case was completed several

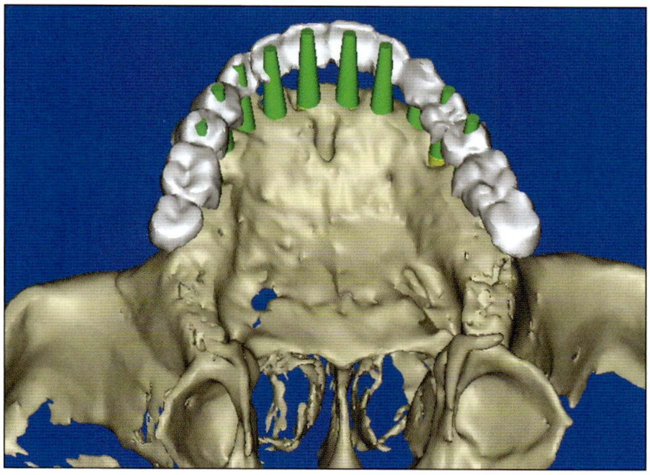

Fig 10-2l Scanning appliance is used at the time of scan acquisition to aid in determining proper implant positioning.

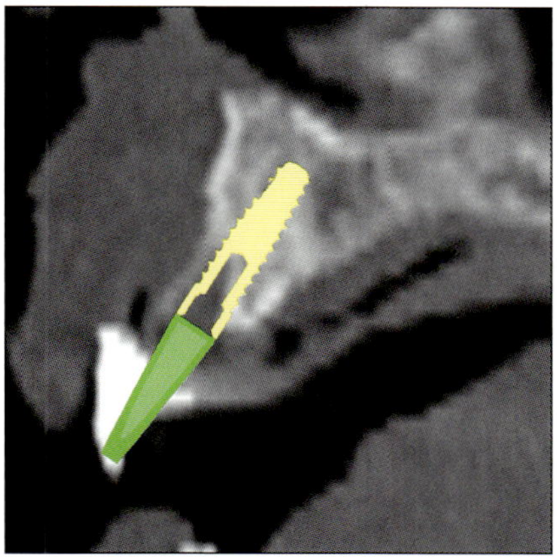

Fig 10-2m Cross-sectional image of the realistic implant with the abutment projection in the envelope of the radiopaque tooth.

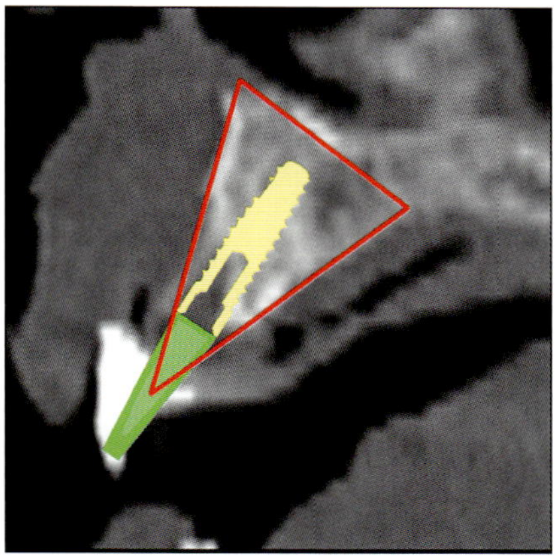

Fig 10-2n The implant position is confirmed to be within the TOB.

years prior to this software innovation, the dataset was still available, and the Virtual Tooth tool was recently used to create a complete maxillary dentition from first molar to first molar (Fig 10-2o). The virtual dentition was then superimposed over the maxillary arch, providing an additional method of evaluating the implant positions in relation to the desired tooth position (Fig 10-2p). Though still in the developmental stages, the virtual tooth tool can be very useful. Using "selective transparency," as described earlier, all of the 3D volumes can be viewed with individualized effects to maximize diagnostic quality (Fig 10-2q). The virtual teeth can be made totally opaque to aid in determining embrasures and implant angulations, or the bone can be made semi-translucent to emphasize the anatomic and implant components (Figs 10-2r and 10-2s). The virtual teeth can ultimately be combined with the scanning appliance to highlight the differences and the preferred position of each implant (Fig 10-2t).

Using the clipping function within SimPlant, the 3D reconstruction can be sliced to reveal the realistic implant, the abutment projection, and the radiopaque scanning appliance (Fig 10-2u). The virtual tooth design closely matched the same tooth represented in the scanning appliance, as illustrated in Fig 10-2v, confirming that the implant was placed within the TOB (Fig 10-2w). Using the feature-rich functionality of SimPlant, the operator can determine the distance between the cervical contour of the virtual tooth to the crest of the bone and the position and angulation of the implants, so that abutment choices can be made in advance. These tools greatly empower the clinician with the ability to evaluate restorative alternatives for the patient, whether for a fixed-detachable hybrid type

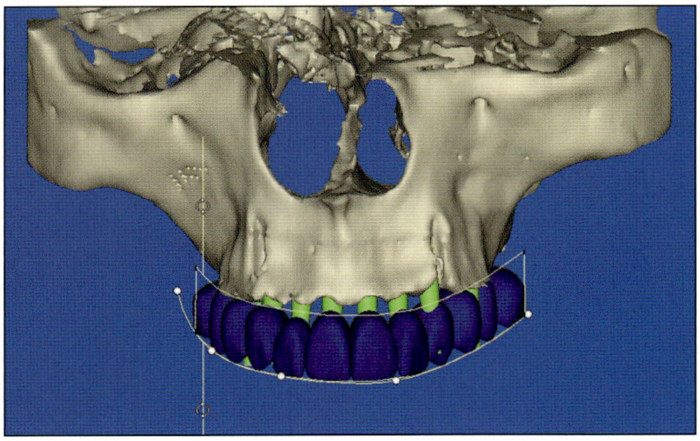

Fig 10-2o A full arch of simulated virtual teeth wrapped around the maxillary arch.

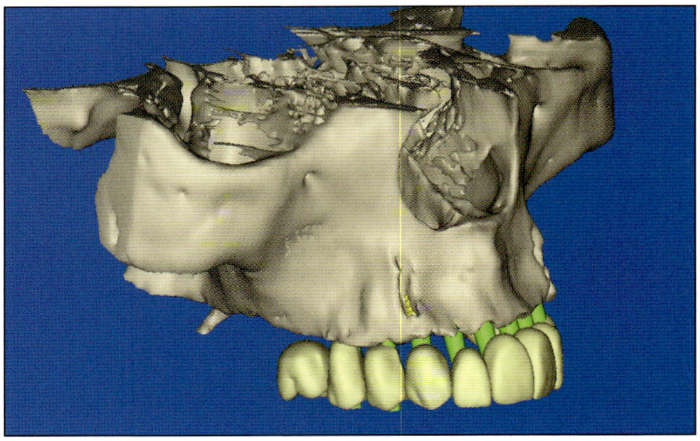

Fig 10-2p The Virtual Tooth set-up over the maxilla and implants.

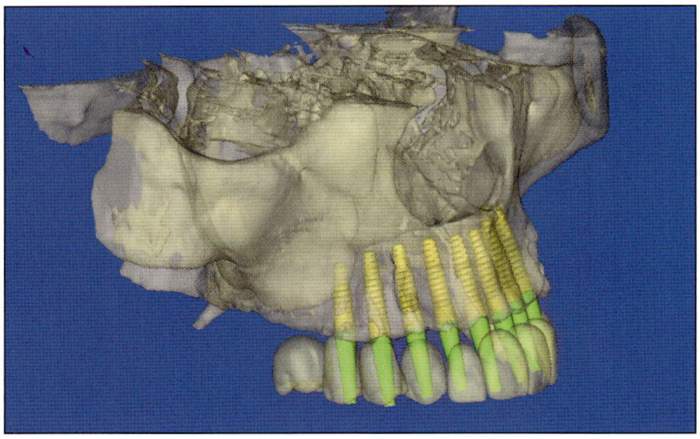

Fig 10-2q With the use of selective transparency, the maxilla and the virtual teeth become transparent.

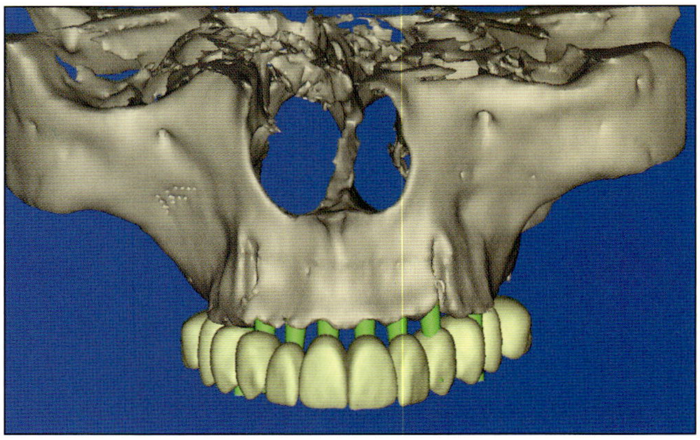

Fig 10-2r Facial view of the virtual maxillary occlusion.

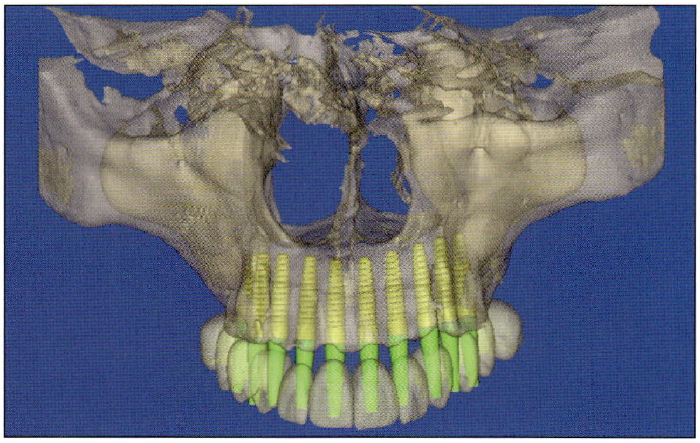

Fig 10-2s Facial view with the maxillary bone and virtual occlusion in the transparent mode.

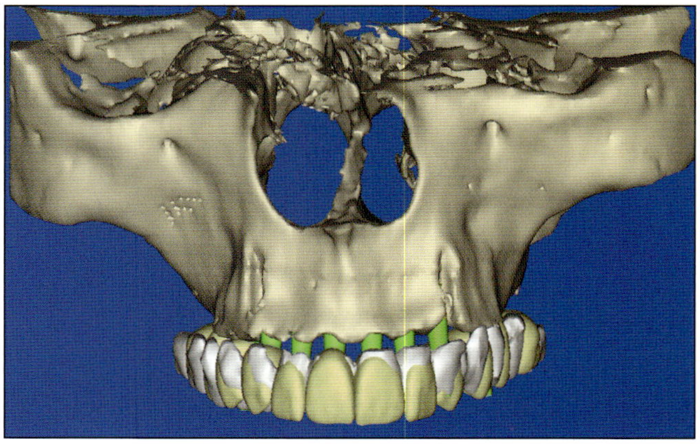

Fig 10-2t Superimposition of the Virtual Tooth set-up over the scanning appliance.

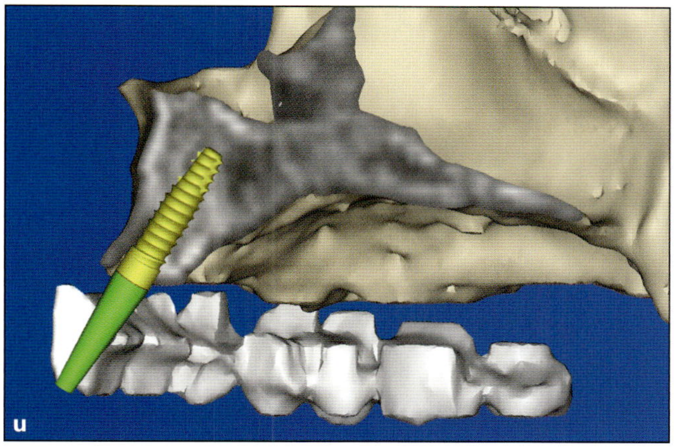

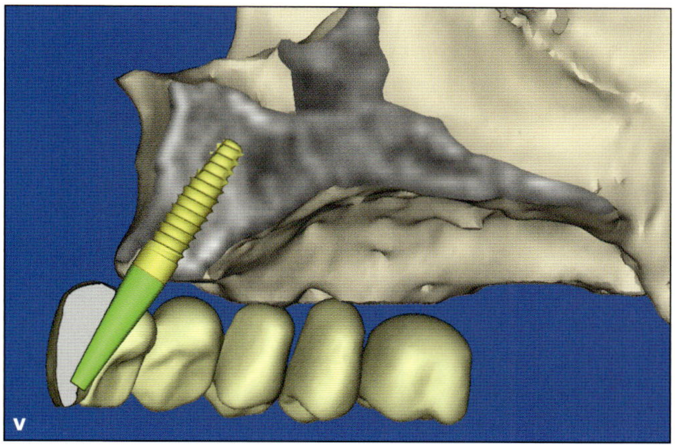

Fig 10-2u and 10-2v With the use of the clipping tool, the 3D reconstruction is sliced through the radiopaque template: *(u)* the virtual tooth set-up; *(v)* the maxillary arch revealing the implant trajectory.

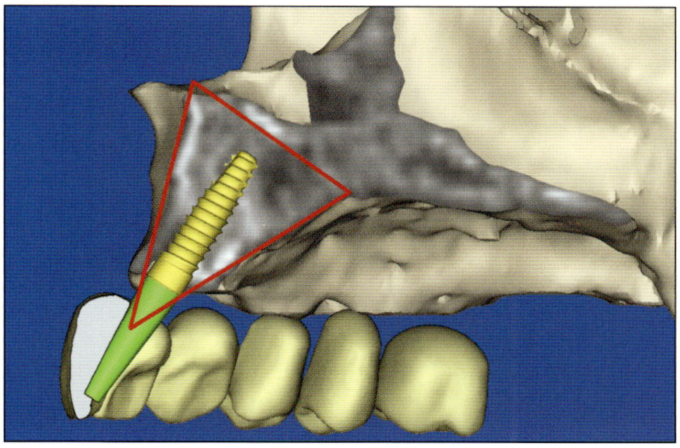

Fig 10-2w The TOB demonstrated on clipping slice of the 3D reconstruction.

prosthesis when an acrylic flange is desired, or for a conventional porcelain-fused-to-metal cemented restoration, which requires greater precision to avoid embrasure areas and to maximize esthetic outcomes. The final treatment plan was to place 10 implants and have the patient leave the office with an immediate conventional fixed bridge restoration supported by the implants.

Surgical phase

Once the final plan is established, the software permits a "preview" of the bone-supported surgical guide. This useful feature allows for a final review of the implant placement, implant-to-implant distances, and the bone coverage required to stabilize the SurgiGuide (Fig 10-2x). If fixation of the template is indicated, this can be planned as well. For this case, the extent of the acrylic flange of the bone-supported guide was sufficient for stabilization without the need for fixation screws. The final SimPlant plan was sent via email to Materialise for the fabrication of the surgical guides. The bone-supported SurgiGuides were created from the CT scan data, incorporating the stainless steel tubes with diameters that conform to the drilling sequence to be used (Fig 10-2y).

The patient was given local anesthesia, and a full-thickness mucoperiosteal flap was elevated to expose the underlying crestal bone. The flap design must allow for the intimate seating of the bone-supported guides (Fig 10-2z). Using the different guides, osteotomies were created and 10 Silhouette IC Laser-Lok implants (BioHorizons) were placed, including four 4.0-mm-diameter internal connection, tapered implants in the anterior maxilla and six 4.5-mm-diameter implants in the posterior sites. These implants have a laser micromachined collar designed to halt vertical epithelial cell migration and generate soft tissue attachment, combined with a secondary zone of grooves designed to improve load transfer and prevent crestal bone loss (Fig 10-2aa).

Temporary cementable abutments were delivered to 8 of the 10 implants (the canine positions were not attached to the provisional bridge). The canine implants received

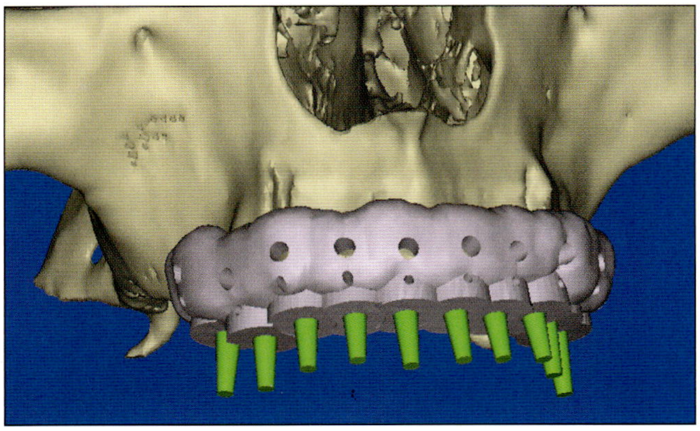

Fig 10-2x Facial view of the SurgiGuide preview showing implant abutment projections.

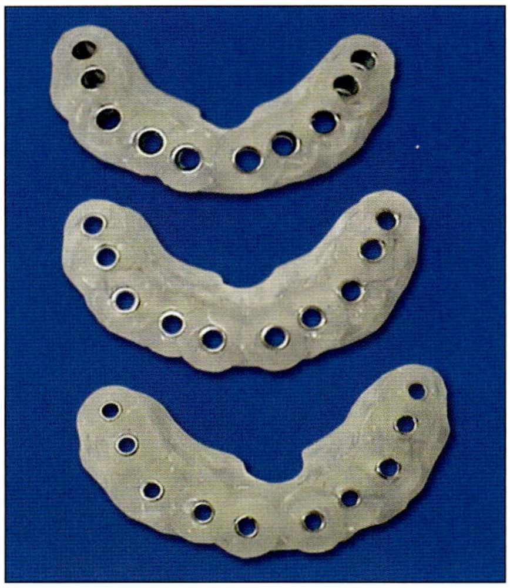

Fig 10-2y Stereolithographic SurgiGuide templates for sequential osteotomy preparation.

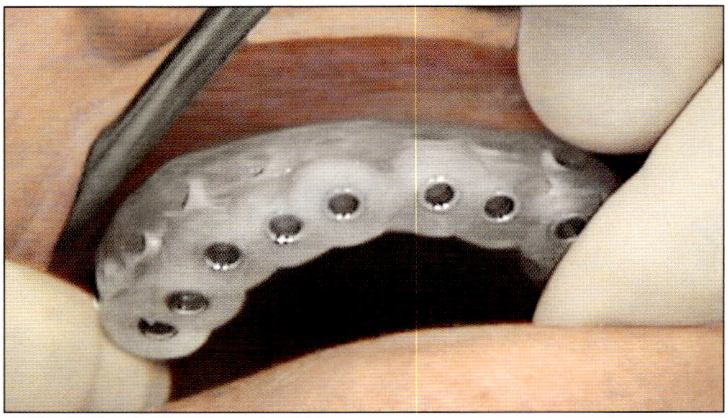

Fig 10-2z Intraoral placement of the SurgiGuide.

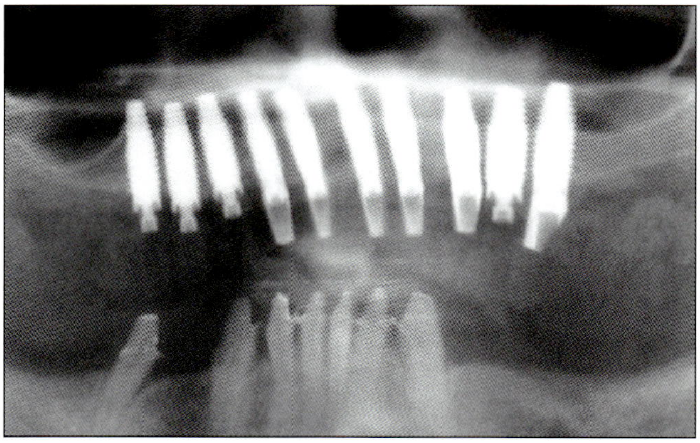

Fig 10-2aa Postoperative panoramic radiograph showing the placement of 10 implants.

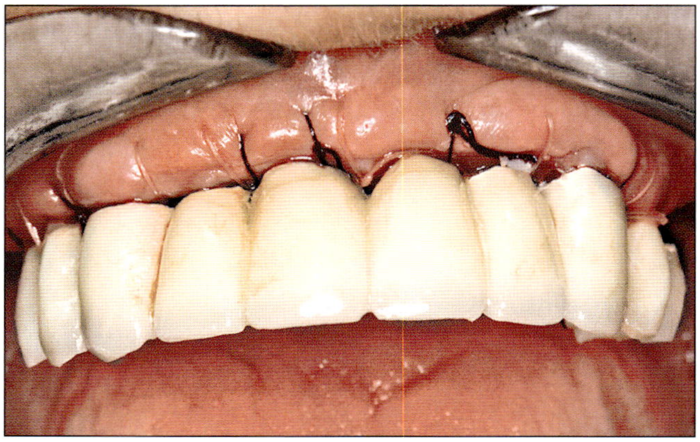

Fig 10-2bb Immediate provisionalization with soft tissue approximation and sutures.

healing collars in a one-stage approach but were left unloaded. The bone defects were filled with cancellous particulate bone graft material (Puros, Tutogen/Zimmer Implant), mixed with platelet-rich plasma (PRP) drawn from the patient's blood (Harvest Technologies) and then covered with a collagen membrane (CollaCote, Zimmer Implant). The soft tissue was then approximated around the transitional abutments and the provisional fixed bridge cemented in place (Fig 10-2bb). The entire site was then sprayed with the PRP solution to enhance soft tissue heal-

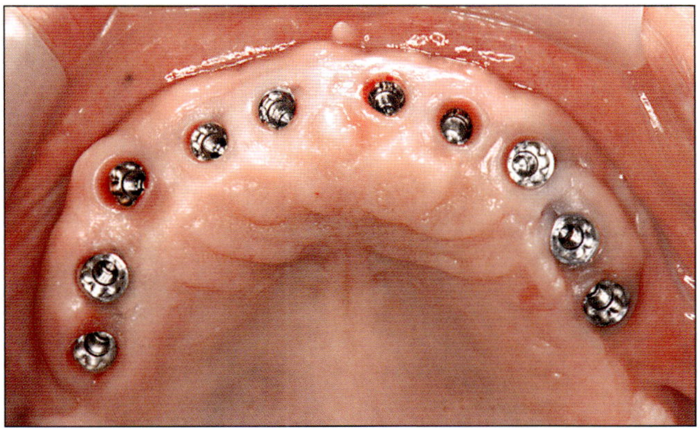

Fig 10-2cc Soft tissue maturation in preparation for impressions.

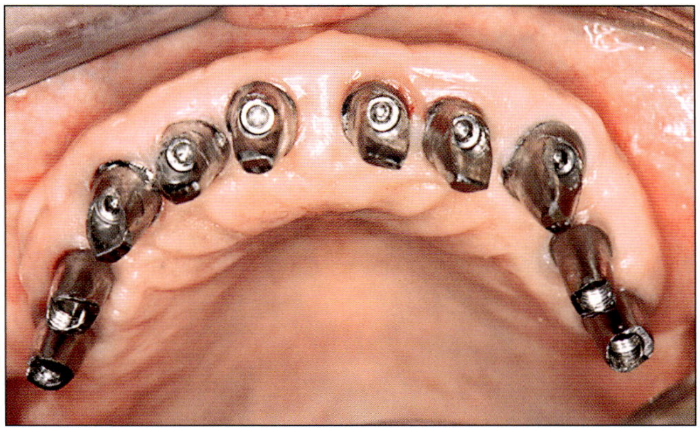

Fig 10-2dd Retracted view of the maxillary implant abutments revealing excellent adaptation and maturation of the keratinized tissue.

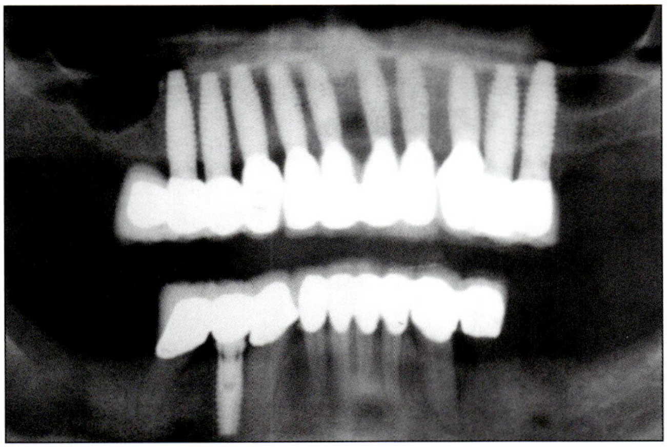

Fig 10-2ee Postoperative panoramic radiograph revealing completed full arch maxillary metal-ceramic restoration.

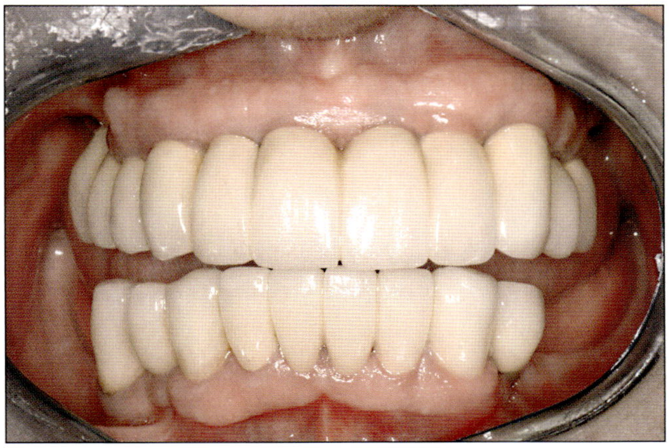

Fig 10-2ff Follow-up 2½ years after placement of the definitive prosthesis shows excellent emergence profile and esthetics.

ing. The patient tolerated the procedure well and was pleased that her palate was freed from the pressures of the complete maxillary denture.

Restorative phase

The fixed transitional restoration was left in place for approximately 10 weeks. During this interim period the patient was seen for routine follow-up for suture removal and then to monitor healing progress. The patient was advised that a soft diet was essential to avoid prematurely overloading the implants. The healing phase was unremarkable, and at 10 weeks the canine implants were activated with temporary abutments fit to the provisional bridge. At 12 weeks the soft tissue had matured sufficiently to allow fixture-level impressions (Fig 10-2cc). Note the increased width of the alveolar crest and keratinized tissue. Impression transfers were attached to the implants and impressions taken to start the final restorative phase. A soft tissue model was fabricated to help determine proper emergence profiles. It was decided that custom abutments would be fabricated for the anterior four implants and prepared stock abutments used for the posterior six implants (Fig 10-2dd). A conventional porcelain-fused-to-metal framework was fabricated in three sections—one anterior and two posterior. The prosthetic seating was verified with the panoramic radiograph (Fig 10-2ee). The completed case met the esthetic and functional needs of the patient. The patient was able to go from a complete denture to an immediate interim restoration in the same day, followed by a fixed, conventional cemented porcelain-fused-to-metal prosthesis within 4 months of implant placement.

The patient has been followed for several years, and the definitive restoration shown in Fig 10-2ff represents the soft tissue quality 2½ years after placement. The relationship of the interdental papillae, emergence profile, and overall esthetic result was made possible through excellent preoperative prosthetic planning afforded by CT technology and SimPlant. When it is possible to replace a complete removable denture with a nonremovable metal-ceramic restoration and achieve this type of precision, it goes beyond esthetics and function and remains a permanent change in the quality of life for the patient.

Conclusion

In the past, 2D imaging was inherently limiting. For single-tooth applications, especially, even today clinicians do not feel the need for 3D volumetric imaging for diagnosis of available bone. However, the acceptance of CT/CBCT has helped clinicians expand beyond their conventional imaging modalities to understand the 3D anatomy of their patients and the importance of this technology even for missing single teeth. This chapter started with a patient who came to the consultation with her CT scan data on a disk. Thus, even patients are becoming more knowledgeable about this important technology. Interactive treatment-planning software can take the CBCT data and reprocess it in a manner that can be readily used for evaluating potential implant receptor sites. The continued development of software applications to incorporate realistic virtual implants, realistic abutments, and virtual teeth takes the technology to new levels of accuracy, allowing for true restoratively driven implant dentistry. This type of assessment represents how these 3D tools can be used to define new paradigms for implant planning and offers an excellent educational opportunity for all members of the implant team.

To complete the process, the placement of simulated implants must then be transferred to the patient via a CT-derived template that aids in surgical accuracy and avoidance of vital anatomic structures. The ability to virtually plan the case, discuss it with the members of the implant team, present the treatment plan to the patient, and execute the plan with a high degree of accuracy using surgical guides has, in the author's opinion, elevated the art of implant dentistry to a science. Although this technology has been available since the early 1990s, it has not been until recently that clinicians worldwide have started to use it to define new paradigms in understanding anatomy and implant planning. Even the dental implant companies have recognized the importance of this modality for proper diagnosis and treatment planning, as evidenced by new software and hardware product offerings.

There is a danger when we are bound by 2D concepts when we live in a 3D world. The evolution will continue.

Acknowledgment

A short version of Case 1 appeared in *Dentistry Today* (2008, vol 27) and is adapted here with permission.

Suggested Reading

Amet EM, Ganz SD. Implant treatment planning using a patient acceptance prosthesis, radiographic record base, and surgical template. Part 1: Presurgical phase. Implant Dent 1997;6:193–197.

Basten CH, Kois JC. The use of barium sulfate for implant templates. J Prosthet Dent 1996;76:451–454.

Basten CH. The use of radiopaque templates for predictable implant placement. Quintessence Int 1995;26:609–612.

Besimo CE, Lambrecht JT, Guindy JS. Accuracy of implant treatment planning utilizing template-guided reformatted computed tomography. Dentomaxillofac Radiol 2000;29:46–51.

Borrow W, Smith Justin P. Stent marker materials for computerized tomograph-assisted implant planning. Int J Periodontics Restorative Dent 1996;16:61–67.

Casap N, Tarazi E, Wexler A, Sonnenfeld U, Lustmann J. Intraoperative computerized navigation for flapless implant surgery and immediate loading in the edentulous mandible. Int J Oral Maxillofac Implants 2005;20:92–98.

Choquet V, Hermans M, Adriaenssens P, Daelemans P, Tarnow DP, Malevez C. Clinical and radiographic evaluation of the papilla level adjacent to single-tooth dental implants. A retrospective study in the maxillary anterior region. J Periodontol 2001;72:1364–1371.

Di Giacomo GA, Cury PR, de Araujo NS, Sendyk WR, Sendyk CL. Clinical application of stereolithographic surgical guides for implant placement: Preliminary results. J Periodontol 2005;76:503–507.

Farr C. Computer assisted planning and presentation. Dent Today 1995 June;14:38–40.

Fortin T, Champleboux G, Lormee J, Coudert JL. Precise dental implant placement in bone using surgical guides in conjunction with medical imaging techniques. J Oral Implantol 2000;26:300–303.

Galluicci GO, Bernard J-P, Bertosa M, and Beiser UC. Immediate loading with fixed screw-retained provisional restorations in edentulous jaws: The pickup technique. Int J Oral Maxillofac Implants 2004;19: 524–533.

Ganz SD. Conventional CT and cone beam CT for improved dental diagnostics and implant planning. Dent Implantol Update 2005; 16(12):89–95.

Ganz SD. CT scan technology—An evolving tool for predictable implant placement and restoration. Int Mag Oral Implantol 2001;1:6–13.

Ganz SD. CT-derived model-based surgery for immediate loading of maxillary anterior implants. Pract Proced Aesthet Dent 2007;19:311–318.

Ganz SD. Defining new paradigms for assessment of implant receptor sites–The use of CT/CBCT and interactive virtual treatment planning for congenitally missing lateral incisors. Compend Contin Educ Dent 2008;29;256–267.

Ganz SD. Presurgical planning with CT-derived fabrication of surgical guides. J Oral Maxillofac Surg 2005;63(9 suppl 2):59–71.

Ganz SD. Restoratively driven implant dentistry utilizing advanced software and CBCT: Realistic abutments and virtual teeth. Dent Today 2008 Jul;27:122, 124, 126–127.

Ganz SD. Techniques for the use of CT imaging for the fabrication of surgical guides. Atlas Oral Maxillofac Surg Clin North Am 2006; 14:75–97.

Ganz SD. The reality of anatomy and the triangle of bone. Inside Dentistry 2006 June;72–77.

Ganz SD. The triangle of bone—A formula for successful implant placement and restoration. Implant Society 1995;5(5):2–6.

Ganz SD. Use of stereolithographic models as diagnostic and restorative aids for predictable immediate loading of implants. Pract Proced Aesthet Dent 2003;15:763–771.

Ganz SD. Using stereolithographic CT technology for immediate functional and non-functional loading. Presented at the Annual Meeting of the Academy of Osseointegration. Orlando, FL, 12 March 2005.

Ganz SD. What is the most important aspect of implant dentistry? Implant Society 1994;5(1):2–4.

Ganz SD, Kraut RA. Perspectives. The ultimate end results of implant dentistry as it is being practiced today. Implant Dent 2003;12:193–197.

Israelson H, Plemons JM, Watkins P, Sory C. Barium-coated surgical stents and computer-assisted tomography in the preoperative assessment of dental implant patients. Int J Periodontics Restorative Dent 1992;12:52–61.

Jabero M, Sarment DP. Advanced surgical guidance technology: A review. Implant Dent 2006;15:135–142.

Jacobs R, Adriansens A, Verstreken K, Suetens P, van Steenberghe D. Predictability of a three-dimensional planning system for oral implant surgery. Dentomaxillofac Radiol 1999;28:105–111.

Kan JY, Rungcharassaeng K, Umezu K, Kois JC. Dimensions of peri-implant mucosa: An evaluation of maxillary anterior single implants in humans. J Periodontol 2003;74:557–562.

Kan JY, Rungcharassaeng K. Immediate placement and provisionalization of maxillary anterior single implants: a surgical and prosthodontic rationale. Pract Periodontics Aesthet Dent 2000;12:817–824.

Klein M, Abrams M. Computer-guided surgery utilizing a computermilled surgical template. Pract Proced Aesthet Dent 2001;13:165–169.

Klein M, Cranin AN, Sirakian A. A computerized tomographic (CT) scan appliance for optimal presurgical and preprosthetic planning of the implant patient. Pract Periodontics Aesthet Dent 1993;5(6):33–39.

Klein M. Implant surgery using customized surgical templates: The Compu-Guide Surgical Template System. Dent Implantol Update 2002;13(6):41–46.

Kois JC. Predictable single-tooth peri-implant esthetics: Five diagnostic keys. Compend Contin Educ Dent 2004;25:895–900.

Marino JE, Arenal AA, Ceballos AP, et al. Fabrication of an implant radiologic-surgical stent for the partially edentulous patient. Quintessence Int 1995;26:111–114.

Misch CA, Yi ES, Sarment DP. Accuracy of cone beam computed tomography for periodontal defect measurements. J Periodontol 2006;77:1261–1266.

Mizrahi B, Thunthy KH, Finger I. Radiographic/surgical template incorporating metal telescopic tubes for accurate implant placement. Pract Periodontics Aesthet Dent 1998;10:757–765.

Nevins M, Camelo M, De Paoli S, et al. A study of the fate of the buccal wall of extraction sockets of teeth with prominent roots. Int J Periodontics Restorative Dent 2006;26:19–29.

Papalexiou V, Novaes AB Jr, Ribeiro RF, Muglia V, Oliveira RR. Influence of the interimplant distance on crestal bone resorption and bone density: A histomorphometric study in dogs. J Periodontol 2006;77:614–621.

Peñarrocha M, Lamas J, Garcia B. Immediate maxillary lateral incisor implants with nonocclusal loading provisional crowns. J Prosthodontics 2008;17:55–59.

Richardson G, Russell KA. Congenitally missing maxillary lateral incisors and orthodontic treatment considerations for the single-tooth implant. J Can Dent Assoc 2001;67:25–28.

Rosenfeld A, Mandelaris G, Tardieu P. Prosthetically directed placement using computer software to insure precise placement and predictable prosthetic outcomes. Part 1: Diagnostics, imaging, and collaborative accountability. Int J Periodontics Restorative Dent 2006;26:215–221.

Rosenfeld AL, Mecall RA. Use of interactive computed tomography to predict the esthetic and functional demands of implant-supported prostheses. Compend Contin Educ Dent 1996;17:1125–1146.

Rosenfeld AL, Mecall RA. Use of prosthesis-generated computed tomographic information for diagnostic and surgical treatment planning. J Esthet Dent 1998;10:132–148.

Salama H, Salama MA, Garber D, et al. The interproximal height of bone: A guidepost to predictable aesthetic strategies and soft tissue contours in anterior tooth replacement. Pract Periodontics Aesthet Dent 1998;10:1131–1141.

Sarment DP, Al-Shammari K, Kazor CE. Stereolithographic surgical templates for placement of dental implants in complex cases. Int J Periodontics Restorative Dent 2003;23:287–295.

Sarment DP, Misch CE. Scannographic templates for novel pre-implant planning methods. Int Mag Oral Implantol 2002;3:16–22.

Sarment DP, Sukovic P, Clinthorne N. Accuracy of implant placement with a stereolithographic surgical guide. Int J Oral Maxillofac Implants 2003;18:571–577.

Scarano A, Assenza B, Piattelli M, et al. Interimplant distance and crestal bone resorption: A histologic study in the canine mandible. Clin Implant Dent Relat Res 2004;6:150–156.

Sonic M, Abrahams J, Faiella R. A comparison of the accuracy of periapical, panoramic, and computerized tomographic radiographs in locating the mandibular canal. Int J Oral Maxillofac Implants 1994;9:455–460.

Tardieu PB, Vrielinck L, Escolano E. Computer-assisted implant placement. A case report: Treatment of the mandible. Int J Oral Maxillofac Implants 2003;18:599–604.

Tarnow DP, Cho SC, Wallace SS. The effect of inter-implant distance on the height of inter-implant bone crest. J Periodontol 2000;71:546–549.

Tarnow DP, Magner AW, Fletcher P. The effect of the distance from the contact point of the crest of bone on the presence or absence of the interproximal dental papilla. J Periodontol 1992;63:995–996.

Van Steenberghe D, Malevez C, Van Cleynenbreugel J, et al. Accuracy of drilling guides for transfer from three-dimensional CT-based planning to placement of zygoma implants in human cadavers. Clin Oral Implants Res 2003;14:131–136.

Van Steenberghe D, Naert I, Andersson M, et al. A custom template and definitive prosthesis allowing immediate implant loading in the maxilla: A clinical report. Int J Oral Maxillofac Implants 2002;17:663–670.

Verde MA, Morgano SM. A dual-purpose stent for the implant-supported prosthesis. J Prosthet Dent 1993;69:276–280.

11

ORAL-MAXILLOFACIAL SURGERY SOFTWARE

Benoît L. Philippe, MD

The conditions for functional, esthetic, and long-lasting implant treatment include a skeletal infrastructure appropriate for placing implants, a sufficient amount of high-density bone volume, orientation of the implants to ensure no or limited angulation of abutments, and maxillary and mandibular skeletal bases with a satisfactory three-dimensional (3D) relationship. Maxillofacial surgery involves reconstructing the bone using the most appropriate autogenous donor site to meet the needs of reconstruction[1,2] and correct any skeletal imbalances,[3–5] which can be either secondary (related to the aging process) or primary (congenital). In the case of fully or partially edentulous patients, there is the same proportion of concealed dysmorphoses compared with dentate individuals. In addition, the desires of esthetically motivated patients wishing to regain an anatomy resembling their profile before edentulism, whether in the buccal area alone or the entire face, must be considered. The edentulous patient is a potential candidate for a complete functional and esthetic rejuvenation of the face.

To meet these objectives, the surgeon must confirm the diagnosis, explore possible donor sites (ramus, symphysis, or parietal), simulate all stages of the planned grafting or osteotomy, and transfer the simulation data to the patient to perform the surgery.

SimPlant oral-maxillofacial surgery (OMS) software provides the tools and functions for diagnosis, simulation, and execution of oral-maxillofacial surgery. The benefits are the same as for dental implant placement. The software allows treatment to be individually adjusted to each patient's needs, because all therapeutic options can be evaluated virtually and all possible risks identified and eliminated before surgery. Furthermore, the stereolithographic guide makes it possible to maintain full control at the time of surgery.

Treatment Plan

Define the final prosthetic outcome

The prosthetic outcome is based on the simulation (number, shape, 3D position, and angle) of the prosthetic crowns and of gingival soft tissues. The prosthesis is integrated into the global buccal and facial esthetic plan, which examines the esthetic relationship between implant-supported crowns and lips, the volume and position of the false gingiva, support of the lips and cheeks, and the facial profile (convex or concave).

In the presence of skeletal discrepancies and before performing osteotomies, the use of semi-adjustable articulators allows the surgeon to confirm the compatibility of the restorative project with the repositioned skeletal infrastructure (Fig 11-1).

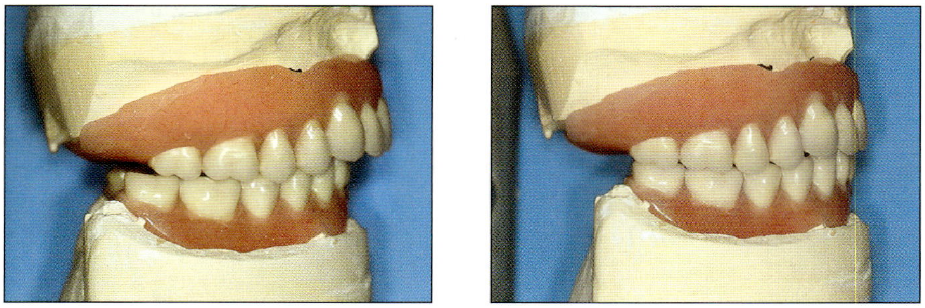

Fig 11-1 Removable immediate prostheses set up on a semi-adjustable articulator. These prostheses are compatible with the initial deformity (Class II, division 1) and with the expected occlusion after the maxillofacial surgery (Class I).

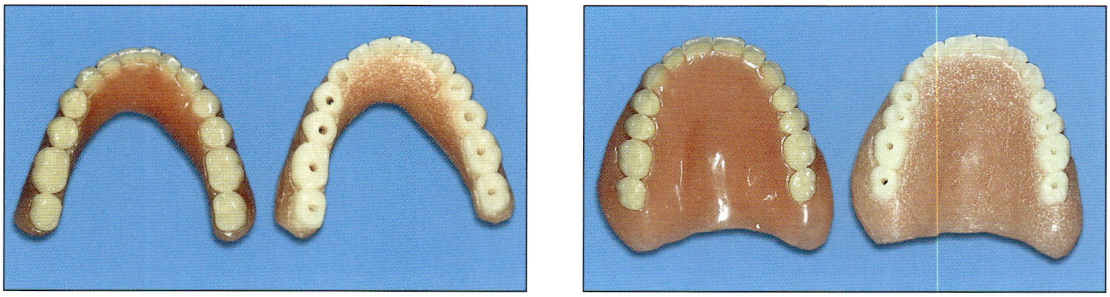

Fig 11-2 Fabrication of the scanning appliance from the provisional removable prosthesis (duplicate). Teeth are loaded with a 30% barium sulfate mix and the base is loaded with a 10% barium sulfate mix.

Manufacture the scanning appliance

The scanning appliance is a duplicate of the restorative plan. It allows for exploration of the entire range of restorative and periodontal parameters, such as implant-retained crowns; defines the axes of abutments and implants; and stabilizes the gingiva during the scan (Fig 11-2).

Obtain a preoperative scan

The computed tomography (CT) scan is based on a defined protocol: cephalic position, acquisition of the complete craniofacial area from the symphysis mandibulae to the vertex, and from the top of the nasal spine to the occiput. Use of this protocol ensures a stable, centered occlusion (no displacement of the scanning appliance), removal of metal artifacts, minimal irradiation, and storage of the data in a suitable file format. The scan data provide all of the information needed to make a reliable diagnosis, to explore mandibular (ramus and symphysis) and cranial (parietal bone) donor sites, to simulate the surgery, and to prepare surgical guides.

Diagnosis

The diagnosis is based on sagittal, frontal, and axial sections as well as 3D views of the facial area (surface or transparent mode). SimPlant OMS offers qualitative and quantitative assessment of bone atrophy and the identification of problems such as skeletal discrepancies, problems in the restorative space, and possible pathologic conditions (apical or cystic pathology, intrasinusal foreign bodies, sinusitis, etc).

SimPlant OMS allows the surgeon to visualize all of the anatomic constituents of cephalic donor sites in 3D space (direct view or transparent mode), specify respective relationships between different anatomic elements (a virtual dissection is offered), and interactively gather patient-specific encrypted data from anatomic landmarks (Fig 11-3).

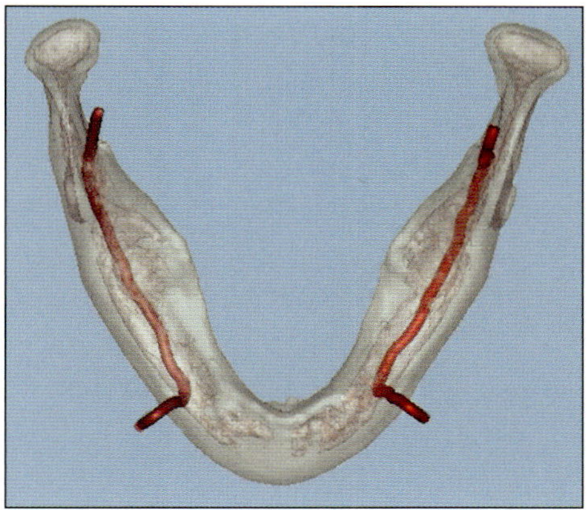

Fig 11-3 Transparence mode. Visualization of dental pedicles.

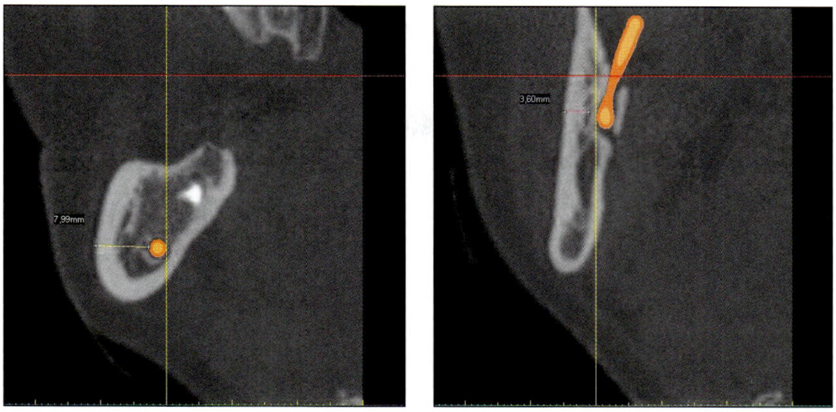

Fig 11-4 Frontal sections. Relationship between external cortex and dental pedicles (ramus and area 47).

Ramus donor site

The software can estimate the bone available at the ramus donor site (volume and density) and determine anatomic relationships with constant individual variations such as age, morphotype, ethnic type, asymmetry of mandibular skeleton, and edentulism with atrophy of alveolar bone.[5]

To make a dissection of a graft that corresponds best to the planned reconstruction, the thickness and density of the cortex and corticocancellous bone can be studied (Fig 11-4).

The mandibular anatomic structures can also be thoroughly examined, particularly the composition of the underlying spongy bone and the course or the limits of the dental channel. Assessing the risk of a fracture should be done before an extended or bilateral dissection in case of skeletal atrophy (slender morphotype) or secondary consequences of an old edentia. SimPlant OMS reduces the risk of fracture by tracking atrophic (at-risk) mandibles.

Symphyseal donor site

SimPlant OMS makes it possible to study the volume and profile of the symphysis and the thickness of the external vestibular table as well as the internal configuration of the symphysis (Figs 11-5 to 11-8). The position of labiomental pedicles and dental apexes of the incisor-canine area can also be systematically studied.

Parietal donor site

An overall study of the calvaria can also be prepared to the global thickness of parietal bone and thickness and density of both external and internal tables as well as the spongy intermediate bone. To perform a separation of the external atraumatic cortex, it is recommended that the degree of respective differentiation of the external cortex and spongy intermediate bone be examined. A thick spongy intermediate substance (low density) is well differentiated with regard to the external cortex (high density) and permits an atraumatic dissection, thus reducing neurologic risks.

Surgical simulation

Bone augmentations and osteotomies may be simulated. The surface mode for soft tissue makes it possible to perform a complete estimation of the effects of skeletal displacements on soft tissues, providing additional important preoperative information.

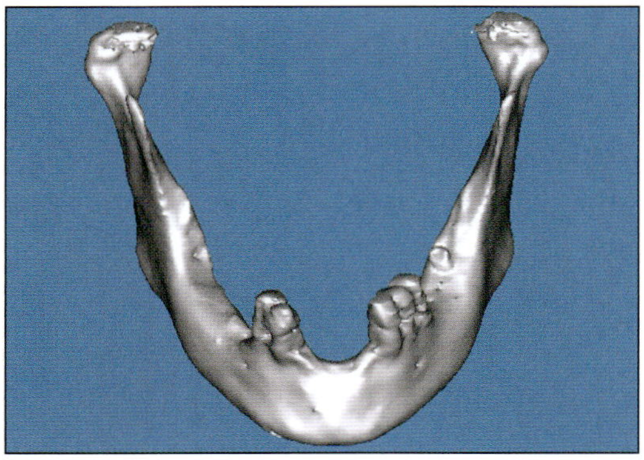

Fig 11-5 Normal morphotype. Surface visualization.

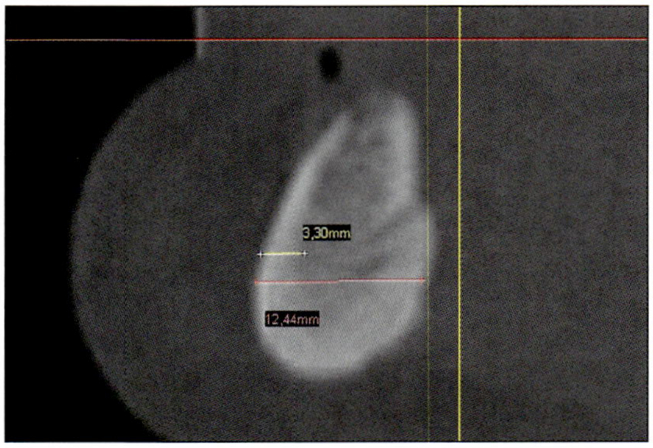

Fig 11-6 Same patient. Parasagittal section of symphysis (area 31). Sufficient available volume.

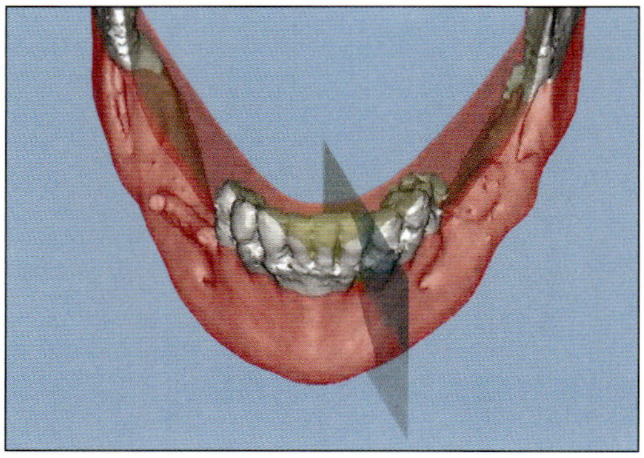

Fig 11-7 Another patient. Slender morphotype. Transparence mode and cut plane selection in lieu of 32.

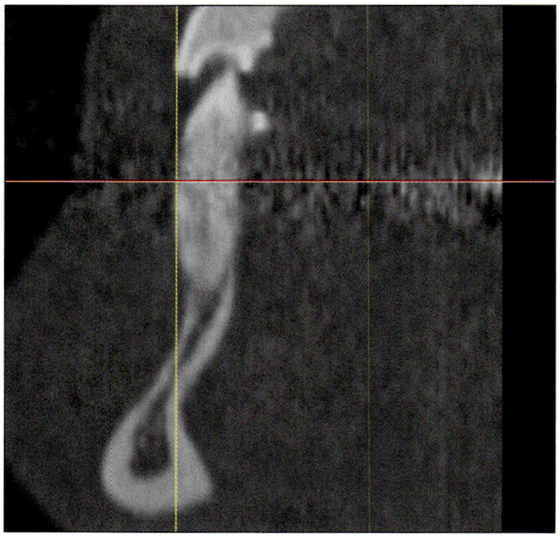

Fig 11-8 Same patient. Parasagittal section (area 32). Insufficient available volume.

Preoperative preparation

The following measurements need to be obtained:

- Quantitative (volume) and qualitative (density) study of the reconstruction
- Simulation of implant placement (type, geometric specifications, and 3D position: orientation, angulation, and peri-implant density)
- Simulation of abutment positions (type, geometric specifications, orientation, and angulation)
- Volume and position of periodontal soft tissues

Manufacture of surgical guide

Surgical guides may be tooth-, bone-, or mucosa-supported.

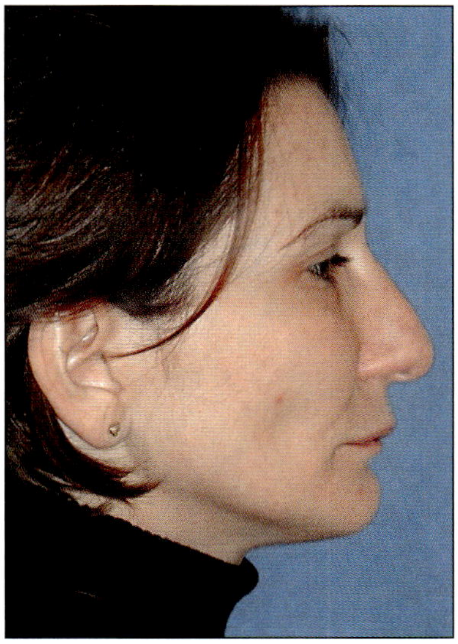

Fig 11-9a Initial profile showing dentomaxillofacial dysmorphosis (Class II, division 1; convex profile).

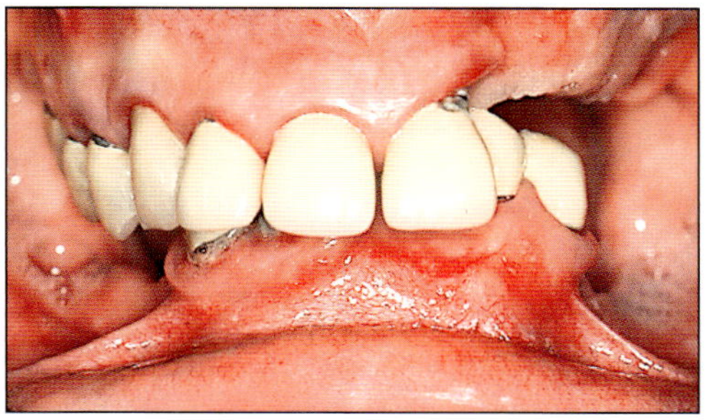

Fig 11-9b Initial intraoral view of occlusion (Class II, division 1; loss of vertical height).

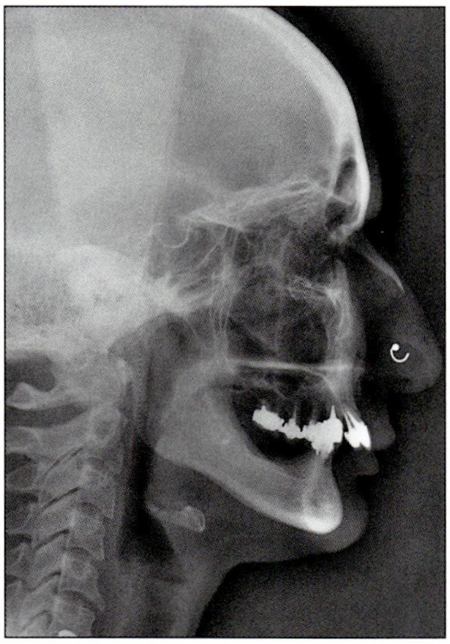

Fig 11-9c Radiographic image of the initial profile (Class II, division 1; loss of vertical height, advanced periodontitis).

Clinical Demonstrations

Case 1

Initial presentation

The patient had advanced periodontitis, which required complete extraction; dentomaxillofacial dysmorphosis (Class II, division 1); a short mandible, severe overbite, and insufficient vertical and prosthetic height; and general maxillary bone atrophy (thin maxillary bone crest anterior and insufficient bone height at sinus level) (Figs 11-9a to 11-9c).

The patient requested maxillary and mandibular fixed dentures. Esthetic concerns included the smile line, rebalancing of facial dimensions, normal profile, and support of lips and cheeks.

The therapeutic objectives were to correct mandibular dysmorphosis with forward movement of the mandible and augmentation of vertical and prosthetic height; reconstruct the maxillary bone; place implants in the mandible and maxilla; and create complete mandibular and maxillary dentures.

Therapeutic intervention was planned, consisting of extracting teeth and constructing provisional mandibular and maxillary denture prostheses. Whether the new vertical dimension was compatible with the prosthesis requests of the patient and the tolerance of the temporomandibular joint (TMJ) needed to be determined (see Fig 11-1). Sagittal osteotomy with advancement of the mandible would be required for mandibular dysmorphosis as simulation on semi-adjustable articulators has shown (see Fig 11-2). Finally, implants would be placed, and an autologous bone graft would be needed for maxillary bone atrophy.

Simulation

Placement of five anterior implants and two posterior implants was simulated in the mandible (Fig 11-9d), as well as sagittal osteotomy of the mandibular rami with advancement of the body of the mandible over a distance of 5.2 mm (Figs 11-9e to 11-9g).

Implant placement in the anterior maxilla and estimation of the exposure in axial and frontal views were simulated (Figs 11-9h and 11-9i). Also, the design and size of the anterior onlay graft (augmentation of the thickness of the alveolar crest) and of the grafts in the sinus region (sinus lift) were determined.

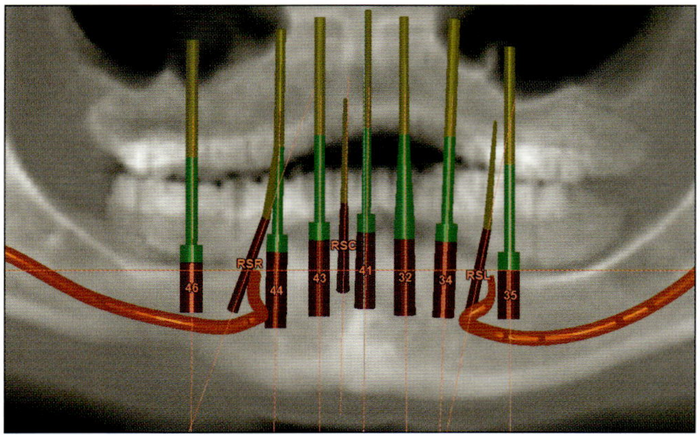

Fig 11-9d Complete mandibular simulation.

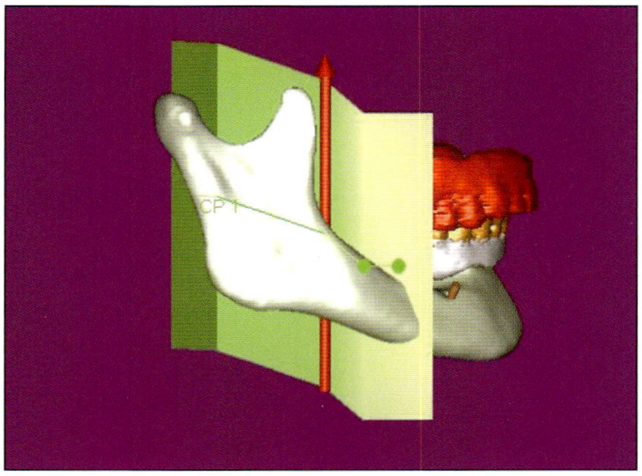

Fig 11-9e Simulation of the sagittal osteotomy of the right ramus (external view).

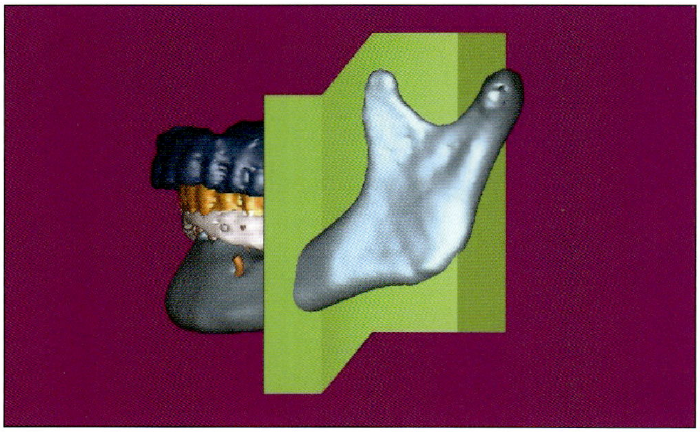

Fig 11-9f Simulation of the sagittal osteotomy of the left ramus.

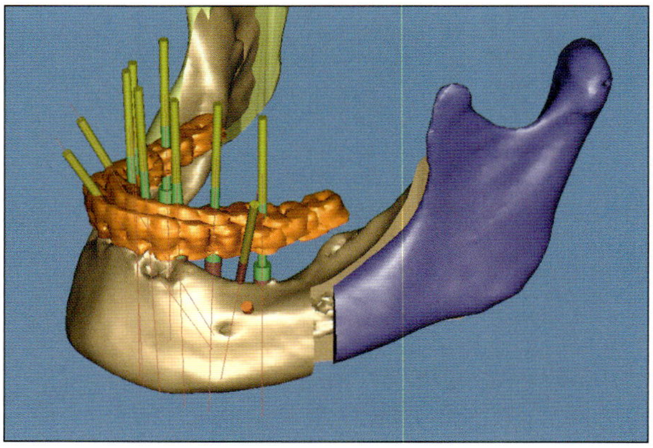

Fig 11-9g Isometric view. Forward movement of the mandible and prosthesis on implants.

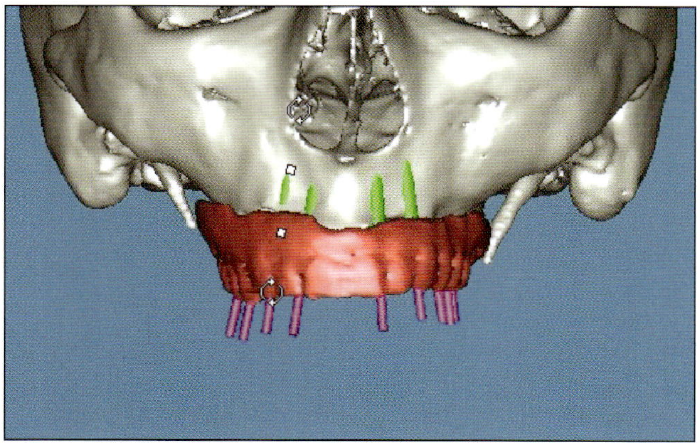

Fig 11-9h Maxillary implant simulation. Observation of the anterior maxillary atrophy.

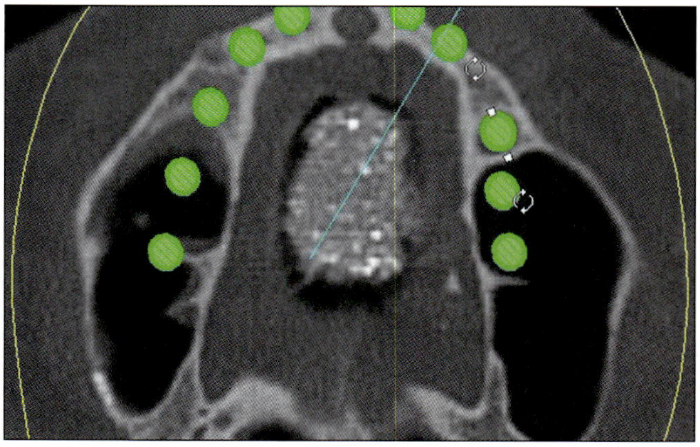

Fig 11-9i Same simulation as in Fig 11-9h, axial view. Thin crest at the anterior maxillary level.

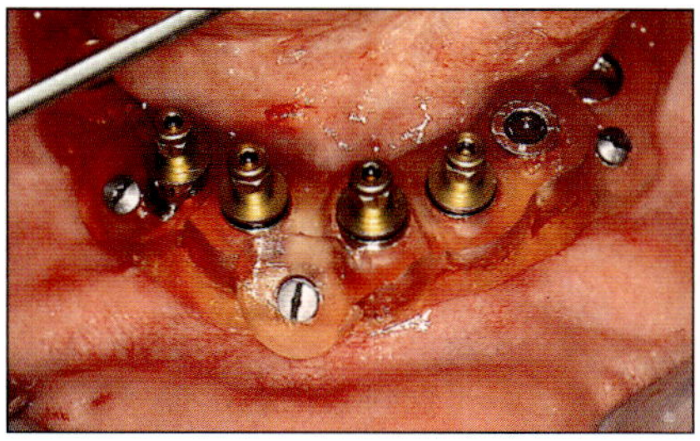

Fig 11-9j Placement of the implants through the guide (SAFE System procedure).

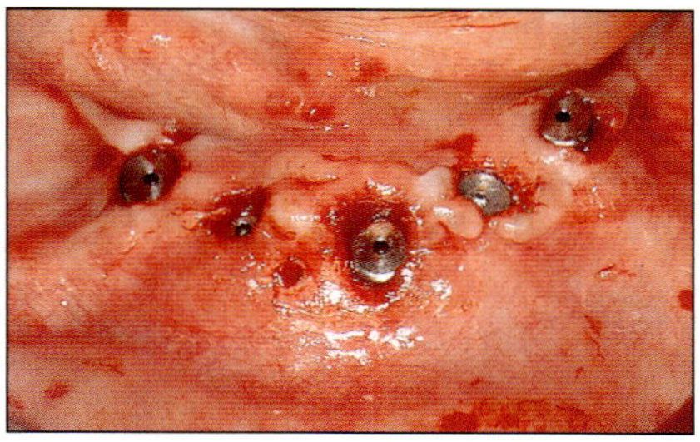

Fig 11-9k Placement of the symphyseal implants. Placement of the two distal implants situated in the proximity of the osteotomy sites was postponed.

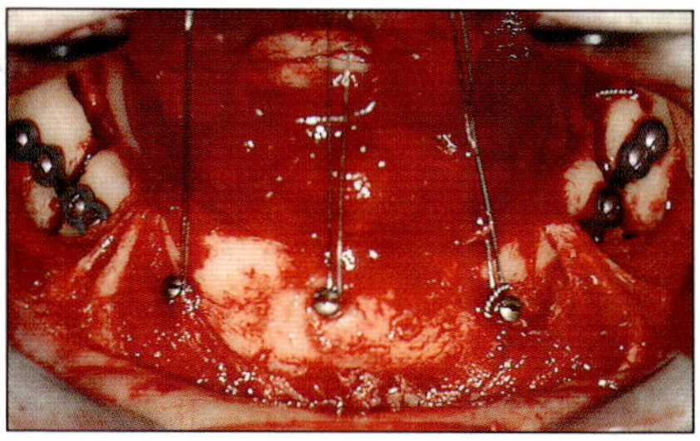

Fig 11-9l Simultaneous mandibular sagittal osteotomy. The bivalve splint allows the placement that was chosen preoperatively (Class I). The steel threads through the perforated screws and the stereolithographic guides assure fixation.

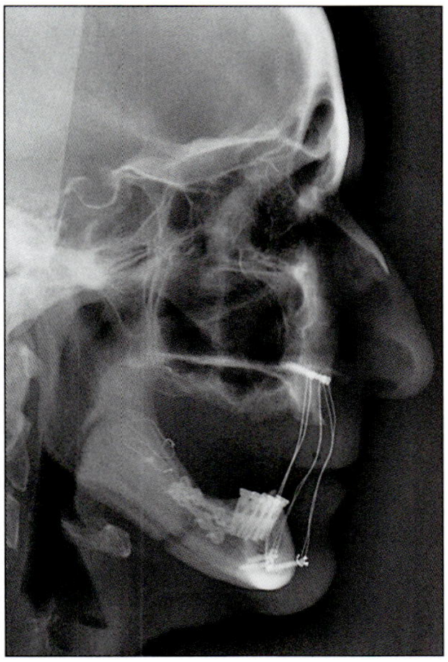

Fig 11-9m Radiograph of the postoperative profile. Physiologic orientation of the implants, forward movement of the mandible, and the new vertical height corresponding to the simulations can be observed.

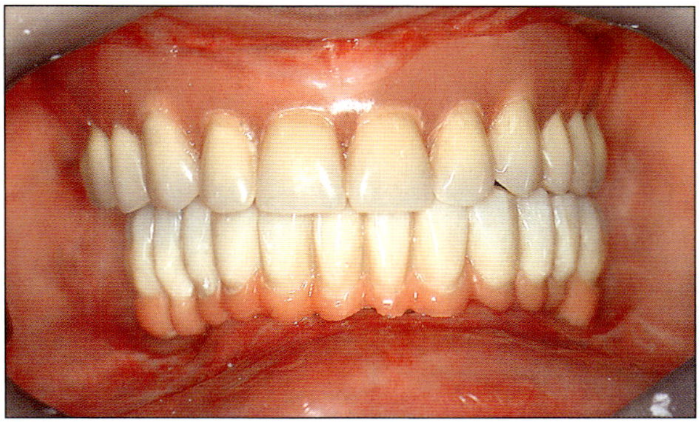

Fig 11-9n Loading of the provisional denture after removal of the fixation.

Treatment

Mandible

Transmucosal placement of the five mandibular implants with the SAFE System protocol was performed (Figs 11-9j and 11-9k). The two mandibular implants distal to the sagittal osteotomy were not placed immediately. Their transmucosal positioning was technically possible but too close to the osteotomy site. In case there was a lack of consolidation, which is always possible with a distal osteotomy (the risk being greater in case of an osteotomy on an edentulous atrophic mandible), it is possible that the lack of ossification would be attributed to the implants. It was therefore decided to place the implants only after consolidation of the sagittal osteotomy.

Simultaneous correction of the dysmorphosis was done, involving sagittal osteotomy of the mandibular rami with advancement of the mandibular body (Figs 11-9l and 11-9m). Maxillomandibular fixation was needed for 4 weeks. One week after the fixation period ended, a provisional mandibular bridge with 12 elements was placed (Fig 11-9n).

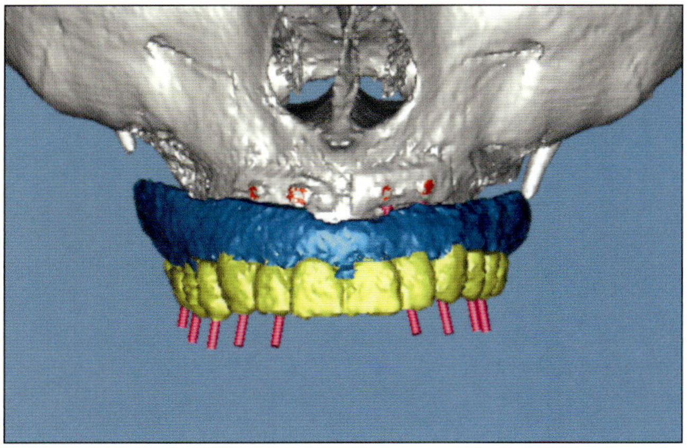

Fig 11-9o Check of the maxillary reconstruction and the implant simulation shows good coverage of the implants.

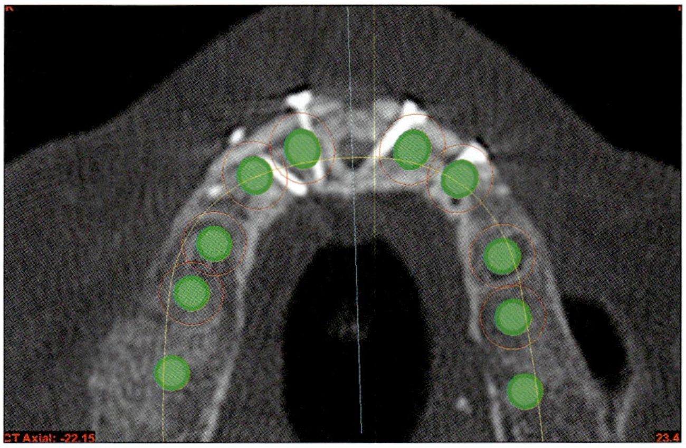

Fig 11-9p Axial view also reveals good coverage of the implants.

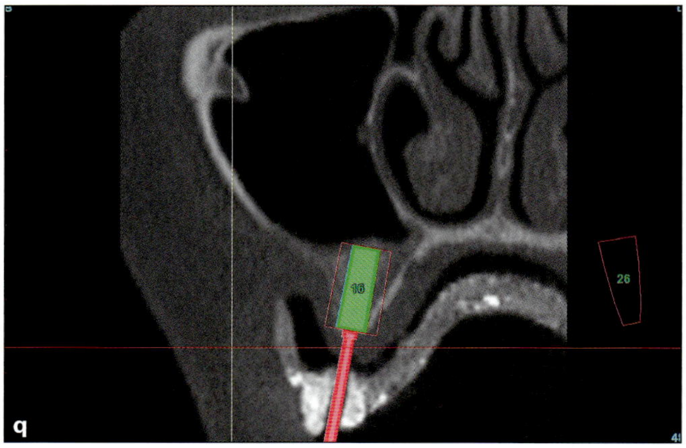

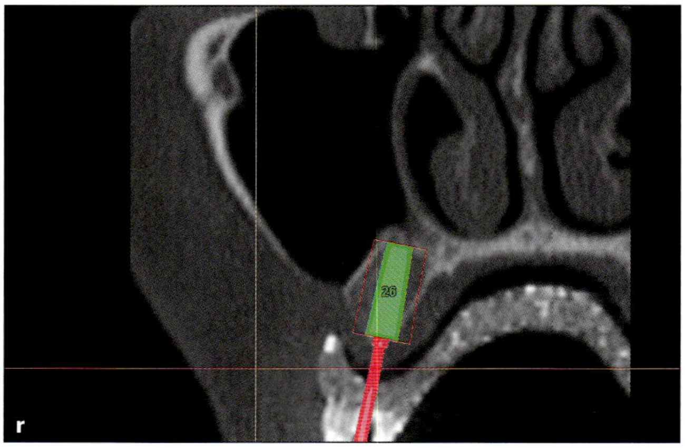

Figs 11-9q and 11-9r Check of the maxillary reconstruction on the right *(q)* and left *(r)* sides.

Maxilla

Complete reconstruction of the maxilla involved enlargement of the anterior maxillary bone crest (symphyseal bone) and bilateral sinus augmentation (iliac crest bone) in addition to the use of platelet-rich growth factors (Figs 11-9o to 11-9r). Implants were placed 6 months after the reconstruction of the maxilla (Figs 11-9s to 11-9u). A bone-supported stereolithographic guide was used. The two distal implants in the mandible were placed simultaneously (Fig 11-9v). Placement of a provisional maxillary bridge was postponed until 2 weeks after surgery (Figs 11-9w to 11-9y).

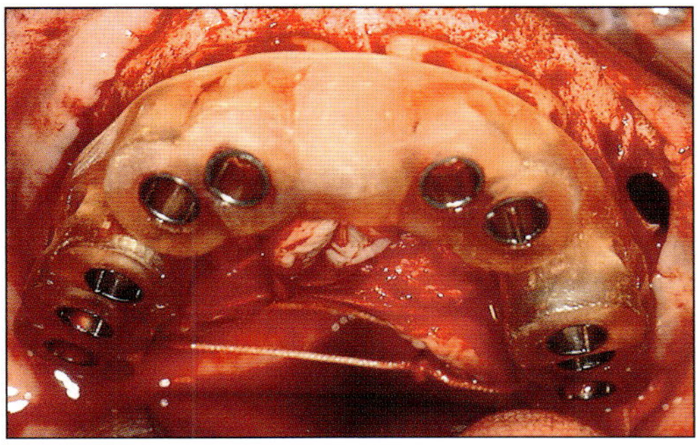

Fig 11-9s Loading of the bone-supported surgical guide during surgery.

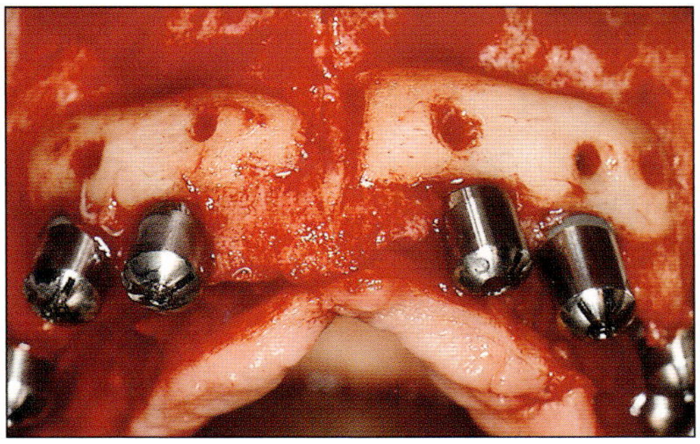

Fig 11-9t Loading of the implants and the healing abutments in the anterior maxilla. Good coverage of the implants.

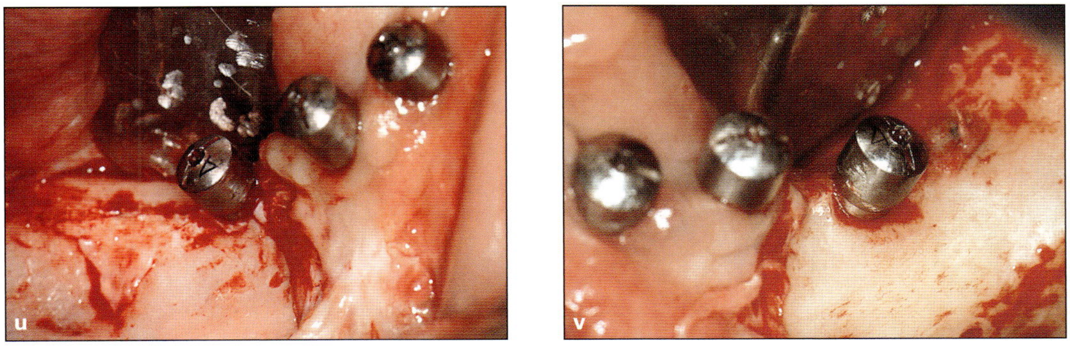

Figs 11-9u and 11-9v Loading of the distal mandibular implants and their transmucosal healing abutments on the right *(u)* and left *(v)* sides.

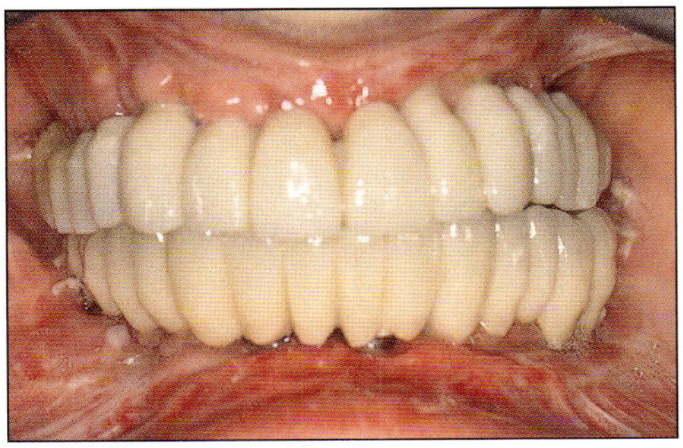

Fig 11-9w Provisional dentures. Normal articulation (Class I). Slightly delayed loading in the maxilla (second week after surgery). Elongation of the mandibular denture with immediate placement of the distal implants.

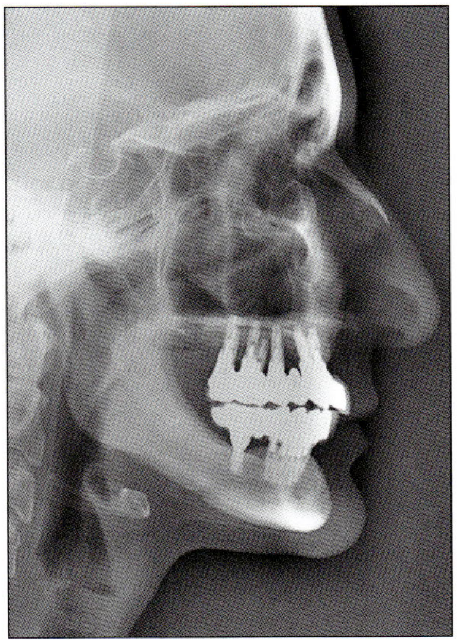

Fig 11-9x Radiograph showing sagittal relationships of the normalized skeletal bases (Class I). Note the new vertical dimension.

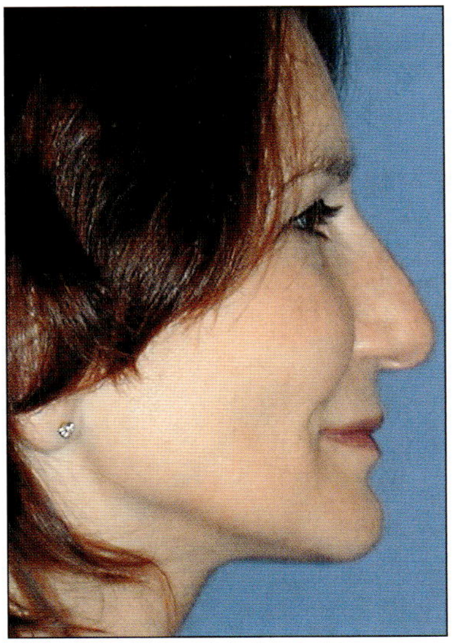

Fig 11-9y Lateral view of the final result. Note the new vertical dimension and harmonization of the profile in the sagittal and vertical dimensions.

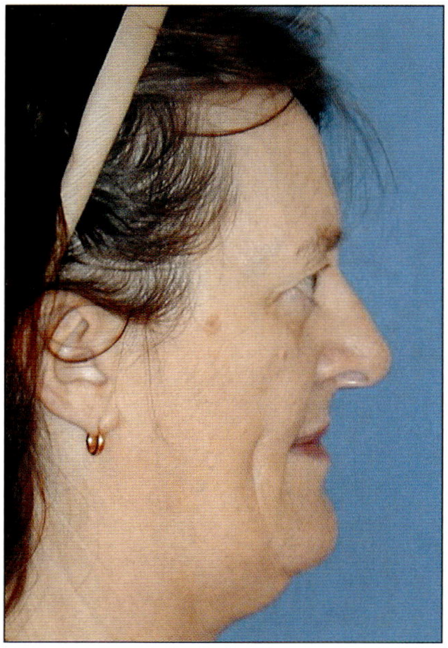

Fig 11-10a Initial profile. Moderate acquired dentomaxillofacial dysmorphosis (Class III). Discretely concave soft tissue profile.

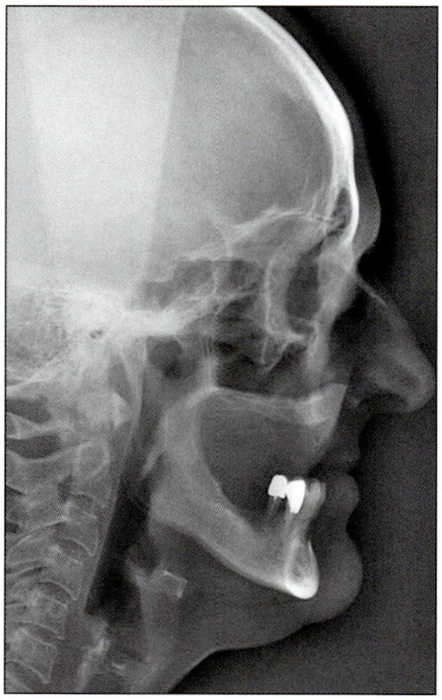

Fig 11-10b Radiographic view of initial profile showing maxillary atrophy and excessive restorative space.

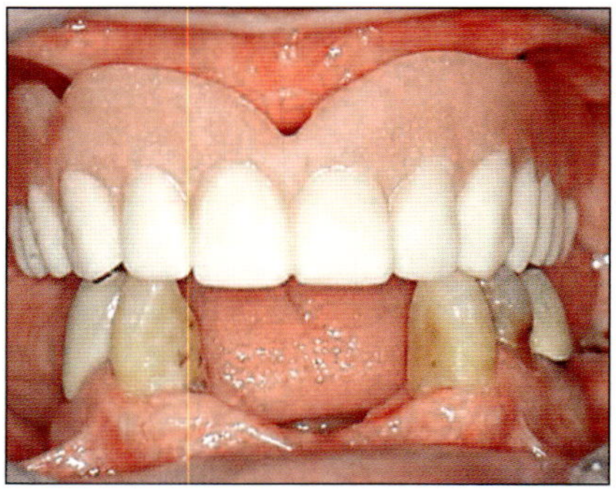

Fig 11-10c Check of the coordination of the scanning appliance with the mandibular arch at rest. Note the space formed between the basal prosthesis surface and the maxillary mucosa.

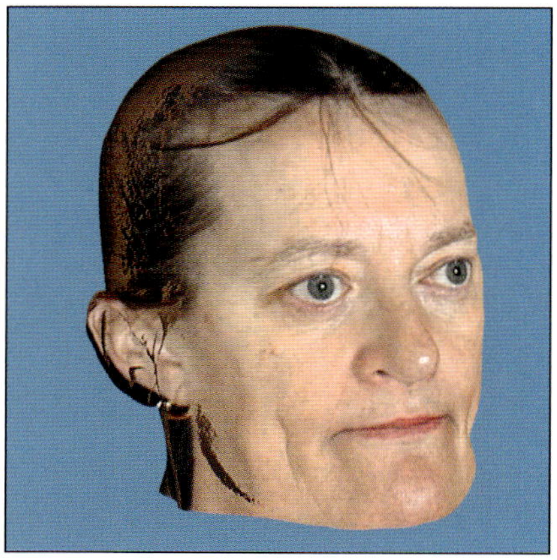

Fig 11-10d Three-quarters profile view before surgery.

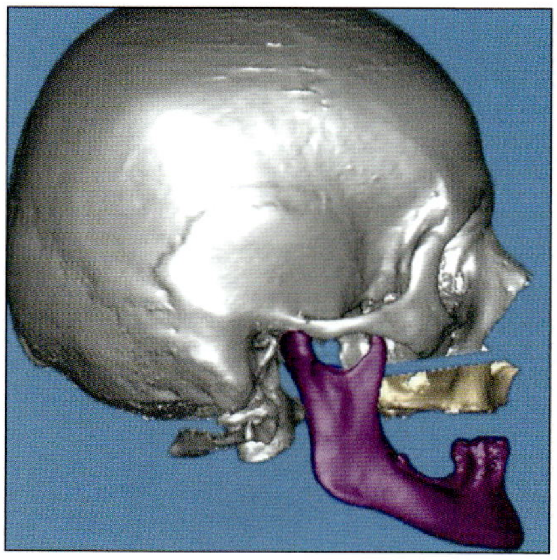

Fig 11-10e Lateral view of the simulation of the Le Fort I osteotomy in surface mode.

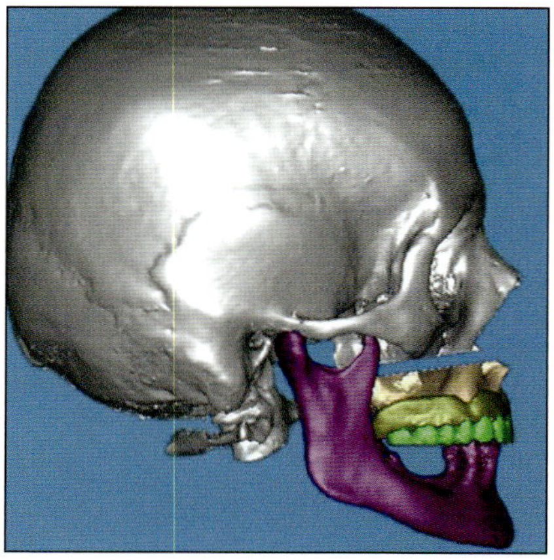

Fig 11-10f Lateral view of the maxilla and scanning appliance after the simulated Le Fort I osteotomy simulation.

Case 2

Initial presentation

The patient was completely edentulous in the maxilla with acquired atrophy (Class III) and partially edentulous in the mandible. In addition, the patient exhibited mandibular periodontitis, moderate maxillary recession with a discretely concave profile, and excessive restorative space (Figs 11-10a and 11-10b).

The patient requested a complete maxillary denture, rebalancing of facial dimensions, a normal profile, and support of lips and cheeks.

Therapeutic objectives included total reconstruction of maxillary skeletal structure (restoration of skeletal structure of the alveolar crest in height and thickness); correction of acquired maxillary dysmorphosis; reduction of the

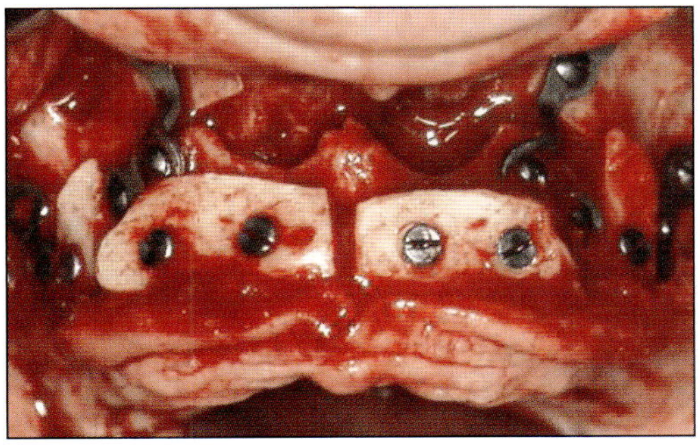

Fig 11-10g Frontal view of the reconstruction.

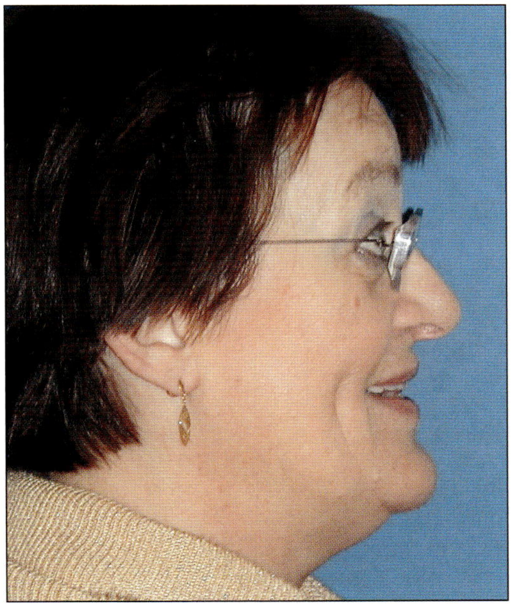

Fig 11-10h Final profile view 2 years after surgery.

hyperprojected mental protrusion; and placement of maxillary implants with a complete maxillary denture.

A total Le Fort I osteotomy was planned with anterior and inferior advancement of the maxilla (Figs 11-10c to 11-10f), together with simultaneous interpositional bone grafting (bilateral sinus grafting), enlargement of the anterior maxillary crest with symphyseal bone (bilateral sinus graft) (Figs 11-10g and 11-10h). The dental implants would be placed in 6 months.

Conclusion

SimPlant OMS is an essential software tool that allows comprehension of the skeletal and mucosal disorders that accompany complete or partial edentulism, and an accurate diagnosis, taking into consideration the surrounding anatomic structures. Thorough knowledge of the distinctive anatomic features of every case is offered through exploration of rami, symphyseal, and parietal donor sites; and surgical procedures (bone grafts and osteotomies) can be simulated, providing incomparable assistance to the surgeon throughout the course of treatment. The stereolithographic guides guarantee the best possible result as well as maximum safety to the patient.

References

1. Philippe B. Reconstructions maxillaires pré-implantaires: critères de choix du site donneur osseux. Implant 1998;4(4):279–292.
2. Philippe B, Tardieu PB, Tran-Minh-Thien JM. Edentement complet maxillaire avec atrophie osseuse: Prise en charge d'un cas. Part 1. Phase chirurgicale: principes thérapeutiques et indications. Implant 2001;7(2):99–111.
3. Keller EE, Van Roekel NB, Desjardins RP, Tolman DE. Prosthetic-surgical reconstruction of severely resorbed maxilla with iliac bone graftings and tissue-integrated prosthesis. Int J Oral Maxillofac Implants 1987;2:155–165.
4. Obwegeser HL. The indications for surgical correction of mandibular deformity by sagittal splitting technique. Br J Oral Surg 1964;1:157–171.
5. Obwegeser HL. Mandibular surgery. Br J Oral Surg 1973;10:251–253.
6. Philippe B,Tardieu PB. Chirurgie reconstructrice préimplantaire. Le site donneur mandibulaire postérieur. Information dentaire. No. 10, March 8, 2006:491–496.
7. Philippe B,Tardieu PB. Mise en place trans-muqueuse des implants dentaires et ostéotomie sagittale assistées par ordinateur (logiciel Simplant et guides stéréolythographiques). A propos d'un premier cas d'édentement complet maxillo-mandibulaire avec classe II. Abstract, 2006 Annual Congress of the French Maxillofacial Surgeons Association, March 24, 2006.

INDEX

Page numbers followed by "f" denote figures; those followed by "t" denote tables

A

Absorbed dose, of radiation, 17
Abutments, temporary, 109f
Advanced generalized caries, 123–127
Advanced masking. *See* Segmentation.
Aggressive periodontitis, generalized, 169–172
Anterior maxillary trauma, 128–131
Anterior teeth retroclination, 93f
Artifacts
  beam-hardening, 14, 14f
  Compton scatter, 14
  definition of, 9–10
  helical, 14f, 15
  limiting of, 65
  motion, 14
  partial volume effect, 14
  starburst, 13, 13f
As low as reasonably achievable (ALARA), 19
Axial views, 10

B

Background equivalent radiation time, 17
Bar connector, 127f
Barium differential gradient ScannoGuide, 81f
Barium-impregnated denture base, 42, 50
Beam-hardening artifacts, 14, 14f
BERT. *See* Background equivalent radiation time.
Bilateral maxillary partial edentulism, 155–159
Bitewing radiographs, 18t
Bone density
  determination of, 103, 103f
  Misch scale of, 9, 9t
Bone fixation pins, 69, 70f
Bone reduction guide, 71, 72f
Bone-supported SurgiGuides
  for advanced posterior mandibular atrophy, 139f
  description of, 69f–74f, 69–73, 75, 83, 106, 107f, 109f, 116
  loading of, 219f
  for mandibular complete edentulism, 147
Broad flap reflection, 109f

C

Caries
  advanced generalized, 123–127
  mandibular anterior advanced nonrestorable, 165–168
Case studies
  advanced generalized caries, 123–127
  chronic periodontitis, 123–127
  mandible
    edentulism of, 118–122, 132–137
    posterior, advanced atrophy of, 137–140
  maxilla
    anterior trauma of, 128–131
    partial edentulism of, 114–117
  maxillary anterior implant reconstruction, 150–154
  scanning appliances
    anterior maxillary trauma, 129f
    mandibular complete edentulism, 119, 133
    maxillary anterior implants, 151, 161
    maxillary partial edentulism, 115f
  SimPlant oral-maxillofacial surgery software, 215–221
Case type patterns, 94, 95f–97f
Cementable abutments, 205
Chronic periodontitis, 123–127
Clinical diagnostic inquiries, 91–93, 92t
Clipping, 196, 197f, 203

Collaborative accountability, 22, 38, 42
Complete denture, 98f, 98t
Compton scatter, 14
Computed tomography
  accuracy of, 100, 100f
  acquisition settings, 18t
  anterior maxilla, 25, 27f
  artifacts
    beam-hardening, 14, 14f
    Compton scatter, 14
    definition of, 9–10
    helical, 14f, 15
    motion, 14
    partial volume effect, 14
    starburst, 13, 13f
  axial views, 10
  background of, 1
  benefits of, 16–19
  case study of, 190, 191t
  in computer-guided implant treatment pathway, 99
  cone-beam. *See* Cone-beam computed tomography.
  contrast resolution, 9
  datasets, 9–10
  distance measurements, 20
  helical, 6
  history of, 21
  images
    noise in, 9
    principles of, 5
    SimPlant-compatible format conversion of, 59, 60f
  maxilla, 25, 27f
  multislice. *See* Multislice computed tomography.
  overrun effect, 6–7
  radiation dose, 17
  radiation risks, 17
  reconstruction settings, 18t
  referral guidelines for, 19
  reformatted images, 10–12, 11f–12f
  root fracture, 31, 31f
  scanners used in, 5–8
  scanning plane
    hard palate, 15t, 16
    lower border, 15t, 16
    occlusal plane, 15, 15t, 16f
    selection of, 15, 15t
  scout views, 10
  single-slice sequential, 6, 7f
  slice, 5
  spiral, 6
  in 3D environment, 22–23
  transaxial images, 9
  treatment planning using, 23–27
  views
    axial, 10
    cross-sectional, 10–11, 12f
    definition of, 5
    panoramic views, 10
    scout, 10
    three-dimensional, 12
Computer-aided implantology, 1–2
Computer-guided implant treatment pathway
  computed tomography scan and SimPlant conversion, 99
  definitive restoration and supportive maintenance, 110, 110f
  eight-step treatment-planning process, 100f–105f, 100–105
  initial diagnostics
    assessments, 91b
    case type patterns, 94, 95f–97f
    clinical diagnostic inquiries, 91–93, 92t
    diagnostic waxups, 97, 97f
    radiographic diagnostic inquiries, 94
  medical modeling, 106, 107f
  overview of, 89, 90f
  scanning appliances, 98
  summary of, 110–111
  surgery, 108, 108f
Cone-beam computed tomography
  clinical uses of, 193
  cross-sectional view using, 194f
  description of, 7–8, 8f
  radiation doses, 18t
  scanning plane for, 15
  SimPlant data and, 193
Congenitally missing teeth, SimPlant case planning for
  maxillary canines, 29, 29f–30f
  maxillary lateral incisors
    description of, 28, 28f, 193
    planning phase for, 193–198
    restorative phase, 199, 199f
    surgical phase, 198f–199f, 198–199
    triangle of bone, 194, 194f, 197f
Connector bar, 136f
Contrast resolution, 9
Convolution and backprojection, 5
Cortical plate fenestration, 103, 103f
Corticocancellous bone
  block graft, 34f
  description of, 213

Crestal bone height, 92
Critical actions, 91, 92t
Cross-sectional views, 10–11, 12f

D

Definitive restoration, 110, 110f
Dentomaxillofacial dysmorphosis, 215f, 220f
Denture base
  barium-impregnated, 42, 50
  fabrication of, 51–52
  impression for, 50, 50f
Depth control, 73
Deterministic effects of radiation, 17
Diagnostic inquiries
  clinical, 91–93, 92f–93f
  definition of, 91
  physical, 104, 104t, 105f
  radiographic, 94
Diagnostic waxups, 97, 97f
DICOM file, 180
Digital cast, 186, 186f
Donor site evaluation, 34, 34f
Drilling cylinders, 177, 178f
Drilling tubes, 71, 72f, 73
Drills, 178, 179f

E

Edentulous patients
  mandible, 118–122, 132–136, 145–149
  maxilla
    bilateral edentulous, 155–159
    case study of, 141–144
    ScannoGuide of, 82f
    segmenting of, 62f–64f, 62–63
  partially. *See* Partially edentulous patients.
  scanning appliances for
    description of, 49
    fabrication, 51–52
    imaging, 52–53, 53f, 60f
    impression, 50, 50f
    positioning, 52
  SurgiGuide application in, 86f
Effective dose, of radiation, 17
Emergence axis, 101, 101f

F

Facial assessments, 92, 93f
Fifth dimension, 196
Filtered backprojection, 5
Final drill, 178, 179f
Fixation pins, 69, 70f
Fixed prosthesis
  description of, 4
  implant-supported, 159f, 164f, 168f, 172f
  maxillary, 144f
Fractured/nonrestorable mandibular first molar, 173–176
Full-contour scanning appliance, 98f–99f, 98t
Full-contour waxup, 97f, 97t

G

Generalized aggressive periodontitis, 169–172
Genetic effects, of radiation, 17
Gingival asymmetry, 96f
Global parameter, 181f
Guided bone regeneration, 128f
Guiding cylinder, 177, 178f

H

Hard palate scanning plane, 15t, 16
Healing abutments, 184f
Healthcare Information Portability and Accessibility Act, 198
Helical artifacts, 14f, 15
Helical computed tomography, 6
HIPAA. *See* Healthcare Information Portability and Accessibility Act.
Horizontal bone loss, 96f–97f
Hounsfield units, 9, 62, 62f

I

i-CAT, 193, 194f
Imaging/imaging techniques
  comparison of, 6t
  computed tomography. *See* Computed tomography.
  ideal characteristics of, 5
  purpose of, 5
Immediate Smile
  components of, 186f
  considerations for, 185
  implant analogues, 188, 190, 191t
  implant planning, 185, 185f
  presurgical laboratory phase of, 186, 186f–187f
  protocol for, 188–192
  provisional prosthesis, 187f–189f, 187–188
  SimPlant planning for, 189f
  summary of, 188
  SurgiGuide placement, 187, 187f
"Immediate Smile," 4

Immediate-load maxillary fixed restoration
planning phase for, 200–205
restorative phase of, 207–208
surgical phase for, 205–207, 206f–207f
Immediate-load provisional restoration, 106, 107f
Impacted teeth
maxillary canines, 29, 29f–30f
third molar, 37f
Implant(s)
anti-rotational feature of, 196
computer-guided treatment planning. *See* Computer-guided implant treatment pathway.
cross-sectional view of, 77f, 101, 101f
loading of, 219f
master model, 106
parallelism of, 102, 102f
planned
cross-sectional view of, 77f
3D reconstruction of, 76f
prosthetically driven
placement of, 47–48, 48f
selection of, 25, 47–48, 48f
site preparation without bone exposure, tooth-, or tooth and mucosa–supported surgical guides for, 74–79
symphyseal, 217f
tapered virtual, 195, 196f
3D viewing of, 102, 102f
treatment planning for
computer-guided. *See* Computer-guided implant treatment pathway.
illustration of, 79f
virtual, 195, 196f
Implant holders, 178, 179f, 180, 186f
Implant-supported fixed prosthesis, 149, 159f, 164f, 168f, 172f
Implant-supported overdenture, 97f
Impression, for scanning appliances for edentulous patients, 50, 50f
Inferior alveolar nerve, 26f, 35, 37f
Influental developmental abnormality, 33
Informed consent, 87
Interdental papillae, 199f
Interforaminal dentition, 27f
International Commission on Radiological Protection, 17

L

Laser photopolymerization, 2–3
Lateral cephalogram, 18t, 21
Lateral entrance sleeves, 84, 84f
Lateral scout views, 10
Le Fort osteotomy, 220f, 221
Lip line, 92, 93f
Lower border scanning plane, 15t, 16
Low-toxicity resin, 3

M

Mandible
edentulism of, 118–122, 132–136, 145–149
posterior
advanced atrophy of, 137–140
description of, 26f, 35, 35f
SimPlant of, 24f, 26f–27f, 42, 42f–44f
3D reconstruction of, 26f
Mandibular anterior advanced nonrestorable caries, 165–168
Mandibular central incisor, 34, 34f
Mandibular denture, implant-supported immediate-load, 44f
Mandibular first molar, fractured/nonrestorable, 173–176
Mandibular implants, 217
Mandibular molars, impacted, 37f
Masking. *See* Segmentation.
Maxilla
anterior, trauma of, 128–131
atrophy of, 220f
computed tomography of, 25, 27f
edentulism of
alveolar ridge, 200f
case study of, 220–221
complete, 141–144
partial, 114–117, 155–159
fixed prosthesis of, 144f
posterior
regional anatomy of, 35, 35f
SimPlant in, 38, 38f–41f
reconstruction of, 218, 218f–219f
3D reconstruction of, 22f, 39f
Maxillary anterior implant reconstruction
case study of, 150–154
failure of, 160–164
Maxillary canines
congenitally missing, 29, 29f–30f, 32, 32f
impacted, 29, 29f–30f
skeletal abnormalities, 32f
Maxillary central incisors, 33f, 78f, 95f
Maxillary complete denture, 44f, 200f
Maxillary implant reconstruction, 150–154
Maxillary lateral incisors
gingival margin position of, 96f
SimPlant case planning for. *See* Congenitally missing teeth.

Maxillary premolars, 25f
Maxillary sinus
  anatomy of, 35f
  computed tomography of, 25f
  perforation of, 35
Medical modeling, 67–68, 106, 107f
Mental foramen, 27f
Metal-ceramic prostheses, 76
Misch scale of bone density, 9, 9t
Motion artifacts, 14
Mouth examination, 92, 93f
Mucosal flaps, 108, 108b
Mucosa-supported SurgiGuides
  description of, 80–83, 81f–83f, 108, 108f, 183f
  development of, 179
  for maxillary complete edentulism, 143f
Multislice computed tomography
  description of, 6–7
  partial volume effect in, 14
  scanning plane in, 15

N

Nasopalatine canal, 33, 33f
Noise, 9
Nonrestorable caries, mandibular anterior advanced, 165–168

O

Occlusal plane, 15, 15t, 16f
"Optimal final tooth position," 21, 24f
Oral-maxillofacial surgery software
  case demonstrations using, 215–221
  description of, 211
  diagnosis, 212–213
  parietal donor site, 213
  preoperative preparation, 214
  prosthetic outcome using, 211, 212f
  ramus donor site, 213, 213f
  scan before, 212
  scanning appliance fabrication, 212, 212f
  summary of, 221
  surgical simulation using, 213
  symphyseal donor site, 213, 214f
  treatment plan, 211–214
Osteotomy
  bone reduction before, 71
  description of, 38
  drilling tube elongation, 83, 84f
  SurgiGuides for preparation of, 43f, 71, 71f
Overrun effect, 6–7

P

Palatal bone, 33, 33f
Palatal root tip, 36f
Panoramic tomogram, 18t
Panoramic views, 10
Partial volume effect, 14
Partially edentulous patients. *See also* Edentulous patients.
  maxillary, 114–117, 155–159
  prosthetically driven implant for, 48f
  scanning appliances for, 53–55, 54f–55f
  stereolithographic surgical guide for, 74
  SurgiGuides in
    algorithm for, 85f
    bone-supported, 70f
Patient consultation, 104
Periapical pathosis, 25f, 35, 35f
Periapical radiographs, 18t, 195
Periodontitis
  chronic, 123–127
  generalized aggressive, 169–172
PHIDIAS project, 2–3
Physical diagnostic inquiries, 104, 104t, 105f
Pilot drill, 178, 179f
PISA project, 3
Pixels, 9
Posterior mandibular atrophy, 137–140
Post–socket grafting, 166
Precision osteoplasty, 148f, 171f, 175f
Proclination, of teeth, 92, 93f
Prosthetically driven implant
  placement of, 47–48, 48f
  selection of, 25, 47–48, 48f
Provisional restoration
  Immediate Smile, 187f–189f, 187–188
  immediate-load, 106, 107f
  scanning appliances, 98f, 98t

R

Radiation
  as low as reasonably achievable principle for, 19
  deterministic effects of, 17
  doses of, 17, 18t, 20
  stochastic effects of, 17, 19
Radiographic diagnostic inquiries, 94
Radiographs
  bitewing, 18t
  periapical, 18t, 195
Radiolucent interocclusal record, 98b
Radiopaque scanning appliance, 185f

Rapid prototyping, 67–68
Ray, 5
Referrals, 19
Reformatted computed tomography images, 10–12, 11f–12f
Region growing, 61, 61f
Regional anatomy, 25, 25f, 35, 35f, 73
Remounting, 106, 107f
Retroclination, of teeth, 92, 93f
Ridge resorption, 94t
Root fracture, 31, 31f
Root resorption, 94f

S

SAFE System
  accuracy of, 180–182
  for advanced caries and chronic periodontitis repair, 126f
  case example of, 182–184, 183f–185f
  description of, 69, 70f, 73, 76, 83
  development of, 177, 179–182
  drilling cylinders, 177, 178f
  drills, 178, 179f
  guiding cylinders, 177, 178f, 179
  height control for, 179–180
  implant holders, 178, 179f, 180, 186f
  for mandibular complete edentulism, 120f–121f, 134f
  mandibular implants, 217, 217f
  for maxillary complete edentulism, 143f
  regulator for, 179–180
  summary of, 184
  Surgical Tray, 177, 178f, 184f
  trephine, 178, 179f, 187
Sagittal osteotomy, 215, 216f
Scan projection radiograph, 10
Scanning appliances
  case studies of
    anterior maxillary trauma, 129f
    mandibular complete edentulism, 119, 133
    maxillary anterior implants, 151, 161
    maxillary partial edentulism, 115f
  complete denture, 98f, 98t
  in computer-guided implant treatment pathway, 98
  definition of, 49
  dual-density mucosal-supported, 43f
  for edentulous patients
    description of, 49
    fabrication, 51–52
    imaging, 52–53, 53f, 60f
    impression, 50, 50f
    positioning, 52
  fabrication of, 49–55, 98t
  full-contour, 98f–99f, 98t
  for partially edentulous patients, 53–55, 54f–55f
  provisional restoration, 98f, 98t
  radiologic, segmenting an edentulous maxilla with, 62f–64f, 62–63
  radiopaque, 185f
  ScannoGuide, 49
  3D viewing of, 102, 102f
  tooth-form, 98f, 98t
  types of, 98f
  virtual teeth, 55–57, 56f
ScannoGuide
  for aggressive periodontitis, 170
  description of, 49, 80–83, 81f–83f, 183f
  for mandibular complete edentulism, 119, 146
  for maxillary complete edentulism, 142f
Scanora, 18t
Scout views, 10
Screw-retained SurgiGuides, 181f
Segmentation
  benefits of, 195
  definition of, 61
  edentulous maxilla with radiologic scanning appliance, 62f–64f, 62–63
  steps involved in, 61, 61f
Selective transparency, 195, 203
Semi-adjustable articulator, 212f
Silicone impression material, 50
SimPlant
  active work environments in, 23f–24f
  advanced case planning with, 193–208
  anatomy imaging using, 195
  clipping, 196, 197f, 203
  collaborative accountability, 22, 38, 42
  computed tomography images converted into compatible format for, 59, 60f, 99
  in computer-guided implant treatment pathway, 99
  cone-beam computed tomography data and, 193
  DICOM file conversion to, 180
  evolution of, 202
  history of, 2, 21
  Immediate Smile developmental testing using, 189f
  immediate-load maxillary fixed restoration case planning using
    planning phase, 200–205
    restorative phase, 207–208
    surgical phase, 205–207, 206f–207f
  information management, 21, 38

mandible, 24f, 26f–27f, 42, 42f–44f
mandibular edentulism, 119, 133f
masks in, 99b
maxillary canines, 29, 29f–30f, 32, 32f
maxillary lateral incisor case planning using
description of, 28, 28f, 193
planning phase for, 193–198
restorative phase, 199, 199f
surgical phase, 198f–199f, 198–199
triangle of bone, 194, 194f, 197f
oral-maxillofacial surgery software
case demonstrations using, 215–221
description of, 211
diagnosis, 212–213
parietal donor site, 213
preoperative preparation, 214
prosthetic outcome using, 211, 212f
ramus donor site, 213, 213f
scan before, 212
scanning appliance fabrication, 212, 212f
summary of, 221
surgical simulation using, 213
symphyseal donor site, 213, 214f
treatment plan, 211–214
overview of, 21
palatal root tip retention, 36f
in posterior maxilla, 38, 38f–41f
regional anatomy evaluations, 25, 25f
root fracture, 31, 31f
sinus disease, 36f
skeletal abnormality, 32, 32f
surgical treatment planning using, 23
Single-slice sequential computed tomography, 6, 7f
Sinus pneumatization, 94t
Slice, 5
Somatic effects, of radiation, 17
Spiral computed tomography, 6
Starburst artifacts, 13, 13f
Stereolithography
description of, 185
in partially edentulous patients, 74
SurgiGuides, 68, 68f, 71f, 206f
Stochastic effects of radiation, 17, 19
Surgery, 108, 108f
Surgical guides
benefits of, 87
description of, 1, 3
tooth-supported, 74–79, 84f, 106, 106f, 156f, 167f, 174f, 183f
SurgiGuides
algorithms for, 85f–86f
benefits of, 87
bone-supported
for advanced posterior mandibular atrophy, 139f
description of, 69f–74f, 69–73, 75, 83, 106, 107f, 109f, 116
loading of, 219f
for mandibular complete edentulism, 147
definition of, 68
depth control and, 73
design of, 68–69
drilling tubes, 71, 72f, 73
in edentulous patients, 86f
guide pins for, 41f
for maxillary anterior trauma, 130f
medical modeling, 67–68
mucosa-supported
description of, 80–83, 81f–83f, 108, 108f, 183f
development of, 179
for maxillary complete edentulism, 143f
osteotomy preparation, 43f, 71, 71f
overview of, 67
in partially edentulous patients, 85f
placement of, 187, 187f
rapid prototyping, 67–68
regional anatomy effects on, 73
screw-retained, 181f
specialized, 83–84
stereolithography, 68, 68f, 71f, 206f
Symphyseal implants, 217f

T

Tapered virtual implants, 195, 196f
Teeth proclination and retroclination, 92, 93f
3D objects, 61, 61f
3D views
description of, 12
implants, 102, 102f
scanning appliances, 102, 102f
Thresholding, 61
Tooth-alveolar housing, 92, 94f
Tooth-form scanning appliance, 98f, 98t
Tooth-form waxup, 97f, 97t
Tooth-supported surgical guides, 74–79, 84f, 106, 106f, 156f, 167f, 174f, 183f
Transaxial images, 9
Transitional abutments, 206
Trauma, 128–131

Treatment planning
computed tomography for, 23–27
eight-step, 100f–105f, 100–105
implants, 79f
SimPlant software for, 23
Trephine, 178, 179f, 187
Trial tooth setup waxup, 97f, 97t
Triangle of bone, 194, 194f, 197f, 203f

V

Vertical bone loss, 96f–97f
Virtual implants, 195, 196f
description of, 10
on 3D images, 12
Virtual Tooth tool, 55–57, 56f, 194, 194f, 202, 204f
Voxel, 9

W

Waxups, 53, 54f, 97, 97f